PSYCHOSOCIAL ASPECTS OF DISABILITY

ABOUT THE AUTHORS

George Henderson, Ph.D., is Professor Emeritus of Human Relations, Education, and Sociology at the University of Oklahoma. He is the author or coauthor of thirty-one books and more than fifty articles. His books include *Our Souls to Keep: Black/White Relations in America* (1999), *Rethinking Ethnicity and Health Care* (1999), *Understanding Indigenous and Foreign Cultures* (2006), *Excellence in College Teaching and Learning: Classroom and Online Instruction* (2007), and Race and the University: A Memoir (2010). Dr. Henderson has taught cultural diversity courses and seminars throughout the world. His Ph.D. in educational sociology is from Wayne State University in Detroit.

Willie V. Bryan, Ed.D., is Professor Emeritus Health Promotion Sciences, University of Oklahoma Health Sciences Center. Dr. Bryan has authored several books on disabilities and helping relationships, including *In Search of Freedom, Multicultural Aspects of Disabilities, Sociopolitical Aspects of Disabilities, and Helping Relationships: The Fundamentals of Being an Effective Helper.* Before his thirty-nine years of service at the University of Oklahoma, he served as a vocational rehabilitation counselor for the state of Oklahoma and Director of Rehabilitation and Personnel for Goodwill Industries of Oklahoma City. Dr. Bryan has degrees in education, psychology, and counseling. Dr. Bryan has taught courses on disabilities and counseling, helping relationships around the world.

Fourth Edition

PSYCHOSOCIAL ASPECTS OF DISABILITY

By

GEORGE HENDERSON, PH.D.

*Professor Emeritus
University of Oklahoma
Norman, Oklahoma*

and

WILLIE V. BRYAN, ED.D.

*Professor Emeritus
University of Oklahoma Health Sciences Center
Oklahoma City, Oklahoma*

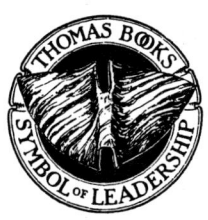

CHARLES C THOMAS • PUBLISHER, LTD.
Springfield • Illinois • U.S.A.

Published and Distributed Throughout the World by

CHARLES C THOMAS • PUBLISHER, LTD.
2600 South First Street
Springfield, Illinois 62704

This book is protected by copyright. No part of
it may be reproduced in any manner without
written permission from the publisher.
All rights reserved.

©2011 by CHARLES C THOMAS • PUBLISHER, LTD.

ISBN 978-0-398-08612-1 (hard)
ISBN 978-0-398-08613-8 (paper)
ISBN 978-0-398-8614-5 (ebook)

Library of Congress Catalog Card Number: 2010032507

With THOMAS BOOKS *careful attention is given to all details of manufacturing and design. It is the Publisher's desire to present books that are satisfactory as to their physical qualities and artistic possibilities and appropriate for their particular use.* THOMAS BOOKS *will be true to those laws of quality that assure a good name and good will.*

Printed in the United States of America
CR-R-3

Library of Congress Cataloging-in-Publication Data

Henderson, George, 1932–
  Psychosocial aspects of disability / by George Henderson and Willie V. Bryan. -- 4th ed.
    p. cm.
  Includes bibliographical references and index.
  ISBN 978-0-398-08612-1 (hard) -- ISBN 978-0-398-08613-8 (pbk.)
  1. People with disabilities--Psychology. 2. People with disabilities--Rehabilitation--Social aspects. 3. People with disabilities--Public opinion. I. Bryan, Willie V. II. Title.
  RD798.H46 2011
  362.4--dc22

2010032507

*This book is dedicated to all persons with disabilities
and their families and advocates.*
W.V.B.

*For the many lessons of compassion, courage, and sacrifice that I have
learned from my students and colleagues who have disabilities,
I dedicate this book to their lives not wasted.*
G.H.

PREFACE

The fourth edition of *Psychosocial Aspects of Disability* strikes what we consider a balance of past, present, and future views of individual, family, societal, and governmental interaction and reaction to persons with disabilities. The past is presented in Part 1, Psychosocial Aspects of Disabilities, in which we present a view of the evolution of societal reactions to disabilities and persons with disabilities. This perspective is important because it explains how some of the beliefs and attitudes toward disabilities and those that have a disability have developed. Additionally, Part 1 makes us aware from a historical perspective why persons with disabilities have been subject to certain types of treatment from family, friends, and society. Although Part 1 primarily deals with explaining philosophical societal views of attitude development with regard to disabilities, there are some hints of attitudinal changes such as in Chapter 1, Psychosocial Aspects of Disability, when we discuss emerging disability models such as sociopolitics and empowerment. Also, in Chapter 4, Growth for People with Disabilities, we discuss changing attitudes of persons with disabilities, their families, and advocates. These positive attitudes, beliefs, and approaches to the world of disabilities and those who possess disabilities serve as a lead into Part 2, Empowerment.

Parts 2 and 3 provide discussion of present situations for persons with disabilities as they move toward better inclusion in society. Chapter 5 discusses the need for empowerment of persons with disabilities and how they can empower themselves. Chapter 6 discusses the need for better employment opportunities for persons with disabilities because this is a significant way of empowering persons with disabilities. Chapter 7 discusses federal legislation that has been developed to facilitate the empowerment of persons with disabilities. Chapters in Part 3, Psychosocial Intervention, discuss how helping professionals can assist persons with disabilities with regard to empowerment.

Part 4, Psychosocial Issues, to a large extent, represents the future for persons with disabilities. The chapters in this section discuss some disability issues that some persons with disabilities will encounter and/or by which they will be affected during the twenty-first century. Additionally, there is discussion of the need for persons with disabilities to attain the full human rights to which they are entitled.

G.H.
W.B.

INTRODUCTION

When the first edition of this book was published in 1984, we discussed some of the negative attitudes and treatments persons with disabilities had received both historically and at that time. This was prior to the development and passage of the Americans with Disabilities Act of 1990. In fact much of the groundwork by persons with disabilities and their advocates was being developed so that they could encourage the United States Congress to pass what would become the previously mentioned Act. Over the years since the publication of the first edition, we have seen significant progress made with regard to the reaction to and treatment of persons with disabilities.

As previously stated when the first edition of this book was published, persons with disabilities had begun to make significant progress with their disability rights and independent living movement. By developing and shaping their organizational and coalition building skill, a national disability agenda was established.

Similar to the Civil Rights Movement of the 1950s and 1960s that produced, among other things, pride of their cultures within ethnic and racial minorities, the Disabilities Rights and Independent Living Movement increased the self- and group pride of persons with disabilities. This self-pride of persons with disabilities has led to their empowering themselves. Many persons with disabilities no longer rely on the non-disabled to determine their agenda with regard to attaining increased inclusion into society. Persons with disabilities are increasingly taking control of their lives and demanding full citizenship and all of the rights and privileges that go with citizenship. Many persons with disabilities are shedding the shame they once felt because of their disabilities and have begun to value themselves as persons who are capable of making significant contributions to the communities in which they reside.

Although significant progress has been made with regard to improved attitudes and treatment of persons with disabilities as well as improved self-esteems of persons with disabilities, this does not mean that there will not be issues and hurdles that persons with disabilities will have to overcome. This simply means that everyone concerned about the human rights of persons with disabilities must continue to demand equal rights for persons with all types of disabilities.

CONTENTS

Page

Preface vii
Introduction ix

Chapter

Part 1: Psychosocial Aspects of Disabilities

1. Psychosocial Aspects of Disabilities 5
2. Beliefs and Treatments 17
3. The Nature of the Problem 31
4. Growth for People with Disabilities 49

Part 2: Empowerment

5. Empowerment 67
6. Employment 79
7. Politics of Disabilities 99
8. Family 119

Part 3: Psychosocial Intervention

9. Human Services Personnel 135
10. Coping Styles 153
11. Helping Professionals 167
12. Cultural Sensitivity 183

Part 4: Psychosocial Issues

13. Human Rights for All 197
14. Psychosocial Disability Issues for the Twenty-First Century 209

Appendices
   Appendix A: Famous Deceased Persons with Disabilities:
     A Brief Sample 219
   Appendix B: Resources for People with Disabilities 223
   Appendix C: Recreation Associations 229
   Appendix D: Disabilities Quiz 233
   Appendix E: Medical Terminology and Definitions 239

Index 259

PSYCHOSOCIAL ASPECTS
OF DISABILITY

Part 1

PSYCHOSOCIAL ASPECTS OF DISABILITIES

Chapters 1 through 4 provide a glimpse at some of the beliefs about persons who have disabilities and their perceived worth to society. These beliefs, attitudes, and perceptions have an impact on how persons with disabilities are treated within a society. In Chapter 1 we present several models that have influenced perceptions of persons with disabilities and have influenced our reactions to them for generations. The aggregate of these perceptions and treatments has, to a large degree, defined the ways persons who have disabilities are incorporated in our society.

Attitudes perceptions, and beliefs play major roles in defining the status and positions persons who have disabilities occupy in our nation. For example, beliefs determine (1) how persons with disabilities are educated, (2) where they are employed, (3) where they live, (4) how they live, (5) with whom they socialize, and (6) types of leisure and recreational activities in which they participate.

Chapter 1

PSYCHOSOCIAL ASPECTS OF DISABILITY

Outline

- Introduction
- Disability Models
- Moral/Religion Model
- Charity Model
- Social Paternalistic Model
- Medical/Functional Limitation/ Rehabilitation Model
- Minority/Cultural Group Model
- Empowerment Model
- Sociopolitical Model
- Summary
- Points for Discussion and Suggested Activities

Objectives

- To introduce several disability models that have influenced attitudes toward persons with disabilities
- To introduce several disability models that have influenced rehabilitation actions toward persons with disabilities
- To introduce several emerging disability models that are having a positive impact with regard to the interaction with persons with disabilities.

INTRODUCTION

The science of human psychology in many ways is devoted to understanding human behavior. To be more specific, a major aspect of human psychology is dedicated to developing a better understanding of why we as humans think and behave in the ways we think and behave. With advancements in our understanding of human behavior we are able to develop techniques and other methods of eliminating, controlling, or changing inappropriate thinking or behaviors. Additionally, we are able to replace faulty thinking and inappropriate behavior with more socially acceptable behavior. Therefore, a significant advantage of human psychology is its ability to focus a spotlight on our behaviors and demonstrate how behavior influences and produces the type of society in which we will live.

As members of a social order, we humans are both the producers and products of our societies. Stated in other terms, to a major degree we humans determine the type of society in which we will live and, based upon those determinations, influence how we live. With regard to persons with disabilities, they are members of every society in the world, and their existence has greatly been influenced by various views of how they fit into society. There are various concepts of why disabilities exist, how persons with disabilities should be managed within a society, and the value, or lack thereof, persons with disabilities have for a society. Some of these concepts have been developed into models that attempt to explain how at various times societys view persons with disabilities. The significance of these models is they reveal various perceptions of how societies view how persons with disabilities should be treated, and in many cases, how they are being treated. The models to which we are referring are the moral/religion model, charity model, social paternalistic model, medical/ functional limitation/rehabilitation model, minority/cultural group model, sociopolitical model, and a relatively new and emerging model the empowerment model.

DISABILITY MODELS

Before we discuss each of the previously mentioned models we will discuss the purpose of these models and the advantages and disadvantages of the models. How to treat and react to persons with disabilities as well as how persons with disabilities fit within a given society have been issues that have never been completely or accurately answered. Throughout human history we have struggled with these issues; consequently, a variety of methods of dealing with persons with disabilities with regard to some of the issues they face have been tried. As is discussed in various chapters of this book, the variety of beliefs about the meaning of disabilities and how disabilities impact the lives of the persons who possess disabilities is vivid testimony to the complexity of societal understanding and dealing with disability issues. Some of the perplexing issues rehabilitation-helping professionals as well as family and friends encounter are social justice, rehabilitation, economics, and inclusion, to mention only four. Although some critics of the development of disability models may exclaim that these models do very little to assist persons with disabilities in their daily lives, the fact is that these models emphasize the various ways in which persons with disabilities are treated and also explain to a large degree why they are treated in certain ways. One might argue that textbooks and personal accounts of persons with disabilities as well as stories in the mass media and information provided by advocacy groups tell the same story that disability models portray. To a large extent this is true; however, the more avenues and methods of presenting the issues, the better the chances are these issues will get attention and hopefully provide opportunities for persons with disabilities to overcome them. The authors of this book have taught for a significant number of years, and both are amazed at students' lack of knowledge and understanding of disability issues. Most students are well-informed with regard to ethnic/racial and gender issues; however, as previously stated with regard to issues impacting persons with disabilities, students tend to be much less informed. A further point being made is that if as students they are inadequately informed, the chances are great that as professionals, unless they are in the medical/rehabilitation field, they will remain uninformed with regard to disability issues. Therefore, the more avenues for presenting disability issues, the better the chances for sharing the message of how persons with disabilities have been and to a major extent continue to be treated and the better the chances are for persons with disabilities their families, friends, and advocates to receive empathetic understanding assistance. With those remarks as justification we will begin our presentation of some disability models.

MORAL/RELIGION MODEL

Moral and religious beliefs are the bedrock foundation of this model. To be more specific, some people, if not many, believe that some disabilities are the result of lack of adherence to social morality and religious proclamations that warn against engaging in certain behavior. To further explain this model, some beliefs are based upon the assumption that some disabilities are the result of punishment from an all-powerful entity. Furthermore, the belief is that the punishment is for an act or acts of transgression against prevailing moral and/or religious edits.

The moral/religion model was a much more common belief in less-enlightened times; however, the philosophy behind this belief rests just below the surface of human emotional reactions and, depending on the circumstances, the belief is subject to reappearance and to the surprise of some becomes a powerful and influential belief for a period of time. Provided as an example, in the not to distant past, when HIV/AIDS began to occur in industrialized developed countries, the moral/religion model of explaining this disability was common, and to some extent remains one means of explaining its cause today. Persons with this disability, during those early days, were stigmatized and ostracized to a much greater extent than they are today. Undoubtedly, as new diseases occur and the exact cause is unknown and the cure or method of containment is unknown, this disability belief model will be used again to explain the cause and to some extent offer an answer or answers to what to do with those who have the disease and/or disability. Not only will this line of thinking reoccur, as previously stated, the fact is that the line of thinking has not totally disappeared. One only has to consider some of the thoughts expressed when someone becomes disabled as a result of substance abuse use or after having an accident while driving under the influence of alcohol.

An extreme form of moral/religion model application is when someone explains that disabilities are caused by transgressions, not of the person with the disability or his/her parents but as a result of transgressions of past ancestors. Some today also tend to believe some emotional and mental disabilities have their grounding in breaking some moral or religious edict. The less we know about a disease and/or situation, the more fear is generated, and we tend to resort to blaming the victim or in some cases ancestors of the victim.

As previously stated, the moral/religion model is one of the oldest models of disabilities and appears to be one of the most enduring models. Fortunately it is not frequently adopted by many people. The concept supporting the model is alive and well in some people's minds, however, and is available for them to resurrect when the next illness and/or debilitating condition surfaces.

CHARITY MODEL

The charity disability model is based upon persons providing what they consider benevolent help to persons with disabilities. The charity model appears to be on the opposite end of the helping spectrum in comparison to the moral/religion model. Whereas the moral/religion model has a decisive negative view of some disabilities, the charity model takes an approach that is intended to benefit persons with disabilities. The charity model in further comparison with the moral/religion model is a good reflection of society as we discuss the reaction to disabilities and those who have a disability. As we view societies, past and present, we notice with regard to beliefs and treatments of persons with disabilities that acceptable and less acceptable approaches to interacting with persons with disabilities exist. In the distant past, while some persons with disabilities were being burned at the stake, there were other groups lobbying for humane/paternalistic treatment of persons with disabilities. Likewise, in the present, there are some who advocate institutionalization and custodial care, while others are petitioning for more inclusion of persons with disabilities in societal activities. Somewhere between the two extremes stands the charity model. The charity model certainly has the benevolent approach of humane treatment of persons with disabilities. However, past methods of obtaining support for persons with disabilities have, in these authors' opinions, caused many persons with disabilities, particularly those with severe disabilities, to be viewed as dependent charity cases. To attract attention to what some supporters of persons with disabilities thought were helping efforts, they resorted to displaying persons with disabilities as helpless, destitute persons. This approach quite often obtained results such as money donated for services needed by persons with disabilities as well as verbal support for the needs of persons with disabilities. However, along with this support came feelings of sympathy and devaluation of the lives of those persons targeted for help. There is very little question that the development of sympathy was intended; however, the devaluation hopefully was an unintended by-product of the charitable/benevolent actions. The by-product of devaluation is what has made the charity model approach an undesirable method of interacting with persons with disabilities. As is discussed in this text, in the not distant past, national telethons designed to raise money for research and other helping methods for persons with disabilities told heart-wrenching stories about persons with disabilities and would display persons with disabilities as happy but helpless persons to gain the sympathy of the audience and encourage that same audience to donate money and other resources to benefit the helpless disabled people. Most of these types of fundraising/awareness programs have either discontinued the previously mentioned approach or have to some extent backed away from displaying persons with disabilities as being helpless. Despite the change in strategies, damage has been done, and it will take considerable time to change the minds of many people to the more productive view that persons with disabilities are capable individuals who can support themselves if given reasonable opportunities to do so.

The approach of displaying and viewing persons with disabilities as victims in need of charity, as previously stated, has diminished; however, it has given way to a similar approach. This approach or model is called the social paternalistic model.

SOCIAL PATERNALISTIC MODEL

The social model is based primarily on a paternalistic approach to dealing with persons with disabilities. Similar to the charity model, persons with disabilities are viewed as persons who are in need of protecting. The underpinning of the concept is that persons with disabilities are weak, unable to withstand the various challenges with which they will be confronted on a daily basis. Because of this perceived weakness, persons with disabilities must be protected by the stronger member of society: nondisabled persons. Most nondisabled persons will not openly subscribe to or acknowledge that they view persons with disabilities in this manner; however, their actions reveal their subconscious beliefs. Employers not hiring persons with disabilities because they believe they will be unable to adequately perform the job requirements and/or because they believe the nondisabled employees will not want to work with the person with a disability is an example of the subconscious paternalistic attitude. Neighbors attending social events who invite some of their nondisabled friends to go with them or meet them at the event but do not invite a neighbor who has a visible disability because they believe the person with a disability would not enjoy the social event and/or would be uncomfortable attending the event is another example of the subconscious paternalistic attitude of protecting the person with a disability. There are numerous other examples.

The social paternalistic model, in most cases, is not intended to be harmful. In most cases, however this approach has two harmful effects on persons with disabilities: one, it creates and encourages dependency and, two, it limits opportunities for personal and psychological growth. With regard to dependency, the history of disabilities throughout the world has been built, to a large degree, upon the foundation of "can't do." Too often when we think of disabilities and persons with disabilities, one of the first things that comes to one's mind is "can't do." The person can't do this, the person can't do that, the person can't learn that, the person can't go there, and the list could continue. After being told numerous times they can't do certain things, too often persons with disabilities begin to believe they are severely limited with regard to what they can do, thus they need to rely on the nondisabled to provide for their activities of daily living. One should be able to easily understand how consistently living on the charity of others can impact one's self-esteem and psychological well-being. With regard to limitation of opportunities, most often when we attempt to protect people from failure, we are also limiting their chances of success and psychological growth. Stated in other terms, persons with disabilities have the same right to fail as nondisabled persons have, because in attempting to protect them from failure we are limiting their chances for succeeding.

The paternalistic attitude is evident in various ways within American society. The high rate of unemployment of persons with disabilities to some extent can be attributed to attempts to protect persons with disabilities from failure. The rate of school children with disabilities being placed in special education classes and/or vocational classes is another example of paternalistic attitudes.

Fortunately, the overall society in the United States is becoming more cognizant of the needs and capabilities of persons with disabilities; thus, more opportunities are opening to them. Additionally, more advance methods of evaluating the capabilities are improving the lives of persons with disabilities and are allowing them to develop stronger and positive self-esteem. With the development of strong self-esteem, many persons with disabilities are refusing to accept the idea that they are a population of people who must be protected from the possibility of failure.

MEDICAL/FUNCTIONAL LIMITATION/ REHABILITATION MODEL

The medical/rehabilitation model is one of the older models, and it is based on the basic foundation of rehabilitation. The foundational concept of this model is that persons with disabilities are broken persons and in need of being fixed. The standard by which most persons with disabilities are compared is the so-called nondisabled person. Stated in other terms, persons without disabilities are viewed as normal persons and are the yardstick by which the less-than-normal person with a disability is to be judged. The obvious problem with this model is the viewpoint that persons with disabilities are broken or are less than the person who is considered nondisabled.

The rehabilitation/functional limitation aspect of this model emphasizes adapting the person with a disability to function within the environment. The functional limitation part of the concept concentrates on the limitations caused by the disability and places considerable emphasis on putting forth efforts to improve the person's functional capabilities so that he or she can fit within the environment. The efforts may take the form of physical and/or vocational adjustments, as well as emotional support. Those that promote this approach point out that one cannot deny that most disabilities create some limitations. Many, especially severe disabilities such as spinal cord injuries and severe mental and developmental disabilities, to mention only two, can cause considerable limitations for the person with the disability. Therefore, it is reasonable to assess the limitation(s) and devise rehabilitation plans that include, if not center around, (1) restoring the person to as much of that person's previous functioning level as possible and (2) assisting the person to adapt to his or her environment. The proponents of this concept can continue their defense by pointing out that, to a large degree, the extent to which the person becomes rehabilitated is predicated on how well these two points are completed. Those who take exception to the functional limitation model do not deny the fact that disabilities may create various levels of changes in the manner in which the person conducts personal activities of daily living. However, their concerns relate to the rehabilitation efforts being primarily devoted to making the person with the disability adapt and adjust to the environment instead of analyzing the environment with the intent of adjusting the environment to help meet the needs of the person with a disability. Those that may take exception to this concept also contend that this leads to not considering law and policy changes that would encourage environmental changes to aid persons with disabilities being better able to master their environments rather than becoming prisoners to them. Another major argument against this concept is that, although it is necessary and useful to pay considerable attention to the cause of a condition that creates a disability, the extent to which medical and other rehabilitation personnel devote attention to the etiology of the condition has tended to segregate persons with disabilities into disease or causal factor groups. Those opposed would argue that this approach separates people with a disability rather than bringing them together to address common concerns such as attitudinal and environmental barriers.

The viewpoint of fixing persons with disabilities, from a medical and rehabilitation standpoints, is to a large extent a reasonable one. The idea that the ultimate goal in life for persons with disabilities is to be as much like persons without disabilities, however, places many persons with disabilities in a self-concept and self-esteem disadvantage because in many instances the person with a disability may never become a person without a disability. Therefore, a problem becomes "if I can't be whole like persons without disabilities, then I am a lesser human." Certainly, this type of thinking is not a healthy approach to building self-confidence and self-esteem.

MINORITY/CULTURAL GROUP MODEL

The minority/cultural group model is a relative new emerging concept that promotes the idea of recognizing persons with disabilities as a minority group with unique cultural issues. The Americans With Disabilities Act (ADA) recognizes persons with disabilities as a minority group, and with the population estimated at one fifth of the U. S. population, this makes persons with disabilities the largest minority/cultural group in the United States.

This concept emphasizes the discrimination persons with disabilities experience and the neglect of some basic right (in many cases nonintentional) that they experience on a daily basis. This model highlights some of the shared discrimination experienced by persons with disabilities and ethnic/racial minority groups in the United States and other industrialized countries. With regard to the United States, a common denominator of discrimination can be seen in the area of employment, where minorities and persons with disabilities of all ethnic/racial backgrounds experience unemployment at a greater rate than the majority population does, sometime at three times the rate. Other comparisons are income and healthcare disparities. Both of these disparities can be traced back, to a great extent, to lack of appropriate employment. Because of inadequate education, many persons with disabilities are relegated to low-paying jobs, if any. The reality is that because of inadequate or no employment some persons with disabilities have to rely on local, state, and/or federal public assistance. Inadequate employment also impacts the type and quality of healthcare that some receive. Unfortunately, for many, healthcare does not occur until health issues become a dramatically serious issue.

This is precisely what too often occurs to low-income ethnic/racial minorities. Further discussion of the minority/cultural aspect of disabilities can be represented by the diversity of groups within the culture of disabilities: women with disabilities; ethnic/racial minorities; and persons with intellectual, emotional, and physical disabilities to mention only a few.

The discrimination of women in the United States is a well-documented fact. The fact that women receive, on average, slightly more than three-fourth the salary as men doing the same job is part of that documentation. Other parts of the documentation include women being excluded from higher salaried jobs, such as executives with major corporations. Although these represent major acts against discrimination, sexual harassment of women represents an even uglier side of discrimination of women. Add to these acts of discrimination against women with disabilities and the exclusion and damage to women's psyche is increased twofold to threefold. Women with disabilities who are able to secure employment experience the previously mentioned acts of discrimination more intensely because the stigma of having a disability is added to the prevailing negative approaches to hiring and promoting women in the work place. Women, in general, are often considered the weaker gender; thus women with disabilities are considered as being weaker than nondisabled women. Because women with disabilities are considered weak and fragile, this too often makes them targets of physical and sexual abuse.

Another aspect of the cultural diversity of persons with disabilities is intellectual disabilities. Persons who learn at a slower or different pace than the majority of other persons, too often are labeled as mentally retarded. The designation of mentally retarded or slow learner, in the case of some public and private school students, brings with it exclusion and separation from the mainstream of the environment in which the person so designated is affiliated. This separation and segregation places them in a similar class as ethnic/racial groups.

Persons labeled as having an emotional disability are similarly excluded; however, their exclusion too often carries extremely debilitating epitaphs, such as crazy, dumb, and idiot, to mention only three. In addition to the unpopular name calling, these persons experience the social discrimination of exclusion from gainful employment and the exclusion from social contacts that would help them feel they are welcome, contributing members of society, to mention only two forms of exclusion.

The discrimination of persons with physical disabilities with regard to employment is a major act of exclusion that is well-known and -documented. Equally as devastating to persons with physical disabilities are other types of exclusion such as those that are the result of architectural barriers. Although much of the discrimination of persons with physical disabilities is unintentional and occurs as a result of societal ignorance and/or oversight, the fact remains that persons with physical disabilities are excluded from many of the goods and services that nondisabled persons freely enjoy.

Ethnic/racial minority group members who have disabilities are significant members of the disability culture. Ethnic/racial minority persons with disabilities experience double discrimination—ethnicity/race and disability—and ethnic/racial women experience triple discrimination by adding gender to the previously mentioned cultural mixture. One only has to think of some of the discrimination and exclusions ethnic/racial minorities and women of color experience to get a true understanding of the expanded problems they encounter as a person with a disability.

Understanding the concept of minority/cultural group model is helpful because it gives professional helpers, rehabilitation helpers, advocates, and the general public a better understanding of some of the barriers persons with disabilities encounter. As previously stated, most persons are well-aware of some discrimination and barriers ethnic/racial minorities and women encounter on a daily basis. To relate that treatment to persons with disabilities should therefore give everyone a new but familiar perspective of what many persons with disabilities encounter daily. Further advantages can be the fact that techniques used to assess needs of ethnic/racial minorities and women can be applied to assessing needs of persons with disabilities.

EMPOWERMENT MODEL

The empowerment model emphasizes the importance of persons with disabilities taking charge of their lives rather than having or allowing nondisabled persons advocate for them. This model points out that one of the major problems persons with disabilities face is not their disability but the attitudes of the nondisabled with regard to what they as persons with disabilities can and cannot do. This model further emphasizes that it is the responsibility of persons with disabilities to correct the misperceptions that nondisabled persons have concerning the worth of persons with disabilities to society.

It is not enough for persons with disabilities to say that society must change and recognize their potential. Persons with disabilities must aggressively advocate for themselves. Persons with disabilities cannot expect society to change its paternalistic approach to dealing with them until they prove that they are not helpless people. It is not logical to think that one can be dependent on someone and expect the person to treat one as a nondependent person. Being nondependent does not mean that persons with disabilities have to do everything for themselves and not expect help from persons without disabilities. The reality of life is that no one is totally independent. Everyone needs assistance. Needing assistance, giving assistance, and receiving assistance binds people together as a community and a society. Therefore, for persons with disabilities to be independent does not mean that they have to do everything for themselves; however, they must, whenever possible, be the leader in identifying their needs and instruct other in ways of helping them accomplish their goals and needs in life. Persons with disabilities must not expect society to change without their forcing the issue of change.

A major part of empowering persons with disabilities requires them to build strong self-esteem. This is not to imply that all persons with disabilities have poor opinions of themselves and their abilities. The various ways persons with disabilities have been treated throughout the years, however, means that one can realistically expect that many persons with disabilities have learned to depend on the various moods of persons without disabilities. The proof of this statement is reflected in the paternalistic approach that many nondisabled persons have when working with persons with disabilities. The reality is that the paternalistic approach would not have survived if persons with disabilities did not accept this manner of the nondisabled interacting with them.

SOCIOPOLITICAL CONCEPT MODEL

The sociopolitical concept views interaction between a person with a disability and the environment, whereas previous approaches have expected the person with a disability to adapt or be adapted to the environment. Until the 1970s, the primary goal of most rehabilitation programs was to prepare the person with a disability for a job. Most legislation during that period supported this effort. Certainly vocational preparation is a worthy objective; however, most of the job preparation revolved around whether the person could adjust to the work environment as it existed. In addition, strict concentration on employability meant that other needs of the persons with a disability, such as independent living, were overlooked. The sociopolitical approach fosters the idea that the environment can and should be adapted to accommodate the needs of the person with a disability. Some rehabilitation specialists and disability advocates, such as Oliver (1990) and Swain, Finkelstein, French, and Oliver (1993), subscribe to the sociopolitical concept. Their points of view are based upon the premise that to hold persons with disabilities responsible for their life situation is the same as "blaming the victim." Finkelstein (1991) emphasizes the point that most research on disabilities recognizes that the inability of individuals with disabilities to adequately function within their environments is a result of the environment that has erected barriers forbidding their participation. He concludes his observation by pointing out that the social model of disability requires that society address barriers to inclusion rather than spend money on segregation of this population. The sociopolitical model concept re- moves the person with a disability from being totally at the mercy of the environment. Stated another way, by adapting the environment to allow persons with disabilities to navigate within the environment, their life activities do not have to be predicated on whether they can make the necessary adjustments to negotiate environmental barriers. Finkelstein, (1991) further elaborates with the following comments:

> Increasingly, however, laws and regulations adopted in the 1970s permitted the formation of a sociopolitical view that considers disability as a product of the interaction between the individual and environment. Whereas prior orientations regarded disability principally as a personal misfortune or limitation, the sociopolitical view stressed the role of the environment in determining the meaning of this phenomenon. Thus disability cannot be defined simply by functional capabilities or by occupational skills. A comprehensive understanding of disability requires an examination of the architectural, institutional, and attitudinal environmental encounter by disabled persons. From this perspective, the primary problems confronting citizens with disabilities are bias, prejudice, segregation, and discrimination that can be eradicated through policies designed to guarantee rights. (p. 38)

The sociopolitical concept does not limit its concentration to removing or adapting the physical barriers, such as steps, stairways, curbs, and narrow doorways, this viewpoint also emphasizes law and policy changes, such as occurred in the Americans with Disabilities Act, which concentrates on requiring employers to identify essential elements needed to perform the jobs at their place of employment so that prospective employees are evaluated only on those elements necessary for adequate job functioning.

The sociopolitical approach represents another way of viewing disabilities and persons with disabilities; more specifically, the thought is the environment, in most cases, can be altered to accommodate persons with disabilities rather than the person being altered to fit the environment. This is the basis for programs such as supported employment, educational inclusion, and deinstitutionalization.

SUMMARY

As one reviews the various disability models discussed in this chapter it should be noted that each has the overall intent of helping persons with disabilities. The intents are honorable; however, the psychological underpinning that supports some of the models creates perception problems with regard to who persons with disabilities are. Provided as an example, the medical/functional limitation/rehabilitation model makes the assumption that persons with disabilities are broken persons in need of being fixed. The charity model, which promotes giving various support, primarily financial support, to assist with rehabilitation of persons with disabilities, certainly does have good intentions; however, the impression that is often the by-product of these efforts is that persons with disabilities are charity cases, persons who cannot help themselves. Likewise, the moral/religious model and the social paternalistic model, despite their noble intents, both have perhaps unintended negative consequences for many persons with disabilities.

In contrast, some of the emerging models, such as sociopolitical, minority/cultural group, and empowerment models, promote equal access, equal opportunities, and equal rights for persons with disabilities without the negative by-products of some other models discussed. These models are reflective of the changing and improved attitudes that American societies, as well as some other societies around the world, are demonstrating with regard to persons with disabilities.

POINTS FOR DISCUSSION AND SUGGESTED ACTIVITIES

1. Compare and contrast the functional limitation/medical rehabilitation model to the sociopolitical model.
2. Discuss some of the negatives of the charity model.
3. Explain your perceptions of the empowerment model.

REFERENCES

Oliver, M. (1990). *The Politics of Disablement.* London: Macmillan.
Quinn, P. (1990). *Understanding Disability: A Lifespan Approach.* Thousand Oaks, CA Sage.
Swain, J., Finkelstein, V., French, S., and Oliver, M. (Eds.). (1993). *Disability Barriers: Enabling Environments.* London: Sage.

SUGGESTED READINGS

Blaxter, M. (1976). The Meaning of Disability. London: Heinemann.
Goffman, E. (1968). *Stigma.* Harmondsworth, UK: Penguin.
Hicks, P.V. (1980). Brief history of the treatment of disabled citizens—since the beginning of written history. *American Corrective Therapy Journal, 34*: 182–183.
Marks, D. (1997). Models of disability. *Disability and Rehabilitation, 19*: 85–91.
Quinn, P. (1991). Understanding Disability: A Lifespan Approach. Thousand Oaks: CA Sage.

Chapter 2

BELIEFS AND TREATMENTS

Outline

- Introduction
- Ancient Beliefs and Practices
- Early American Views
- Humanitarian and Rehabilitation Activities
- Social Cleansing
- Summary
- Points for Discussion and Suggested Activities

Objectives

- To identify early American beliefs and treatment with regard to persons with disabilities
- To identify sources that have influenced early American beliefs and treatment with regard to persons with disabilities
- To identify early American humanitarian efforts
- To identify early American rehabilitation efforts

INTRODUCTION

The United States of America arguably has the best record of any country with regard to treatment of persons with disabilities. This assertion can be supported by the various pieces of federal legislation designed to assist persons with disabilities (*see* Chapter 6). Additionally, it can be supported by viewing the goals of the many social and civic organizations established to further the independence of persons who have disabilities, some of which will be discussed in this and other chapters of this text. Having the best record of providing services to persons with disabilities does not mean that life for them in the United States is without problems. To the contrary, many people who have a disability can attest that they encounter numerous obstacles as they attempt to obtain an education and training and subsequently gainful employment. Also, parents of and advocates for persons who have disabilities frequently are frustrated when they attempt to navigate what, at times, seems like a maze of uncoordinated agencies and organizations.

The negative treatment of persons who have disabilities is directly correlated with erroneous beliefs that community leaders have had, and in some cases continue to have, with regard to the usefulness of persons with disabilities and societal responsibilities for helping them. The evolution of beliefs about persons who have disabilities and their treatment in the United States is very interesting. These things have at times been very contentious. They have evolved from ancient beliefs, and have been influenced by European norms, and further shaped with American humanitarianism.

ANCIENT BELIEFS AND PRACTICES

During the early period of American nationhood, there were programs to provide public assistance and some rehabilitation for persons who had disabilities. However, the inescapable fact remains that most of those persons were considered to be dependent and a drain on the society in which they lived. The programs of assistance were also too few and too poorly designed. Referring to colonial views of persons with disabilities, Lenihan (1977) stated, "The physically and mentally disabled were treated sympathetically as blameless victims of fate but were nevertheless considered financial burdens" (p. 2). Rubin and Roessler (1978) further noted that early American beliefs with regard to persons with disabilities emphasized that disabilities were "perceived as the result of God's punishment" (p. 4). By reviewing some of the ancient beliefs and treatment of persons with disabilities, we will discover the origins of the early American notions of disabilities and persons who had them. Also, by understanding ancient beliefs and the treatment of people who had disabilities, we gain a better understanding of the foundation of current beliefs and rehabilitation practices.

Based in part on the need to survive, primitive societies were intolerant of physically weak persons. The welfare of a group, not individuals, came before all other needs (Apton, 1959). Anyone who was not physically strong enough to contribute to meeting group needs was expendable. This was certainly a period of survival of the fittest. In primitive societies, persons with disabilities were economic, military, and social liabilities that few groups could afford or, at least, thought they could afford (Hinshaw, 1948).

Religious Beliefs

The religious beliefs and practices of primitive societies were, for the most part, animistic and reflected preoccupation with *mana*, a term adopted by anthropologists. Mana encapsulates the primitive beliefs in a powerful, invisible, all-pervading force at work in the universe that could cripple and kill at will. Thus mental illness and physical disabilities were generally viewed as the work of evil mana or spirits. If after considerable coaxing, the spirits did not leave a possessed body, this was believed to be indisputable evidence that the afflicted individual was being punished. To prevent contamination, people possessed with evil spirits were either avoided or killed.

There was no single regional or ethnic treatment of people who had disabilities. Buscaglia (1975) wrote that the Masai Indians murdered such individuals. The Chagg of East Africa believed that people who had disabilities were endowed with special powers and could use them to ward off evil spirits. The Jukum of Sudan believed that people with disabilities were the work of evil spirits. The Sem Ang of Malaysia used men with disabilities, whom they considered to be "wise men," for settling tribal disputes; the Balinese made them taboo. The Hebrews defined them as sinners; the Nordics called them gods.

Abandonment and Death

Historical records reveal that as civilization replaced primitivism, other ways to deal with people with disabilities evolved. They were accepted and treated well in a few ancient societies. In France, during the Middle Ages, blind individuals occupied a place of privilege. Some physicians in the Mediterranean region and Asia demanded that people who had physical disabilities be treated in a humane manner. However, in most countries, people who had disabilities were still treated much the same way as their ancestors were. In general, whatever human enlightenment was occurring in these countries, little of it was extended to the treatment of people who had disabilities.

In the Far East, infants who had disabilities were abandoned to die in the wilderness. In India, they were drowned in the Ganges River. Roman fathers ritualistically displayed children who had disabilities and, after at least five persons concurred that the children would be of no benefit to society, killed them. In later times, Roman fathers were authorized to make this decision without consultation. Small baskets sold in markets were used as death boats so that children who had disabilities could be set sail on the Tiber River. Infants of Sparta suffered a similar fate. If, after being examined by a committee of elders, certain infants were judged as incapable of contributing to society, they were killed. Infanticide was a popular method used by the nobility to eliminate persons whose disabilities might weaken their family's bloodlines. In Athens, special clay pots were used as depositories for abandoned infants.

Many of the children with disabilities who were spared such fatal judgment roamed the villages and countrysides as gypsies and beggars. Some of them were taken in by other families and subjected to conditions of slavery; others were forced into prostitution. Although a few persons who had disabilities were treated well, they were not immune from abandonment, savage beatings, or death as punishment for being different. In a somewhat macabre turnabout, some societies considered it honorable for children to kill, cook, and eat or to bury alive their aged parents or their relatives who were considered unfit for work or war (Koestler, 1976).

Not all treatment of persons who had disabilities was destructive; in India, there were hospitals that were fully equipped for treating people who had disabilities. A hospital in Baghdad offered the most modern treatment of the period. Similarly, the Egyptians and Greeks began to build hospitals and convalescent centers to care for people who had disabilities. One hospital in Cairo provided free treatment, and, upon discharge, patients were given money to sustain them until they could secure work. Albrecht, Seelman, and Bury (2001) confirmed and elaborated on the enlightenment and compassion of the Arabs with regard to persons who had disabilities:

> During the Middle Ages, Greek and Roman medical and philosophical traditions were introduced into Europe by the Arabs, who had conquered most of the continent and penetrated Spain and France. Asylums for people with mental disabilities had been established by the Arabs in Baghdad, Fez (Morocco), and Cairo in the eighth century, and subsequently in Damascus and Aleppo in 1270. Since the Arabs held the general belief that mental disability was divinely inspired and not demonic in origin, care in these facilities was generally benevolent. (p. 19)

As one can see from that brief review, there was, as is the case today, no universal belief about or treatment for persons who had disabilities. Primary influences on how a given society reacts to persons who have disabilities are their folklore, spiritual beliefs, and, in today's societies, media portrayals of people who have disabilities.

Literature Influences

Many of the ancient myths and stereotypes of people who have disabilities were carried over to subsequent periods of history. Although few persons currently subscribe to abandoning or killing people who have disabilities, many of them still associate disabilities with sin and the devil. They either consciously or subconsciously think that "disabilities" is a synonym for "bad." Thurer (1980) said that persons with disabilities have received negative literary press. She further contended that "physical deformity, chronic illness, and any outer defect have come to symbolize an inner defect" (p. 12). Thurer supported her hypothesis with the following comments:

> What becomes obvious from even a cursory examination of literature is that bodily intactness and glowing health are almost exclusive characteristics of the good and noble, while physical infirmities are reserved for the evil and malevolent. It is hardly ever the arthritic, nearsighted crone that is endowed with virtue and a sunny nature, but the archetypal Snow White, the fairest of them all, who is blessed—as if the character's moral temperaments were predetermined by the outcome of a medical check-up.
>
> The point is that physical deformity in literature and art is almost never unencumbered by the trapping of metaphor. There are almost no average or ordinary and "by the way" physically aberrant characters. While the metaphoric use of disability may seem innocuous enough, it is in face a most blatant and pernicious form of stereotyping. I suspect that the metaphoric use of disability is so entrenched that it is not noticed. (p. 12)

Thurer concluded her comments by giving examples of how authors have used disabilities to explain the evilness of their literary characters. Chaucer's Summones is as loathsome physically as his actions were morally. Shakespeare etches Richard III, an insidious devil who is guilty of wholesale murder in his ruthless ascent to the throne, as a hunchback. In *Of Human Bondage*, Somerset Maugham contrives Philip's clubfoot to symbolize his bitter, confused, warped nature. Metaphoric usages of disabilities as evil and being able bodied as goodness ap- pear abundantly throughout the Bible. Ko- kaska, Woodward, and Tyler (1984) counted forty-six incidents in the Bible in which disabilities and persons who had them are referred to in a negative sense. Weinberg and Sebian (1980) offered the following ex- cellent overview of passages from the Bible that support negative views of people who have physical disabilities:

> Throughout the Bible the notion recurs that disease and physical disabilities are punishment sent by God for sins or immoral behavior. God reveals His law through the writings of prophets and disciples. Those who obeyed God's law thrived in good health; those who transgressed against his commandments were severely punished. In the Old Testament, Deut. 27:27, God admonished people to obey all His commandments or He would inflict them with blindness. The New Testament restates the same sentiments that physical illness and disability are punishments for some religious transgression. In John 5:14, Jesus, upon healing a man said, "See, you are well. Sin no more, that nothing more befall you." In Matthew 9:2, Jesus said to a man with palsy, "My son, your sins are forgiven."
>
> These teachings imply that the sick and disabled deserve to suffer as a punishment for having sinned. Not only can the individual sinner be punished, but divine retribution can be directed toward the innocent offspring of a sinner. This is demonstrated in an incident from the Book of Samuel: David said to Nathan, "I have sinned against the Lord and Nathan said to David, The Lord also has put away your sin; you shall not die. Never-the-less, because by this deed you have utterly scorned the Lord, the child that is born to you shall die." And the

Lord struck the child that Uriah's wife bore to David and it became sick and on the seventh day, the child was dead. (p. 273)

Perhaps no one really knows whether these and other passages accurately represent God's will with regard to disabilities and people who have disabilities; however, because these passages represent the writers' interpretation of God's law and will, this presents a picture of their views of disabilities. Relatedly, these views have influenced millions of people through the ages.

As has been documented previously, metaphoric usage of disabilities and persons who have disabilities are also ingrained in the writings of ancient and contemporary literature and indeed are symbolically woven into almost every reference to health. More often than not, being able bodied is associated with good, cleanliness, and virtue. Conversely, persons who have disabilities have been associated through the ages with all that is bad. A review of literature reveals that at various times, physical disabilities have stood for sin and evil. Positive images of nondisabled persons and negative images of persons with disabilities have been deeply etched in the minds of most people throughout history, and many able-bodied persons have nourished these images to maintain their own self-esteem. Much like the English child in William Blake's poem, the able-bodied perceive themselves as angels, whereas persons with disabilities can only yearn for wholeness through their deeds, hoping to become like able-bodied persons so that they will at last be accepted as worthy beings. This socially perverse arrangement is communicated through social status, peer relationships, education, and job opportunities. This concept is carefully and religiously injected into children through school texts, television, programs, and catechism.

Other forms of literature have also contributed to the negative image of people with disabilities. For example, the Talmud and other Hebrew commentaries refer to the blind as the "living dead." A Talmudic commandment urges those who meet a blind person to say the same prayer as would be said upon the death of a close relative. The belief that disability is synonymous with worthlessness, shame, and pity is displayed poetically in numerous writings, including John Milton's (1671) poem "Samson Agonistes":

Now blind, disheartene'd, shame'd, dishonoured quelled,
To what can I be useful? wherein serve
My nation, and the work from Heave'n imposed?
But to sit idle on the household hearth,
A burdenous drone; to visitants a gaze,
Or pitied object; . . .

In *Lady Chatterley's Lover*, D. H. Lawrence (1930) perpetuated the idea of disability as equivalent to uselessness. In it, Sir Clifford, after being injured in war, becomes impotent; therefore, he is depicted as not being a "whole" man. All myths and stereotypes do not necessarily depict persons who have disabilities negatively. Unfounded positive images are also part of their mystique. For example, it is commonly believed that nature automatically compensates individuals who are blind by sharpening their other senses. Helen Keller was assured by her friends that people who are blind could identify color by touch. Many other positive traits are attributed to persons with disabilities solely on the basis of the "automatic" compensation myth. Some of the more desirable mystical traits are cheerfulness, patience, and extraordinary musical skills. Although these myths positively characterize disabilities, they are nevertheless as inaccurate and as distorted as are the negative ones. Persons who are deaf have no better eyesight that the nondeaf have; they learn to pay attention to things. Persons who are blind have no better hearing than the sighted have; they learn to use their ears more efficiently. Even so, the myths persist.

EARLY AMERICAN VIEWS

During the colonial period, for the most part, the treatment and/or care of persons who were sick, disabled, and indigent was the responsibility of the family and the local community. If the family was unable to provide the needed care or service, generally speaking the community would take the responsibility of providing such care. Sometimes the payment for providing care was indentured servitude. In the following comments, Lenihan (1977) provided a succinct description of this practice: "Farming out a dependent to a family might involve a period of indentured servitude as payment for services rendered. A disabled person not wholly without means might receive public aid on condition that he or she relinquish to the town all existing holding" (p. 3). Because local communities had to assume responsibility for persons who were indigent or disabled, most community leaders were reluctant to accept as residents anyone they believed to be dependent. Again, Lenihan provided us with a glimpse of community behaviors:

> Local communities were likewise reluctant to accept as residents anyone suspected of being dependent. Following British legal precedents, each colony enacted settlement laws. These laws required persons to live and work three months to one year in a particular town for legal residency. During this trial period, a town could worm out any newcomer. A town might allow a prospective dependent to stay if a resident in good standing assumed financial sponsorship. If moving a seriously disabled or sick person were to further compromise the person' health or prove fatal, the town would take charge. The town would attempt to find a private benefactor or seek out the person's family. If this failed, the town would bill the origin town or residence or colonial authorities. (pp. 2–3)

To guard against exportation of sick and dependent persons, some seaboard colonies enacted legislation that required shipowners to post a bond that could be used to help pay for services rendered to passengers or shipmates who required community aid. This practice became law in 1798 when the U.S. Congress passed the Seaman's Sickness and Disability Act. It levied tax of 20 cents a month on each seaman for the purpose of providing temporary health care to those who needed the same. The money could only be spent in the city that collected it, and surplus funds were used for building separate hospital facilities to care for sick seamen (Campbell, 1974). Colonial governments attempted to avoid providing public assistance but, in those instances in which such services were necessary, they generally were guided by the Elizabethan Poor Laws system.

Elizabethan English Poor Laws

The Elizabethan English Poor Laws were a group of laws enacted in Great Britain from 1697 to 1701. They were created to provide financial support for involuntarily unemployed citizens, which included persons who had disabilities. Persons who were unemployed for reasons other than their unwillingness to work were allowed to beg for their daily existence. This group included individuals who moved from one landlord's property to another in order to secure employment. When England shifted its economic base from feudalism to capitalism, workers were free to move around for employment without the permission of their feudal lord. Individuals unable to find employment often resorted to begging. As a growing number of individuals found it more profitable to beg for a living than to work, begging began to be a problem on city streets, Consequently, the English Poor Laws were enacted to determine who was allowed to beg, and people who had disabilities were included in this category. Relatedly, begging became associated with disabilities. It has been said the word "handicap" originated from the act of begging with cap in hand.

Although most American colonists did not subscribe to begging as a way of providing public assistance, according to Lenihan localization of public relief was based on the Elizabethan Poor Laws (1977, p. 3). Using them as a guide, some towns levied taxes and delegated to town personnel the responsibility of administering the required services. Rubin and Roessler pointed out that most of the able-bodied colonists were preoccupied with sustaining their daily lives, and this precluded them from providing much more than basic public relief for persons who had disabilities (1978, p. 4).

The Pioneering Spirit

After the Revolutionary War, the ex-colonists engaged in building a nation. Included in that effort was the westward expansion of the country. During this expansion era, individualism and self-reliance became a familiar theme. As was the case during the colonial period, each family was expected to care for its members who were ill or had a disability. When towns were developed and grew in population, minimal community services were provided to persons with disabilities. In fact, as Lenihan noted; "What did materialize was a great emphasis on institutional almshouses, work houses or indoors as opposed to outdoor relief. The able bodies would be sent to workhouses where they could be rehabilitated into hard working useful citizens. Almshouses would be ideally reserved for the indigent poor to include the physically and mentally disabled" (1977, p. 19). Therefore, if families could not or would not provide support for their members who had disabilities, they were too often placed in a jail or a home for the poor. In the case of persons who were considered to have a mental disability, many of them were placed in jails too. This situation spawned humanitarian rehabilitation treatment initiatives in the 1800s.

HUMANITARIAN AND REHABILITATION ACTIVITIES

Despite progress in the early formation of America, severe limitations in the medical knowledge and inadequate resources available to people with disabilities resulted in a lack of effective treatment in homes or private charity houses. Generally speaking, the quality of medical care in the colonies precluded significant rehabilitation. Although the state of the art of medicine was a considerable improvement over primitive methods, such as casting spells, there was still little scientific knowledge about germs and almost nothing was known about the cause of some disabilities. Colonial physicians, often self-trained, usually tried to rid the body of diseases such as typhoid fever and influenza by inducing nausea. Bleeding, used to cleanse the blood of infections, was another widespread "advanced" method of medical treatment.

Fortunately, medical knowledge and therefore treatment of patients improved in the nineteenth century. Medical schools began requiring their students to study in laboratories and prove their competency by passing examinations. As medical personnel learned more about the cause of disabling conditions, they required better facilities for those patients. Citizens such as Dorothea Dix became public advocates for people who had disabilities. They demanded that mentally ill people be treated humanely. Dix began her crusade in 1841 after she found deplorable living conditions for mentally ill persons confined to asylums. Lamb (1994) provided the following overview of Dix's crusade:

> In the midst of the moral treatment era, in 1841, Dorothea Lynde Dix began her 40-year crusade, devoted principally to the goal of building enough "insane asylums" to accommodate all mentally sick persons then confined in penal and pauper institutions. The shocking conditions that she found in jails and almshouses led her to personally investigate such places of confinement. She made a great point of contrasting the widely prevalent brutality toward and neglect of the mentally ill in jails and almshouses with the humane therapeutic atmosphere of the few mental hospitals in operation at the time. (p. 1015)

Because of the deplorable living conditions and paucity of adequate treatment of persons with mental disabilities, Dix urged states and the U.S. Congress to build helpful, not punitive, institutions to house individuals who needed treatment. She is credited with influencing at least thirty-two states to establish mental institutions. She was also successful in convincing Congress to pass a bill that included land and money for institutions to house persons with a wide range of disabilities. Unfortunately, President Franklin Pierce vetoed the bill on the basis that the responsibility of caring for these persons belonged to the states. Although Dix's national efforts were not successful, she won numerous victories at the state level. Relatedly, she planted public opinion seeds for national attention to be paid to the needs of persons with mental disabilities.

It is noteworthy that Dix's crusade on behalf of the mentally ill was waged as a morality issue. Given the problems that occurred in the twentieth century regarding the institutionalization of mental patients, one may question the value of her efforts. However, if we view them within the context of the living conditions and the treatment that existed prior to her efforts, it is easy to see the value and benefits of her tireless work. A major thing was missing in Dix's humanitarian efforts: there was no attention given to postinstitutionalization. Little thought was focused on patients released from the institutions into the communities and, for some of them, their need for gainful employment. This omission would plague mental institutions well into the twentieth century. It would be many years later before the deinstitutionalization movement would begin.

Dix's efforts were an example of only one of several early American humanitarian efforts. In 1813, Thomas Gallaudet traveled to Europe to learn the latest methods of educating persons who were deaf (Rubin & Roessler, 1978, p. 5). After returning from Europe in 1817, he became the first director of the American Asylum of Hartford, Connecticut, which was also the first school in the United States dedicated to educating persons who were deaf. Gallaudet used the success of this school to encourage other states to establish similar institutions. By the time he died in 1851, there were fourteen institutions dedicated to educating persons who were deaf. In 1857, the first college established to educate persons who were deaf was opened in Washington, DC, and it later became Gallaudet University.

A few years before Dix began her efforts on behalf of persons with mental disabilities, the first school for the blind in the United

States, the Massachusetts Asylum for the Blind, opened in 1832. The name was later changed to the Perkins Institute. Samuel Gridley Howe, Harvard University Medical School graduate, became the director. He believed that persons who were blind could be trained for employment. Although the school prepared students to be employable, it had little success in placing them in gainful employment. To help alleviate this problem, the faculty established a sheltered workshop that employed their graduates. This became one of the earliest sheltered workshops in America.

Before the Civil War, three hospitals in New York and Philadelphia provided care for people with disabilities. Toward the end of the nineteenth century, a group of Cleveland, Ohio, women, known as the Sunbeam Circle, made and sold handiwork and used the profits to help children of Cleveland who had disabilities. In 1918, the Sunbeam Circle became an association for persons with disabilities and later developed a workshop program, an orthopedic center, and a social service center (Bitter, 1979, p. 27). In 1938, the name was changed to the Cleveland Rehabilitation Center, and it became the forerunner of modern rehabilitation centers. Although the center's initial efforts focused on helping children who had disabilities, it later expanded to include adults.

Other well-known private organizations began during this period. For example, the Salvation Army began in England in 1878 and expanded to the United States in 1880. In 1902, the Goodwill Industries was organized in America by Edgar J. Helms, a Methodist minister. It was primarily individual religious groups that initiated major programs to get persons who had disabilities into the mainstream of society. The first totally American state-supported institution designed to aid the poor was established in 1897; it was the Minnesota State Hospital for Indigent and Dependent children. Although it was not established exclusively for patients who had disabilities, the hospital treated a substantial number of such persons who could not afford private care. Much has changed since those early days. Even so, much remains unchanged. For example, there are still social cleansing movements.

SOCIAL CLEANSING

At various times throughout recorded human history, there have been conflicts among humans. Sometimes, the conflicts have been between differing religious views; at other times, the serious disagreements have related to moral or philosophical issues or concerned racial, ethnic, and nationalistic issues. Sometimes the conflicts have led each side to attempt to destroy the other. When the attempt at destruction reaches the point of trying to totally eliminate the opposition, the effort is called "cleansing," or some similar name that implies that one group has as its goal the total eradication of the opposition, or at the very least, rendering it ineffective and of no significance. In the case of persons who have disabilities, particularly those who are considered mentally challenged or physically useless, there have been two attempts at social cleansing in more recent times: social Darwinism and eugenics.

Social Darwinism

In the latter part of the nineteenth century, the English philosopher Herbert Spencer espoused a theory he called "Social Darwinism." Similar to Darwin's theory of evolution, which basically states that animals evolve through the process of survival of the fittest, Spencer's theory says that if commerce had few restrictions and interferences from governmental agencies, this would allow unrestricted competition. Thus, those who survived would represent the strongest and fittest individuals and organizations. Spencer believed an "ideal society" would develop through unbridled competition (Bryan, 2002). It should be noted that Spencer's efforts were not exclusively directed at persons who had disabilities; rather, it pertained to anyone who was poor and considered unproductive. He believed it was better for society to let weak and unfit people perish rather than be supported by public assistance.

Perhaps today it is difficult to conceive of such a heartless approach to life becoming an acceptable community practice. However, as Rubin and Roessler (1978) have pointed out, during the latter part of the 1800s and early 1900s, Spencer's concepts were favorably discussed throughout the United States. Fortunately, moderate voices, particularly the clergy, spoke against his theory, denouncing it as promoting a "cruel society" rather than an "ideal" one. Even though Spencer's theory lost much of its appeal, the basic theme would become part of the second social cleansing effort—eugenics.

Eugenics

The term eugenics, which was popularized by Sir Frances Galton in 1883, means "well born." Gardella (1995) and Kuhl (1994) remind us that Galton viewed eugenics as a science intended to improve the inborn qualities of a race. Bryan (2002) points out that Galton believed that the most intellectual persons would be those without major physical limitations, and that superior persons should be encouraged to reproduce. Conversely, those of lesser intelligence, "feebleminded", and the physically disabled should be discouraged from reproducing because they would produce defective persons like themselves. Galton's theory is based on the belief that individuals inherit good and bad qualities; therefore, intellectual and able-bodied people would pass good qualities to the next generation. Likewise, persons with mental and physical disabilities would pass their attributes to their offspring. In summary, able-bodied and intellectual people should be encouraged to produce and persons with physical and mental disabilities should not be allowed to reproduce.

To support this theory, Galton promoted two "laws of inheritance": first, he postulated that physical and mental traits are derived from all of one's ancestors and the magnitude of those traits diminished in proportion to the degree of ancestral removal. Second, according to Galton, outstanding traits such as genius tend to revert toward mediocrity in successive generations. The major point Galton attempted to make is this: to maintain outstanding physical and mental characteristics in successive generations, one must mate with someone who has desirable traits (Bryan, 2002). To encourage this type of interaction, he suggested that governments promote marriage among gifted persons and provide financial rewards to those who produce children. A primary goal of Galton's proposal was to segregate and sterilize "undesirable" subgroups, which included the mentally disabled, and criminals.

Bambrick and Roberts (1991) informed us that the myth that all people with mental disabilities possessed excessive, uncontrollable sexual urges supported Galton's belief that persons with mental disabilities had to be restrained with regard to their sexual activities. The most effective and permanent way was through sterilization. Kevies (1985) wrote that the belief in eugenics was responsible for the passage of compulsory sterilization laws in many American states during the mid-1920s. Saunders (1998) noted that the eugenics movement extended well into the 1930s. By 1931, compulsory sterilization laws had been passed in twenty-seven American states; by 1935, Denmark, Norway, Sweden, Switzerland, and Germany had similar laws. To get the point of view across, eugenic supporters resorted to hateful propaganda, such as the following examples cited by Shaw (1994):

> Eugenics groups sponsored Fitter Family contests at county fairs around the country and set up exhibits like this at the Sesquicentennial Exposition in Philadelphia. The American Eugenics Society exhibit included a board which like the population counter of a later day, revealed with flashing lights that every fifteen seconds a hundred dollars of your money went for the care of a person with bad heredity, that every forty-eight seconds a mentally deficient person was born in the United States, and that only every seven-and-a-half minutes did the United States enjoy the birth of a high grade person. . . . Who will have the ability to do creative work and be fit for leadership. (p. 24)

The issue of forced sterilization was controversial. Fortunately, there were people who spoke against this form of population control. Even so, as noted earlier, some states enacted sterilization laws. However, challenges in state and federal courts either delayed implementation or struck down the laws (Webb, Marshall & Lombardo, 1998). According to Bryan (2002), in an attempt to resolve constitutional issues, Priddy, an official in the Colony of Epileptics and Feebleminded in Lynchburg, Virginia, developed what the eugenics supporters believed to be a model law of compulsory sterilization. The statute was passed by the Virginia legislature. It was correctly believed by eugenic supporters that the law would undergo legal challenges and ultimately it would be adjudicated in the U.S. Supreme Court. Indeed, the case chosen for review by the U.S. Supreme Court was *Buck v. Bell*. Carrie Buck was a patient at the Virginia Colony for the Epileptic and Feebleminded. She was placed there by her foster parents after she became pregnant as a result of an alleged rape by a relative of her foster parents. She gave birth to a girl, who the courts declared feebleminded based on a psychological examination administered to her when she was approximately six months old. Carrie's birth mother had given birth to several children out of wedlock, including Carrie, and she too was institutionalized and diagnosed as being feebleminded. The eugenic supporters believed this to be the ideal case because it represented three generations of "feeblemindedness," thus from their viewpoint, it was proof that feeblemindedness was inherited. The court upheld the Virginia law by a majority of eight to one. Justice Oliver Wendall Holmes issued the following majority opinion:

> We have seen more than once that the public welfare may call upon the best citizens for their lives. It would be strange if it could not call upon those who already sap the strength of the state for these lesser sacrifices . . . it is better for the entire world, if instead of waiting to execute degenerate offspring for crime, or to let them starve for their imbecility, society can prevent those who are manifestly unfit from continuing their kind. The principle that sustains compulsory vaccinations is broad enough to cover cutting the Fallopian tubes. Three generations of imbeciles are enough. (Cited in Webb et al., 1998, p. 390)

These comments from the highest legal body in the United States represented popular opinion with regard to the reproductive rights of people in America who had a mental disability. It also indirectly represented the view some citizens held about the worthlessness of other persons who had disabilities. It has been estimated that between 1907 and 1970, as many as 60,000 persons considered to have a mental disability were involuntarily sterilized in the United States (Webb et al., 1998). Garver and Garver (1991) pointed out that many of the persons involuntarily sterilized were in fact not mentally retarded. A few years after the *Buck v. Bell* case, it was determined by agency officials that Carrie's birth mother was not mentally retarded. Apparently she was given that label because she had children out of wedlock. Also, it was determined from later interviews that Carrie Buck was not mentally retarded. A review of her daughter's school records revealed she earned grades of A, B, and C while in school and once was placed on a school's honor roll.

Decline of Eugenics

One of the reasons for the decline in the eugenic movement was the extent to which Germany's Nazi government applied the principles of eugenics. Whereas eugenic supporters in the United States attempted to attain their goals primarily through legal sterilization of persons they considered unfit, the Nazi government carried its efforts to the extreme: not only were "inferior" persons sterilized, but also hundreds of thousands of them were killed. The list of inferior people included Jews, Gypsies, and persons with mental disabilities. Germany's euthanasia program began with the elimination of children who were considered to be mentally retarded or born with some type of "birth defect." No one knows exactly how many children were killed. On August 7, 1929, Adolph Hitler spoke publicly of systematically killing approximately 700,000 children annually (Gallagher, 1990; Garver & Garver, 1991).

The German Law on Preventing Hereditarily Ill Progeny passed July 14, 1933, allowed for the sterilization of persons with mental and physical afflictions (Kuhl, 1994). The law stated that any persons suffering from a hereditary disease may be rendered incapable of begetting children by means of a surgical operation conducted by a scientific medical expert if it was highly probable that any offspring of such a person would inherit some serious physical or mental defect. It is estimated that between 350,000 and 400,000 Germans were sterilized, and at least half of them were persons who had disabilities (Gould, 1984; Gallagher, 1990; Saunders, 1998).

SUMMARY

Throughout recorded history persons with disabilities have had to endure ambiguous societal treatments. In some instances, they have been treated as special persons to be honored; in other instances, they have been treated as demons or persons to be destroyed. Historically, the beliefs about and interactions with persons who have disabilities have been many and varied. Many persons have expressed difficulty accepting as sincere the statements of respondents who publicly proclaim their pride in having a disability, because such persons often discover that pride alone cannot overcome disability barriers. Not even rewriting the literature can do that. The conflicts that result from having a disability do not lead to a single response: some individuals withdraw, others clown, some become aggressive or highly suspicious of people without disabilities, and still others assume proud mannerisms. Those who are able to accept the label "disabled" do not find utopia; community bigots prevent them from being treated like first-class citizens (Phillips, 1990).

Indeed, today's biases against "disabilities" to a large degree have as their foundation ancient beliefs about the worth or lack thereof regarding persons who had disabilities. Some of the negative beliefs have survived several generations even though textbooks and medical treatments have been altered to conform to enlightened views. Unfortunately, harsh treatments such as abandonment and death have in many instances been replaced with segregation and isolation, which in some sense can be equated to social or emotional death. There are a few instances of state-sanctioned abuse, but there are still many instances of persons who have disabilities being treated like social pariahs. The cumulative effect of negative beliefs and inhumane treatment is the devaluing of disabilities and those who possess them.

While the treatment of persons who have disabilities has ranged from neglect, to punishment, to paternalistic protection, there is a noticeable movement toward enlightened believers and helpful rehabilitation programs. Added to these trends are persons with disabilities who have begun to speak out in larger numbers and demand fair treatment, thus forcing entire communities to reevaluate some of their negative beliefs. Progress has been slow, but as a nation, we have ceased many of the practices that characterized the "old days."

POINTS FOR DISCUSSION AND SUGGESTED ACTIVITIES

1. Research some health practices from the American colonies carried out to control or rid the human body of disease.
2. Research Dorothea Lynde Dix's background and her crusade to provide moral treatment to persons with mental disabilities. Discuss the impact Ms. Dix's movement has had on the field of mental health. Also in this discussion, identify the pros and cons of her efforts, particularly the issue of institutionalization of persons with disabilities.
3. Research some of the early American institutions that were established to assist persons who had disabilities, such as Goodwill Industries, the Perkin's Institute, Gallaudet University, and the Sunbeam Circle.
4. Discuss some of our nation's—and your own—current beliefs with regard to persons with disabilities. What was their origin?
5. List several ways persons who have disabilities are depicted in television programs, movies, and newspapers. Have there been improvements over the past twenty-five years in the way they are portrayed?
6. Do further research on how and why Social Darwinism came into existence.
7. Does your state allow sterilization of humans? If yes, what are the conditions under which it is allowed?
8. Do you believe sterilization is a necessary and helpful form of birth control? Why or why not?
9. Discuss whether you think a philosophy similar to eugenics could become acceptable in your community.

REFERENCES

Albrecht, G. L., Seelman, K. D., and Bury, M. (Eds.). (2001). *Handbook of Disability Studies*. Thousand Oaks, CA: Sage.

Apton, A. A. (1959). *The Handicapped*. New York: Citadel Press.

Bambrick, M., and Roberts, G. E. (1991). The sterilization of people with a mental handicap:

The view of parents. *Journal of Mental Deficiency Research, 35*: 353–363.

Bitter, J. A. (1979). *Introduction to Rehabilitation.* St. Louis: C. V. Mosby.

Bryan, W. V. (2002). *Sociopolitical Aspects of Disabilities.* Springfield, IL: Charles C Thomas.

Buscaglia, L. C. (Ed.). (1975). *The Disabled and Their Parents: A Counseling Challenge.* Thorofare, NJ: Charles B. Slack.

Campbell, H. L. (1974). The Congressional debate over the Seaman's Sickness and Disability Act of 1798: The origins of the continuing debate on the socialization of American medicine. *Bulletin of History of Medicine, 48*: 423–426.

Gallagher, H. G. (1990). *By Trust Betrayed.* New York: Henry Holt.

Gardella, J. E. (1995). Eugenic sterilization in America and North Carolina. *NCMJ, 56*: 106–109.

Garver, K. L., and Garver, B. (1991). Historical perspectives of eugenics: Past, present and the future. *American Journal of Human Genetics, 49*: 1109–1118.

Gould, S. J. (1984). Carrie Buck's daughter. *Natural History*, Vols. 14-18: July.

Hinshaw, D. (1948). *Take up Thy Bed and Walk.* New York: G. P. Putnam & Sons.

Kevies, D. J. (1986). *In the Name of Eugenics.* Los Angeles, CA: Penguin Hamondsworth.

Koestler, F. A. (1976). *The Unseen Minority.* New York: American Foundation for the Blind.

Kokaska, C. J., Woodward, S., and Tyler, L. (1984). Disabled people in the Bible. *Rehabilitation Literature, 45*: 20–21.

Kuhl, S. (1994). *The Nazi Connection: Eugenics, American Racism and German National Socialism.* New York: Oxford University Press.

Lamb, H. R. (1994). A century and a half of psychiatric rehabilitation in the United States. *Hospital & Community Psychiatry, 45*:1015–1020.

Lenihan, J. (1977). Performance: A history of disabled Americans: *The President's Committee on Employment of the Handicapped, 27*: 6–7.

Phillips, M. J. (1990). Damaged goods: Oral narrations of the experience of disability in American culture. *Social Science & Medicine, 30*: 849–857.

Rubin, S. E., and Roessler, R. T. (1978). *Foundation of the Vocational Rehabilitation Process.* Baltimore: University Park Press.

Saunders, D. E., Jr., (1998). Lessons from eugenics for the neoeugenic era. *Journal of the South Carolina Medical Association, 9*: 383–388.

Shaw, B. (1994). Eugenics then and now. *The Disability Rag & Resource, Jan/Feb,* 23–25.

Thurer, S. (1980). Disability and monstrosity: A look at literary distortions of handicapping conditions. *Rehabilitation Literature, 41*:12–15.

Webb, S. A., Marshall, M. F., and Lombardo, P. A. (1998). Eugenic in the South: The Carrie Buck case. *The Journal of the South Carolina Medical Association, 9*: 389–391.

Weinberg, H., and Sebian, C. (1980). The Bible and disability. *Rehabilitation Counselor Bulletin, 23*: 273–281.

SUGGESTED READINGS

Allan, W. S. (1958). *Rehabilitation: A Community Challenge.* New York: John Wiley.

Allport, G. W. (1958). *The Nature of Prejudice.* New York: Doubleday.

Beutsch, A. (1949). *The Mentally Ill in America: A History of Their Care and Treatment from Colonial Times.* New York: Columbia University Press.

Bower, E. M. (Ed.) (1980). *Handicapped in Literature.* Denver, CO: Love.

Bryan, W. V. (1996). *In Search of Freedom.* Springfield, IL: Charles C Thomas.

Edgerton, R. B. (1967). *The cloak of competence: Stigma in the lives of the mentally retarded.* Berkeley, CA: University of California Press.

Farrell, G. (1956). *The Story of Blindness.* Cambridge, MA: Harvard University Press.

Fiedler, L. (1978). *Freaks, Myths and Images of the Secret Self.* New York: Simon & Schuster.

Goffman, E. (1963). *Stigma: Notes on the Management of Spoiled Identity.* Englewood Cliffs, NJ: Prentice-Hall.

Haj, F. A. (1970). *Disability in Antiquity.* New York: Philosophical Library.

Chapter 3

THE NATURE OF THE PROBLEM

Outline

- Introduction
- Why Are We Prejudiced?
- Who Are Persons With Disabilities?
- What is Considered a Disability?
- Why is the Population of Persons With Disabilities Increasing?
- Brief Review of Related Literature
- Attitudes and Behaviors
- Summary
- Note to Helpers
- Points for Discussion and Suggested Activities

Objectives

- To describe the number and distribution of persons with disabilities in the United States
- To describe reasons people develop prejudices
- To identify how basic attitudes are formed
- To describe how attitudes impact the way some individuals interact with persons with disabilities

INTRODUCTION

There are numerous reasons for the attitudes some Americans have with regard to persons with disabilities. Our prejudices have an impact on our attitudes and our behaviors, which represent the "acting out" of our attitudes, that too frequently display discrimination of persons with disabilities. As Bryan (2002) reminds us, "The act of prejudging a person or a group of people is the foundation for developing a bias for or against the individual or group. The opinions about the individual or group generally are not derived from actual evidence but based on a combination of myths, rumors, and second- and third-hand information" (p. 71). This lack of factual information leads to perpetuating myths and rumors, thus widening the gap between fact and fiction. Therefore, prejudice is the genesis of the oppression of persons with disabilities."

Prejudice of persons with disabilities is often quite different than prejudice of ethnic and racial groups. Whereas prejudice of the latter group too frequently is grounded in hate and dislike, prejudice of persons with disabilities generally has a paternalistic foundation. To be more specific, when behaviors are based on misguided attempts to protect persons with disabilities from being disappointed or experiencing failure, needless limitations are set on their economic, social, or psychological drives. They are seldom consulted before being saved.

WHY ARE WE PREJUDICED?

The same things that perpetuate prejudice of ethnic and racial groups is true for prejudice of persons with disabilities: ethnocentricism, lack of significant contacts, and preference for categorization. Ethnocentrism is the belief that one's own culture is superior to all other cultures. Although most nondisabled persons do not openly admit to feeling superior over persons with disabilities, their actions reveal that they do. Segregation of persons with disabilities in education and housing, as well as the institutionalization of persons with disabilities, are examples of distancing oneself from people who are considered to be inferior, namely persons with disabilities. The authors acknowledge that in some cases blatant acts of these types of exclusion are fewer each year. The exclusion or segregation of persons with disabilities, in whatever form, reinforces the lack of understanding of persons with disabilities. Spicer (1989) points out the negative influences resulting from lack of contact: "Throughout the world many people tend to value their way of life and reject other lifestyles. Our sense of belonging and social harmony can be disrupted when we encounter other cultures and we often seek to maintain our equilibrium by viewing these other people as inferior and even dangerous. Because our prejudices are largely unconscious, this negative stereotype can persist and, without our knowing it, has an impact on our interaction with other people" (p. 2).

Our need to classify people according to categories perpetuates our prejudices. It is difficult to refute the benefits of identifying things according to their appropriate group. Conversely, there is a negative side to categorization when we attach negative labels to certain groups. One only has to look at the negative labels sometimes attached to ethnic and racial groups to understand the destructive human relations born from those acts. In the case of persons with disabilities, negative labels of "inferior" and "dependent" can diminish aspirations and immobilize the recipients.

As previously stated, prejudice influences our attitudes and the acting out of those attitudes is the behavior of discrimination. With regard to persons with disabilities, the legacy of discrimination has been inadequate educational and employment opportunities for them. Unless prejudice is recognized, discriminatory behaviors are likely to stand uncorrected. Recognition is the first step toward minimizing unfair treatment and maximizing fair treatment.

WHO ARE PERSONS WITH DISABILITIES?

As a group, persons with disabilities are the most diverse minority group in the United States. The universe of persons with disabilities consists of membership in every ethnic and racial group, gender, gender orientation, economic category, and religious sect. In fact, for almost any group of which one can think, persons with disabilities have membership. At anytime, anyone can join the ranks of people with disabilities. These facts make persons with disabilities the largest minority group in the United States. The exact number in the United States is not known; currently the estimates range from 49 million to 54 million. Despite the ambiguity with regard to the numbers of persons with disabilities, it is safe to say that one fifth of the U.S. population has some type of disability.

There are understandable reasons for the differing estimates of the U.S. population. Perhaps the most important reason is the fact there are few estimates based on the overall population of persons with disabilities. To be more specific, many estimates are based on a census of a specific population of persons with disabilities, such as persons in the age group of eighteen to sixty-four (the prime work age). In many instances, persons who are institutionalized are not counted. Therefore, to truly understand an estimate of the population of persons with disabilities, one must know the methodology used in the survey. Considering this information, we believe that most estimates of the numbers of persons with disabilities in the United States are too low. An additional reason for our belief is that most surveys use self-identification and too often persons with some forms of heart disease and hypertension, to mention a few, do not report that they have a disability. Closely related to this is the fact that some persons with disabilities do not consider their condition as being a disability. To illustrate this point, one of the authors asked approximately twenty-five students in his class how many of them had a disability. Four students raised their hands. After reviewing with the class a list of conditions considered disabilities, he repeated the question, and two thirds of the class raised their hands.

WHAT IS CONSIDERED A DISABILITY?

Similar to the confusion about the number of persons with disabilities, there are several definitions of what constitutes a disability. Indeed the definition depends on an agency's or organization's reason or need for a definition. As an example, the U.S. Social Security Administration has a somewhat different definition of a disability than seen in the ADA. With regard to the ADA's definition, which is widely accepted as a guide to defining what is a disability, the act identifies a disability in the following ways: A person with a physical or mental impairment that substantially limits one or more major life activities such as walking, seeing, hearing, speaking, breathing, learning, working, or caring for one's self, or a person is considered to have a disability if that person has a record of such a physical or mental impairment, or a person is considered as having a disability if that person is regarded as having such an impairment.

WHY IS THE POPULATION OF PERSONS WITH DISABILITIES INCREASING?

In 1984, the population of Americans with disabilities was estimated at 35 million and, as noted earlier, it is currently estimated to be 49 million to 54 million. What has caused the increase? There are several answers:

1. People are living longer because of improved health care, exercise, and better nutrition information. As our population ages, more limitations that cause disabilities become likely.
2. Because of medical advances, the most significant of which occurred in the past fifty years, people are surviving illness and accidents that in previous times would have resulted in death. In some instances, survival itself may be a disability.
3. Because some of the stigmas attached to disabilities have been removed and because of the fact that there is more

legal protection for persons with disabilities as well as rights and benefits available, more persons are disclosing that they have a disability than there were in previous years.
4. Additional conditions such as learning disabilities and chronic fatigue syndrome are now considered disabilities.

BRIEF REVIEW OF RELATED LITERATURE

Numerous studies have shown commonalities in the social and physical conditions of people who have disabilities and the psychological reactions and negative attitudes toward them. In addition to negative conditions, however, there are also positive ones.

Seminal work focusing on different sources of negative attitudes toward people with disabilities showed that attitudes determine the treatment of an individual; in turn, treatment shapes the individual's personality (Gellman, 1959; Mussen & Barker, 1944; Raskin, 1956; Roeher, 1961; Siller, 1963; Storey & Homer, 1991; Wright, 1960). Each source cited clearly pointed out that negative societal attitudes toward a person with a disability produce devastating results. Such attitudes are seen in avoidance, pity, segregation, and overprotection, as well as other behaviors. Thus, negative attitudes are a main deterrent to the rehabilitation of people with disabilities.

There are some fairly well-prescribed, informal role expectations of persons with disabilities. It is not enough to have a disability; an individual must also *behave as though* he or she has one. The person with a disability is expected to grieve the loss of his or her body part or function, which reflects the value that persons without disabilities place on their own body parts or functions (Dembo, Leviton & Wright, 1956; Sussman, 1969; Thorenson & Kerr, 1978). Individuals who reject the "suffering role" are likely to be verbally or physically punished. Interestingly, guilt is also attached to being ablebodied (Siller, 1963; Wright, 1960). Atonement generally manifests itself in people's contributions to charitable activities for those with disabilities.

The uneasiness that characterizes the interaction between persons without disabilities and those who have disabilities often represents fear of the unknown. Heider (1944) and Hebb (1944) noted that persons in unfamiliar situations become anxious and confused. Certainly, encountering someone who has a disability represents an unfamiliar situation for those who do not have disabilities. Human bodies with missing pieces or individuals whose movement deviates from the norm tend to cause fearful and negative reactions in nondisabled observers. The lack of factual information about a disabling condition facilitates anxiety and withdrawal (Anthony, 1972; English, 1971). Feelings of repulsion and discomfort are felt when people who do not have disabilities come in contact with persons who have certain visible disabilities, for example, skin disorders, amputations, body deformities, and cerebral palsy (Janelle, 1992; Richardson, Hastorf, Goodman & Dornbusch, 1961; Safilios-Rothschild, 1968; Siller, 1963). This is referred to as *aesthetic-sexual aversion.* Related to this concept is Schilder's (1935) concept of *body image,* which states that seeing a person with a physical disability causes discomfort because there is incongruence between an expected "normal" body and the actual perceived body that does not fit the expectation. This may lead to the fear of losing one's physical integrity (Ansello, 1992).

Central to the rehabilitation process is how a person adjusts to his or her disability. The terms *adaptation, coping, mastery,* and *adjustment* have been used at various times to identify the process of handling disabilities, with *adjustment* being the most utilitarian term (Russell, 1981). Shontz (1978) traced the various theories of adjustment over the past three decades and divided them into three categories: (1) *person oriented*, (2) *socioenvironmental*, and (3) *integrative*. Something of value can be found in each of these approaches.

Person-oriented approaches consist of behavioral adjustment, for example, classical conditioning and operant conditioning, and mental adjustment (individual stages of internal processes of adjustment). Although many writers (e.g., Davis, 1963; Fink, 1967; Kerr & Thompson, 1972; Kubler-Ross, 1969; Shontz, 1978) have traced mental adjustment to disabilities through stages that range from shock to acceptance, few empirical data support these stages-of-adjustment theories. Even so, a large number of practitioners have found stages useful, mainly for conceptualizing processes through which persons with disabilities learn to accept their conditions. As Nickerson (1971) observed, adjustment to a disability means being able to function satisfactorily within the limits imposed by it, or, as Linkowski and Dunn (1974) concluded, acceptance of a disability is related to a positive self-concept.

Socioenvironmental approaches focus on factors that are external to the person with the disability; that is, the attitudes of other persons and the physical barriers they erect must be overcome if the person with a disability is to adjust in a socially functional way. Part of this adjustment requires abandoning or readjusting what Parsons (1951) called the *sick role* and Gordon (1966) called the *impaired role*. Some people adjust by hiding their disability. Goffman (1963) called this *passing*. Ultimately, adjustment to socioenvironmental conditions means that instead of ignoring or hiding his or her disability, a person utilizes social and environmental resources to live a productive life.

Lewin (1935) exemplified the integrative *approaches* to adjustment to disabilities. From his perspective, adjustment is relative to the individual and his or her external forces. Specifically, factors such as age, emotional maturity, nature of physical barriers, religious beliefs, and previous coping experiences interact to affect the type of adjustment. Strategies used in the rehabilitation plan should, integrative theorists believe, relate to as many relevant approaches as possible.

Based on the studies reviewed, it should be evident that the task of understanding and abating negative attitudes is formidable. However, it is not impossible or unmanageable. Above all else, helpers who are well-informed, well-trained, and optimistic are needed.

ATTITUDES AND BEHAVIORS

Because human beings are creatures of culture, attitudes, feelings, and values make objective thinking difficult. However, behavior, not attitudes, creates the major problems in human relations. There are many laws against discriminatory behavior, but there are none against prejudicial attitudes. Human rights activists maintain that it is not what people think about those with disabilities that hurts or helps them but how people act out those thoughts. Some individuals act out their prejudices by denying people with disabilities adequate education, jobs, and housing. Because popular writings and the news media have focused on conflicts and confrontations between blacks and whites, prejudice involving other groups is inadequately reported or not reported at all.

Prejudice is not limited to color. There is prejudice against social classes, women, and many other groups. In the long list, there is prejudice against people with mental and physical disabilities. The following statement was made by a visually impaired black man: "I think that disabled people want the same rights as blacks–human rights. I want to be able to go any place I want to go. I want to be able to go to any school. I want to be able to go to any public place. I want to be able to go to any restaurant" (Roth, 1981, p. 189).

Prejudice is a conclusion drawn without adequate knowledge or evidence. It can multiply and spread to areas that are unrelated to the initial object of concern. The bigot blames others for various social misfortunes: floods; high taxes; inflation; wars; and, interestingly, bigotry. Such prejudgments are easier to make than are objective judgments, which require more energy, knowledge, integrity, and time. In their efforts to make expedient decisions, bigots react to concepts rather than to people.

To abate prejudices, people must know their own strengths and weaknesses, understand how people become prejudiced, and empathize with the many groups that are targets of discriminatory behaviors. In short, they must understand not only their own beliefs and behavior but also the beliefs and behavior of others. People usually get back the kind of human relations they give. Acceptance fosters acceptance, and rejection brings rejection. Because each individual's personality reflects his or her intrapersonal and interpersonal experiences, some personalities can be described as ugly and stunted, whereas others are beautiful and dynamic.

Effective human relations result when each individual accepts and respects the differences of others. This basic principle is frequently taught but less frequently practiced. Whether positive or negative, social behavior spreads in a contagious manner. Unfortunately, only a few people living in heterogeneous environments realize that their differences are assets that provide them with an opportunity to learn from others. Many people waste the major portion of their lives rejecting potential friends who look different. Kate Hoffman (Roth, 1981), a woman born without one hand and "normal" in every other aspect, certainly knows how it feels to be physically different: "I became increasingly less popular till seventh grade, when I totally withdrew after the spring dance. I remember it well. Everyone was pairing off, and the popular kids dated the popular kids. I was an outsider, I was not invited. By that time, it was very, very clear that I was totally at the bottom of the social caste" (p. 29).

Americans are exposed daily to mass media programs that characterize this nation as a country dominated by physically able people. Citizens with disabilities who accept this exaggerated view of the United States become willing parties to a prophecy that fulfills itself; they become losers by default. When this happens, individuals without disabilities maintain their positions of power and pass on the socially myopic prophecy from one generation to the next. For these and other reasons, prejudice against people with disabilities is one of the most pressing human relations problems in today's society. Such prejudice is found in neighborhoods, schools, and jobs, and it comes from two main sources: the values and attitudes people learn from others and the tensions and frustrations that are experienced while trying to cope with others, especially strangers.

A social attitude is a degree of readiness to behave in a given manner toward an object or situation. Much could be added to this definition to make it more scientifically precise, but it is adequate for this discussion. There are three implications of this definition for the chapters that follow:

1. A social attitude is a *degree of readiness*. This is a vague statement. However, if it is

thought of as the ability to perceive certain objects and situations and the quickness to respond, motivation to respond, and experience in responding, then degree of readiness can stand the test of further scrutiny. An example of this process is provided by a teacher who experiences anxieties derived from of the thought of having to teach children with disabilities.

2. A social attitude is a degree of readiness to behave *in a given manner.* An attitude is not an overt response. It is a response, to be sure, but an implicit or mental one. Therefore, an attitude is a readiness to act, not an act itself. The crucial human relations question that arises here, then, is "Under what conditions does an attitude elicit overt expression?" Even the most general answer to this question must include at least two variables:

A. *An attitude is likely to result in overt expression in direct proportion to rewards and in inverse proportion to punishments.* Behavior cannot always be predicted on the basis of whether it will be rewarded or punished. A weakly held attitude will produce action if the gratification for doing so is great enough.

B. *Overt behavior is likely to result when there is a degree of readiness.* Some individuals act out their attitudes, no matter how negatively the community reacts to their behavior. These individuals become martyrs for various causes such as those of citizens with disabilities or women. On the other hand, some individuals cannot, under any circumstance, muster sufficient readiness to act out their attitudes. They say, "I know what I should do, but I can't." Technically, the degree of readiness must rise and resistance must lower to a crucial point in order for attitude to result in action. There are thresholds at which the degree of readiness (perception, motives, and response) must be sufficiently developed and the situation must be sufficiently rewarding for at least part of the attitude to result in overt behavior.

Overt behavior can mean anything, from making marks on an attitude questionnaire to dying for a cause. It is generally assumed in psychology experiments that when most variables in a situation are held constant, the degree of action taken toward an object is a function of motivation, the desire to achieve a goal. Although this assumption may be correct in most instances, there is more to the degree of readiness than motivation. There is also a *response system*—the means used to achieve the goal. For example, two individuals, X and Y, may be equally motivated to succeed in getting children with disabilities into their youth clubs, but the response of X is to wait for applicants to call, whereas Y tries to obtain the names of prospective members. In a similar manner, two state legislators may be equally motivated to enact barrier-free housing legislation, but the behavior of one involves only a verbal response, whereas the other writes bills. Thus there are talkers, doers, and talkers who are doers.

3. A social attitude is a degree of readiness to behave in a given manner toward an object or situation. Here, object and situation are used in the broadest senses. Object refers not only to individuals but also to their beliefs. Within this definition, any group of people or their behavior is considered socially significant and may become embodied in social attitudes. A social attitude toward people with disabilities, then, is a degree of readiness to behave in a given manner toward some perceived aspect of them. Whether this readiness will result in overt behavior is determined by certain conditions internal and external to the individuals involved. This is the basic foundation for dealing with the problem of how social attitudes toward people with disabilities are formed.

People Learn to Dislike People

There are four hypotheses about attitudes that are now generally accepted: (1) attitudes are learned; (2) attitudes are learned mainly from other people; (3) attitudes are learned mainly from other people who have high or low prestige for a particular individual; and (4) once attitudes have been learned, they are reinforced.

The first three hypotheses focus on the perception of social objects and the development of motivational and response systems appropriate for these perceptions; the fourth hypothesis suggests that attitudes are difficult to change.

1. Attitudes are Learned.

Attitudes are learned; they are not innate. A mother talking about her child's prejudice against children with disabilities said, "Tina has always played with well children. She never plays with crippled children. I didn't have to teach her that." She reflects the assumption that powerfully held attitudes such as disability prejudices are part of an individual's inherent being. The mother apparently believed that she did not have to teach her daughter to discriminate against children with disabilities. There is evidence to the contrary.

Antidisabled attitudes have been detected in children as young as three years old (Gellman, 1959; Roeher, 1961; Weinberg, 1979). However, studies have shown that even these attitudes are not very well-developed in most children until age ten or eleven. Young children begin to use hate words before they fully understand their connotations. Social scientists have documented thousands of cases illustrating that attitudes are learned. Tina's mother believed that Tina knew instinctively not to associate with "crippled" children, but her third-grade son suggested other reasons for the attitude:

"Mother told me not to play with them [children with disabilities] because they are sick. . . . I had a crippled friend in school. I liked him, but Mother didn't want me to play with him." The mother had taught her children to reject children with disabilities.

Once negative attitudes are learned, children can be very cruel to peers with disabilities (Darrow & Johnson, 1994; Kishi & Meyer, 1994). They mock them and in the process either break them down or steel them to their impairments. One can walk onto almost any playground where large numbers of children gather and hear them taunting others for their physical disabilities–simulating crossed eyes, mocking slurred or stammering speech, and pantomiming epileptic seizures. It is not that children want to be cruel but that they want to be in with the in-group, just as their parents do. Much like their ancestors during the 1692 witch trials in Salem, they must have their sport.

It is not just what people without disabilities do to people with disabilities that constitutes the problem (Gouvier, Coon, Todd & Fuller, 1994). There is a pecking order, or rank order of preference, among people with disabilities. Doe West (Roth, 1981), who must spend some of her time in a wheelchair, described prejudice from within:

> If I meet a disabled person and I'm not in the chair and we're talking and I say, "Yeah, we disabled people," they sort of look at me and think, she doesn't look very disabled–she must have epilepsy or she must have a learning disability or diabetes, or something. And then as we're talking later and I say, "Yeah, you know, when I'm in the chair," they say "When you're in the chair?" I get this ambivalent feeling from disabled people in terms of–well, God, you're a lucky stiff; you can get out of the chair. And sometimes I'll meet anger or bitterness at the fact that I can get out of the chair. And it hurts me, because they don't understand the seriousness of my own disability. (p. 176)

The most insidious prejudices are negative attitudes directed toward groups of people. They take the form of assumptions or generalizations about all or most members of a particular group ("You know how *those* people are!"). Such in-group versus out-group hostility threatens the very existence of this nation. People are employed, housed, married, and buried with one major criterion in mind: group affiliations. The behavior, customs, and habits of out-group people are labeled strange and inferior. Most aspects of growing up with a physical disability add to the probability of societal rejection.

The learning of attitudes is seen when adults change their commitments as they move into situations in which new attitudes are more functional, for example, when they join a club or move into an "exclusive" neighborhood. Thus new attitudes are part of a wide range of adjustment devices that every human being acquires. Attitudes of acceptance must be learned in much the same manner that people learn to reject people. It is hypothesized by many writers that most American children are taught to reject rather than to accept people who are culturally and physically different. In the insightful words of Jung (1968); "We still attribute to the other fellow all the evil and inferior qualities that we do not like to recognize in ourselves, and therefore have to criticize and attack him, when all that has happened is that an inferior soul has emigrated from one person to another. The world is still full of *betes noires* and scapegoats, just as it formerly teemed with witches and werewolves" (p. 65).

Researchers have noted that as children grow older, they tend to forget that they were instructed in attitudes by their parents (Horowitz & Horowitz, 1938). Around the age of ten, most children regard their attitudes toward people with disabilities as their own. Seldom do they recall having been coached by their parents. *Attitude amnesia* develops, and elaborate rationalizations are presented to account for the learned attitudes, with the result that most people believe that they came by their attitudes "naturally."

2. Attitudes are Learned Mainly From Other People.

Most attitudes are learned from other people. As ego deflating as it may be to accept, it is a fact that few people invent their attitudes. An attitude is a complex perceptual invention, and most people are not perceptual inventors. For example, "That man has paraplegia, and, therefore, he is inferior to me" is a seemingly simple perception, but it is a straightforward attitude that includes the man and his label and, therefore, requires considerable rationalizing. Individuals who perceive persons with paraplegia as inferior have to think beyond individuals with paraplegia, who may be adequate by almost every objective standard, in order to define the group of *persons with paraplegia* as inferior.

The superiority or inferiority of a group (as contrasted to that of an individual) is not obvious; not many casual observers can perceive significant group differences. To illustrate, the existence of physical disabilities as a social problem is by no means obvious. Most people simply cannot think of liking or disliking physical disabilities per se but only of liking or disliking particular disabilities, for example, the loss of eyesight, hearing, or use of legs. Before an attitude can be formed about an object, something must be perceived as its characteristic. Because most people are not very adept at inventing new ways (or even old ways) of perceiving the world, there seems to be a sound basis for believing that attitudes, like most things, are invented by a few and used by many.

There are other reasons for assuming that attitudes are learned largely from other people. Autobiographies and case histories illustrate that an individual's attitudes toward disabilities tend to be those of his or her relatives, sex group, peers, officemates, school group, region, religion, and nationality. Certainly, some attitudes are developed independently of significant others, but significant others are the foremost determinants of most social attitudes. Thus the tendency of individuals to hold the same attitudes toward disabilities as the people with whom they interact is so consistent as to make independent acquisition unlikely. This does not necessarily mean that individuals learn their attitudes about disabilities only from the individuals or groups with whom they live, but it certainly suggests the importance of relatives, friends, and social institutions.

Some people will ask, "Is it true that people hold the same attitudes as those with whom they live simply because they are all exposed to similar conditions?" In other words, "Do people learn the same attitudes independently simply because they all have the same experiences?"–of course not. Although many people may look at the same phenomenon, they depend on a few "important" people to tell them what they have seen. Consequently, stereotyped attitudes toward various persons with disabilities are found among people who have had no contact with them. Furthermore, it has been found that initial attempts to change negative social attitudes through personal experience are not always successful.

The unlikelihood that individuals will invent attitudes for themselves, the correlation of their attitudes with those of the people with whom they live, and the low level of correlation between attitude and personal experiences all point to the conclusion that attitudes are learned from other people. However, attitudes are not learned from just anyone, which leads to the third theory of attitudes.

3. Attitudes are Learned Mainly From Other People Who Have High or Low Prestige.

Investigators have been testing this hypothesis for several decades. In a typical experiment, subjects respond to one or more attitude scales. Then they are told the attitudes of 98 percent of the nation's leading educators, of certain authorities, or of the majority of their own reference group on the same scales. Later, they are retested with equivalent tests. In most cases, the retest scores move significantly in the direction of the educators, authorities, and peers, leading inevitably to the conclusion that most people tend to match their attitudes with persons or groups important to them who have high prestige.

There are, of course, exceptions. Some individuals will not shift their attitudes to match those of an admired person if the attitude attributed to the latter is diametrically opposed to theirs. There is, nonetheless, a strong tendency for people to reinterpret their role models' statements in line with their own views rather than admit the role models are wrong. "The press distorted his views," a son replied when asked about antidisability quotes attributed to his father, whom he worshipped.

The second part of the hypothesis is that people tend to adopt attitudes opposite to those of groups with low prestige. Such attitudes are likely to be held for one of two reasons: (1) Certain groups may have low prestige for people because they have rejected those people who adopt attitudes opposite to theirs as a means of rejecting them in turn, or (2) certain groups are poor role models for people, and, thus, the people elect not to imitate them.

4. Once Attitudes Have Been Learned, They Are Reinforced.

If one assumes that the first three theories are correct, the initial formation of attitudes is the result of a desire to be like individuals who are held in high esteem. Once formed, however, an attitude may serve various other motives. For example, although most persons in a community learn negative attitudes toward people with disabilities from their friends, the attitudes of some persons center on economic motives. Most individuals, for instance, initially adopt antidisability attitudes in order to conform to social pressures but maintain those attitudes in order to exclude qualified job competitors with disabilities.

The economic motives that reinforce attitudes are relatively obvious. Clearly, in the short run, it is economically advantageous for one group to keep another group out of certain kinds of work, to deny them adequate legal protection in bargaining for their labors, to keep their aspirations low, or even on occasion to exterminate them. The questions that economic interpretations of social attitudes fail to answer, however, are "Why are repressive methods used against one group but not another?" and "Why are certain attitudes enforced even to the point of national disaster?" Some critics observe that as a nation, America seems to be willing to waste the human resources of people with disabilities.

Group prejudices are expressed in terms of *stereotypes*, false images of out-groups. Some stereotypes are given a typical verbal expression such as "Cripples are pushy," "Deaf people are lazy," "Amputees are sneaky," or "Poor handicapped people are trashy." These images are clearly false, but they trigger the premature social and psychologic deaths of the people so labeled. In most instances, these images can be destroyed only after the prejudiced person has had a positive experience with a person in the stereotyped group. However, it is likely that a positive experience will only cause the prejudiced person to discount its general significance by saying, "That person is different, exceptional, not like the others:" That is, people tend to refence their prejudices to exclude a few token members of the oppressed group.

> In casual contacts with the handicapped, normals tend to measure them against the stereotype, and such contacts reinforce common stereotypes. An example may help to demonstrate this process. Recently, a number of typical skiers observed a blind skier coming down the slope. They spoke about him and his "amazing feat." They commented on how "truly remarkable" that he could have the courage and fortitude to do what must be exceptionally difficult for a person with no eyesight. From the tone of their comments, it was clear that they did not perceive this person as any ordinary blind person. The sighted skiers did not question their stereotypes of the blind as physically inept. Instead, they confirmed the stereotype by classifying this skier as an exception to the rule–as "amazing." (Bogdan & Biklen, 1981, p. 19)

How Attitudes Are Formed

There are several ways in which attitudes are formed. Being aware of these processes will better enable people to alter their negative attitudes. Some popular ideas about how attitudes are formed have been refuted in scientific experiments.

Attitudes Are Seldom Formed by Logic.

It is very difficult to find circumstances in which attitude change has come about as a result of logical argument or additional information (Rees, Spreen & Harnadek, 1991;

Wilson & Alcorn, 1969). When students in classroom experiments are confronted with logic or new information, they do not tend to change their attitudes. For example, racist students who receive intensive instruction in anthropology do not as a rule abandon their belief in innate racial differences. Instead, they give nonracist answers on tests in order to get passing grades. Individuals who register changes in attitude because of such information consistently fail to maintain the new attitudes as the prestige of the person presenting the logical arguments or imparting the information decreases. Therefore, not simply *what* is said but also *who* says it are important variables influencing whether an argument or information will change attitudes. Bankers and real estate developers influence housing patterns for citizens with disabilities more than college professors and factory workers.

There is the general finding that attitudes acquired by logical argument are not acted out very logically (Hafer & Narcus, 1979). For example, a college student's attitude toward people with disabilities may become more tolerant during a course in vocational rehabilitation but show very little carryover into the job. In fact, some vocational rehabilitation trainees adopt what they perceive to be "correct" answers in order to get a diploma but revert to polar attitudes and behaviors when they are employed as rehabilitation counselors. There is not only little evidence that important attitudes are changed by logical information inputs but also considerable evidence that a great amount of information, particularly on controversial topics, actually hardens or freezes whatever attitude is already in the making.

Techniques such as an exceedingly emotional religious appeal or a relatively unstructured workshop focusing on physical disabilities often are more effective than highly structured scientific lectures. Elaborate conferences and professional seminars with "experts," situations in which opposing interests are presented in great detail, tend to produce little shift in attitude but instead add to the confusion about what attitude should be taken. The unqualified assumption that information will improve attitudes in one way or another is based on the questionable assumption that what is true and what is desirable are one and the same.

Important attitudes are seldom influenced by logic because in most cultures, including this one, logic is valued as a means but seldom as an *end* in life. The desired end tends to be some visible sign of success, and when the choice is between logic and success, success generally prevails. This is not to imply that most people want to seem illogical. On the contrary, most people would like to project an image of being very logical, but not if such an image will cause them to fail to achieve certain goals, especially economic ones. In some settings, little prestige accrues to individuals who associate with persons with disabilities.

The power of logic (and information) can easily be tested by following these simple steps: (1) select an individual who is fairly neutral; (2) determine an attitude toward disabilities that he or she holds with considerable strength but that happens not to be based on logic and fact; (3) objectively and unemotionally try to alter his or her attitude by pointing out the illogical aspects of it; and (4) observe the effect. This exercise is likely to illustrate that logic and information have little to do with attitude formation. There are, however, at least two special instances in which this may not be the case. Attitudes may be formed by logic and information if the attitude to be formed or changed does not conflict with motives more powerful than the desire to be logical or if the individual in whom the attitude is to be formed or changed is one of those rare persons for whom "having it right" is more important than "having it his or her own way."

Attitudes Are Seldom Formed as a Function of Intelligence.

In this day of loose and careless logic, it has been claimed that some people become radicals (or liberals) because they are more (or less) intelligent than those who become conservatives. Studies investigating intelligence and attitudes have shown correlations between intelligence and liberalism or conservatism ranging from low positive correlation to no correlation at all. There is little scientific support for attributing attitudes to intelligence (Katz, 1960). Interestingly, there is a tendency for people to believe that those who share their values are intelligent and that those who do not are stupid.

Ignorance leads people without disabilities to assume that they are superior to those with them. Nondisability is thus equated with high intelligence, whereas disability becomes synonymous with *low intelligence.* Persons engaging in such assumptions have not learned that (1) all people are of the same genus and species; (2) there are more differences within groups than among them; and (3) apparent group differences are largely attributable to environmental conditions, training, and opportunities.

Attitudes are Seldom Formed by Personal Experience.

It is often heard that integration of persons with disabilities would become a way of life if people of the various groups would only live together. Placing bodies together is not enough. One factor that reduces the importance of personal experience on attitude formation is the tendency of people to perceive and remember only what they are socially and psychologically prepared to see and recall. A person's friends predetermine not only how he or she reacts to a given stimulus but indeed whether he or she perceives it in the first place. Consider then the difficulty of changing the attitude of persons without disabilities toward those with them by getting them together, if those without are prepared to see only negative characteristics in people with disabilities.

A second factor that may reduce the importance of personal experience in shaping attitudes is the possibility that personal experiences may actually reinforce the negative attitudes that they are supposed to change. Prejudiced persons will not develop a favorable attitude when they interact as neighbors with individuals having disabilities if the behavior of the newcomers fits their existing stereotypes about people with disabilities. It is difficult for many social reformers to accept the fact that some members of groups actually reinforce the very attitudes that the reformers are eager to eradicate; in other words, some people with physical disabilities are behaviorally disconcerting. Myers (1969) provided an illustration:

> The child's arm flailed, her head wobbled, and her eyes rolled. Before her, on the school recreation table, were the sickening shambles of a lunch. The table had been crowded around by many children. Now every one of them had beat a retreat and clustered again at a safer distance, to watch and even cruelly to mimic the helpless youngster rooting so dreadfully in her food. . . . Bits of cookie, sandwich, fruit littered the table, and the little girl gagged like a little beast. (p. 59)

Does all of this mean that personal contacts are entirely without value? Certainly not. Negative attitudes toward people with disabilities can be formed or changed by personal experience if (1) the attitudes are not in conflict with more powerful motives,

(2) the experience is carefully selected to represent people with disabilities in the best possible light, (3) the persons who are to experience changed attitudes are prepared to experience the best in the situation, or (4) the attitude involves perceptions that are so simple as to be obvious examples of empirical contradiction.

New attitudes toward people with disabilities can be learned if such experiences with them are rewarding, providing that more punishing experiences do not follow. When a couple is ridiculed by parents, peers, and others for moving into a housing unit largely occupied by persons with disabilities, they are less likely to associate with persons with disabilities, even friendly ones.

SUMMARY

Being against someone or something is not necessarily a prejudice. When based on facts, an attitude opposing someone or something is a *bias*, which does not violate democratic principles. For example, an individual is not behaving prejudicially if she concludes after interacting with a neighbor who has a disability that she does not like him. It is also important to note that not all prejudices are harmful or negative. Some, such as clothing preferences, are both harmless and a source of amusement to others. Prejudicial attitudes can support a group rather than oppose it. Black, Brown, and Red Power advocates, for instance, state that they are for their people and not against other groups. These individuals are not interested in integration.

The most insidious prejudices are negative attitudes directed toward groups of people. They take the form of assumptions or generalizations about all or most members of a particular group. Being identified with an out-group adds to the probability of societal rejection of individuals with disabilities.

NOTE TO HELPERS

Efforts to bring about attitudinal and behavioral changes can and often do result in strong resistance to those changes. Zander (1950) outlined several reasons for this resistance:

1. Resistance to change can be expected if the change is not clear to the people who are going to be influenced by the change. Most people want to know exactly what they must do in order to help persons with disabilities. It is not enough to say, "The change is because of new laws" or "It's the right thing to do."

2. Different people will see different meanings in the proposed change. There is a tendency for people to see in proposed changes the things they want to see; in other words workers with disabilities may see equal opportunities, whereas workers without disabilities may see "reverse discrimination." Complete information can be distorted just as easily as incomplete information, especially if the persons to be changed are insecure.

3. Resistance can be expected when individuals in power positions are caught between strong forces pushing them to make the change and strong forces opposing the change. If trying to bring about change, the individual or group must be able to show that there is a greater payoff for the organization to make the change rather than not make it. Little energy should be spent trying to destroy opponents' reputations.

4. Resistance can be expected to increase to the degree that the persons in the organization influenced by the change (rank and file workers) have pressure put on them to change and decrease to the degree that these same persons are involved in the nature or direction of the change. It is true that behavior can be legislated or mandated, but it is also true that forcing people to accept persons with disabilities can be a fleeting victory for the organization and persons with disabilities.

Change is almost always accepted and institutionalized in a nondestructive manner when the decision-making process is shared. However, ultimately, someone must be responsible for carrying out the change.

5. *Resistance may be expected if the change is made on personal grounds rather than impersonal requirements or sanctions.* After the individuals to be affected by the change have had a chance to discuss it, if they still do not want to make it, then it is not prudent for the administrator in charge to say, "I think we should do this." Who really cares what he or she thinks? A better approach is, "This change is consistent with this organization's equal opportunity/affirmative action objectives." The change should be grounded in organizational objectives and commitments.

6. *Resistance may be expected if the change ignores established group norms.* There are formal as well as informal ways changes are made within organizations. An effective change will neither ignore old customs nor abruptly create new ones. For example, if it is an informal custom for new workers to be given certain workspaces or schedules, then new workers who have disabilities should be given these spaces or schedules, too.

In summary, coworkers are likely to accept persons with disabilities when the newcomers prove that they are basically the same as persons without disabilities. Anyone who wishes to alter the status quo of organizations and positively influence the quality of life for people with disabilities would be well advised to heed Zander's warning.

POINTS FOR DISCUSSION AND SUGGESTED ACTIVITIES

1. List on a piece of paper at least three prejudices that you have (they do not have to relate to disabilities or persons with disabilities) and under each one try to identify how you acquired them.
2. Identify and discuss some of the attitudes that currently prevail with regard to persons with disabilities.
3. Identify at least three negative attitudes society has with regard to persons with disabilities and discuss some possible ways to alter them.

REFERENCES

Ansello, E.R. (1992). Seeking common ground between aging and developmental disabilities. *Generations, 16,* 9–15.

Anthony, W.A. (1972). Societal rehabilitation: Changing society's attitudes toward the physically and mentally disabled. *Rehabilitation Psychology, 19,* 117–126.

Bogdan, R., and Biklen, D. (1981). Handicapism. In A. D. Spiegel, S. Podair & E. Fiorito (Eds.), *Rehabilitation People with Disabilities Into the Mainstream of Society.* Park Ridge, NJ: Noyes Medical.

Bryan, W.V. (2002). *Sociopolitical Aspects of Disabilities.* Springfield, IL: Charles C Thomas.

Darrow, A.N., & Johnson, C.M. (1994). Junior and senior high school music students' attitudes toward individuals with a disability. *Journal of Music Theory, 31,* 266–279.

Davis, R. (1963). *Passage Through the Crisis: Polio Victims and Their Families.* New York: Bobbs-Merrill.

Dembo, T., Leviton, G.L., and Wright, B.A. (1956). Adjustment to misfortune: A problem of social psychology rehabilitation. *Artificial Limbs, 3,* 4–62.

English, R.W. (1971). Combatting stigma toward physically disabled persons. *Rehabilitation Research & Practice Review, 2,* 1–17.

Fink, S.L. (1967). Crisis and motivation: A theoretical model. *Archives of Physical Medicine & Rehabilitation, 48,* 592–597.

Gellman, W. (1959). Roots of prejudice against the handicapped. *Journal of Rehabilitation, 40,* 4–6.

Goffman, E. (1963). *Stigma: Notes on the Management of Spoiled Identity.* Englewood Cliffs, NJ: Prentice Hall.

Gordon, G.A. (1966). *Role Theory and Illness: A Sociological Perspective.* New Haven, CT: College & University Press.

Gouvier, W.D., Coon, R.C., Todd, M.E., & Fuller, K.H. (1994). Verbal interactions with individuals presenting with and without disability. *Rehabilitation Psychology, 39,* 263–268.

Hafer, M., and Narcus, M. (1979). Information and attitude toward disability. *Rehabilitation Counseling Bulletin, 23,* 95–102.

Hebb, D.O.H. (1944). On the nature of fear. *Psychological Review, 51,* 259–276.

Heider, F. (1944). Social perception and phenomenal causality. *Psychological Review, 51,* 358–374.

Horowitz, E.L., and Horowitz, R.E. (1938). Development of social attitudes in children. *Sociometry, 1,* 301–338.

Janelle, S. (1992). Locus of control in nondisabled versus congenitally physically disabled adolescents. *American Journal of Occupational Therapy, 46,* 334–342.

Jung, C.G. (1968). *Civilization in Transition.* Vol. 10. Princeton, NJ: Princeton University Press.

Katz, D. (1960). The functional approach to the study of attitudes. *Public Opinion Quarterly, 24,* 163–204.

Kerr, W.G., and Thompson, M.A. (1972). Acceptance of disability of sudden onset paraplegia. *Paraplegia, 10,* 94–02.

Kishi, G.S., and Meyer, L.H. (1994). What children report and remember: A six-year follow-up of the effects of social contact between peers with and without severe disabilities. *Journal of the Association for Persons with Severe Handicaps, 19,* 277–289.

Kubler-Ross, E. (1969). *On Death and Dying.* New York: Macmillan.

Lewin, K.A. (1935). *A Dynamic Theory of Personality.* New York: McGraw-Hill.

Linkowski, D.C., and Dunn, M.A. (1974). Self-concept and acceptance of disability. *Rehabilitation Counseling Bulletin, 18,* 28–32.

Mussen, P.H., and Barker, R.G. (1944). Attitudes toward cripples. *Journal of Abnormal & Social Psychology, 39,* 351–355.

Myers, J.M. (1969). The linneth on the leaf. In W.C. Kvarceus and E.N. Hayes (Eds.), *If Your Child is Handicapped.* Boston: Porter Sargent.

Nickerson, E.T. (1971). Some correlates of adjustment by paraplegics. *Perception & Motor Skills, 32,* 11–23.

Parsons, T. (1951). *The Social System.* New York: Free Press.

Pfeiffer, D. (1993). The problem of disability definition: Commentary. *Journal of Disability Policy Studies, 4,* 77–82.

Raskin, N. J. (1956). *The Attitude of Sighted People Toward Blindness.* Paper presented at the National Psychological Research Council on Blindness, Denver, March.

Rees, L.M., Spreen, O., and Harnadek, M. (1991). Do attitudes toward persons with handicaps really shift over time? Comparison between 1975 and 1978. *Mental Retardation, 29,* 81–86.

Richardson, S.A., Hastorf, A.M., Goodman, N., & Dornbusch, S.M. (1961). Cultural uniformity in reactions to disabilities. *American Sociological Review, 26,* 241–247.

Roeher, G.A. (1961). Significance of public attitudes on the rehabilitation of the disabled. *Rehabilitation Literature, 22,* 66–72.

Roth, W.E. (1981). *The Handicapped Speak.* Jefferson, NC: McFarland.

Russell, R. (1981). Concepts of adjustments to disability: An overview. *Rehabilitation Literature, 42,* 330–337.

Safilios-Rothschild, C. (1968). Prejudice against the disabled and some means to combat it. *International Rehabilitation Review, 14,* 8–10.

Schilder, P. (1935). *The Image and Appearance of the Human Body.* London: Kegan Paul, Trench, Trubner.

Shontz, E.C. (1978). Psychological adjustment to physical disability: Trends in theories. *Archives of Physical Medicine & Rehabilitation, 59,* 251–254.

Siller, J. (1963). Reactions to physical disability. *Rehabilitation Counseling Bulletin, 7,* 12–16.

Spicer, J. (1989). *Counseling Ethnic Minorities.* Minneapolis, MN: Hazeiden.

Storey, K., and Homer, R.H. (1991). An evaluative review of social validation research involving persons with handicaps. *Journal of Special Education, 25,* 352–401.

Sussman, M.B. (1969). Dependent disabled and dependent poor: Similarity of conceptual issues and research needs. *Social Service Review, 43*, 383–95.

Thorenson, R.W., and Kerr, B.A. (1978). The stigmatizing aspects of severe disability: Strategies for change. *Journal of Applied Rehabilitation Counseling, 9*, 21–25.

Weinberg, N. (1979). Preschool children's perception of orthopedic disability. In B. Bolton & M.E. Jacques (Eds.), *The Rehabilitation Client*. Baltimore: University Park Press.

Wilson, E.O., and Alcorn, D. (1969). Simula- tion and development of attitudes toward the exceptional. *Journal of Special Education, 3*, 303–307.

Wright, B.A. (1960). *Physical Disability: A Psychological Approach*. New York: Harper & Row.

Zander, A. (1950). Resistance to change: Its analysis and prevention. *Advanced Management, 15*, 10.

SUGGESTED READINGS

Allport, G. (1958). *The Nature of Prejudice*. New York: Doubleday.

Bryan, W.V. (1996). *In Search of Freedom*. Springfield, IL. Charles C Thomas.

Eisenberg, M.G., Giggins, C., and Duval, R.J. (Eds.). (1982). *Disabled People as Second-Class Citizens*. New York, Springer.

Gartner, A., and Joe, T. (Eds.). (1987). *Images of the Disabled*. New York: Praeger.

Mackelsprang, R.W., and Salsgiver, R.O. (1987). People with disabilities and social work. *Social Work, 41*: 7–14.

Ponterotto, J.G., and Pedersen, P.B. (1973). *Preventing Prejudice: A Guide for Counselors and Educators*. Newbury Park, CA: Sage.

Rubin, S.E., & Roessler, R.T. (1978). *Foundations of the Vocational Rehabilitation Process*. Baltimore: University Park Press.

Stone, D.A. (1984). *The Disable State*. Philadelphia: Temple University Press.

Yuker, H. E. (Ed.). (1988). *Attitudes Toward Persons With Disabilities*. New York: Springer.

Chapter 4

GROWTH FOR PEOPLE WITH DISABILITIES

Outline

- Introduction
- Feelings
- Social Development
- Self-Acceptance
- Positive Thoughts
- Realism
- Responsibility
- Effective Communication
- Pride
- Self Improvement
- Summary
- Note to Helpers
- Points for Discussion and Suggested Activities

Objectives

- To encourage persons with disabilities to have pride in themselves
- To identify ways persons with disabilities can effectively express themselves
- To emphasize how persons with disabilities can be responsible for their own feelings and actions and ultimately be the major force in their own rehabilitation

INTRODUCTION

"Laugh and the world laughs with you, cry and you cry alone" is an old saying that describes two reactions to problem-solving behaviors. The authors are not suggesting that people should take their disabilities lightly, because having a disability is a serious matter. However, they are suggesting that instead of viewing a disability as an end to life, it is much more productive to view it as an aspect of living. This is a proactive, as opposed to a reactive, approach to disabilities. It is true that crying over one's disability is likely to generate sympathy, but feelings of sorrow and pity soon give way to antagonism or indifference, especially when individuals do little to overcome their impairments. Sadness is not a solid foundation upon which to build relationships (Stuifbergen & Becker, 1994).

Similar to a child who feels anger and temporary hatred for his mother following an argument, persons with disabilities often experience feelings of guilt, self-consciousness, inadequacy, depression, and shame following behavior to elicit sympathy. Persons without disabilities tend to send out mixed messages with regard to their feelings about the situation, and their interaction becomes less helpful. On the one hand, they may treat people with disabilities as dependent persons who do not have the full range of feelings, emotions, wants, and responsibilities of able-bodied people. On the other hand, they may send signals that say to people with disabilities that they should feel good about themselves because, despite their physical limitations, they are worthwhile human beings. These mixed messages confuse and greatly affect both parties.

FEELINGS

No matter how positive the self-image of persons with disabilities, there will be times when they will feel inadequate. These negative feelings may be partially due to their disability and partially due to the fact that all people periodically have doldrums. This is normal behavior. Too often, people with disabilities are made to feel guilty because they become unhappy with their lives. Books and articles written by "experts" frequently chide people with disabilities for being human. When one takes a careful look at what these authors are saying, it is a message of Spartan self-discipline. This regimen is not realistic, and it most certainly is not achievable.

A person with a disability should not believe that he or she is emotionally ill if there are times when feelings of inferiority and shame, to mention just two, take hold. It is not easy living in a human fishbowl; persons staring or making comments about an individual's disability draw attention to his or her limitations. It is not abnormal or a sign of emotional instability to react negatively to being the object of attention, but it is abnormal to spend an inordinate amount of time feeling inferior or ashamed. Many individuals with disabilities forget that *all* humans, regardless of their physical condition, experience these feelings. For example, an able-bodied man who is in good physical condition may feel inferior when he sees a person with a physique that in his estimation is more developed than his own. The same is true for a woman who observes another woman who she thinks is better looking. There will always be someone with more or fewer attributes that a person values, and individuals who compete to be number one run the risk of losing self-esteem.

The authors' message to persons with disabilities is this: Do not think that because of your disability your life must be considerably different than that of other people. We acknowledge and have discussed in previous chapters that a disability imposes limitations that may require special attention. However, at the other end of the continuum—and equally wrong—is the idea that an individual has to be Mr. or Ms. Superdisabled in order to be accepted. On the contrary, people with disabilities are entitled to be as average as people without disabilities. Not only are they entitled, but in reality they are.

More important than trying to excel in all behaviors is the need to express the broad range of feelings and emotions, as long as an individual abides by moral, social, and legal standards that restrict infringement on the rights of others. At this point, it is important to repeat what has been stated in previous chapters: A physical disability should neither restrict an individual from expressing himself or herself nor be a license to abuse others. A brief discussion of the stages of development and expression of feelings and social competence follows.

SOCIAL DEVELOPMENT

Information about child development has accumulated so rapidly that it is now subdivided into intellectual, physical, emotional, and social areas of research. This separation does not negate the fact that no one phase of development takes place independently of the others. For example, physical impairments frequently interfere with school adjustment; the effective use of language is closely related to social relationships; emotionally disturbed children are not likely to do well in school; and acceptance by the peer group is an important factor in a child's success in school. There are many ways to tell if a person with a disability is having growth problems, including observing the stages and periods listed in the following.

Certain motor behavior patterns are common in all children. Experimental evidence indicates that physical maturation determines the rate and pattern of mental growth. Little skill has developed until the child has matured sufficiently to engage in a particular activity, and each child's developmental pattern is unique. The internal growth process of the body organs and functions is called maturation. Specific organs do not function until minimum growth has taken place. For example, a sighted child does not learn to read until his or her nervous system has developed sufficiently for language capacity, eye control, and ability to concentrate. Obviously, eye control is not a factor in blind children learning to read Braille.

The age at which children are ready to read and write is determined by their level of development—neuromuscular, physical, and intellectual—and by their earlier experiences. Children with physical and social disabilities tend to be slower in learning to read and write, but all children tend to move in their learning from concrete to abstract. Therefore, children who have disabilities should be actively involved with materials, substances, tools, and concrete situations.

Piaget (1954) demonstrated that the very young child is easily and quickly confused by apparent changes in sizes and objects. Preschool children have not yet learned some of the basic physical constants of their environment. That is, they do not know that the weight, volume, length, and quantity of objects remain constant despite changes in their shapes or the contexts in which they appear. Thus, a two-year-old will acknowledge that two identical glasses contain the same amount of milk, but if the contents of one glass are emptied into a taller glass, he is likely to decide that the taller glass has more milk. His understanding of the concept is not yet stable and abstract.

Bruner (1966) emphasized four factors related to maturation: linguistic skills are best taught at an early age; mental growth is based not on gradual increases of associations or stimulus-response connections but rather on sudden sharp rises and stops as certain capacities develop; children are in a state of readiness at an earlier age than previously had been thought; and the emphases in education should be on skills and areas related to learning skills, with a curriculum based on self-reward sequences.

Although social development begins slowly at birth, it is greatly accelerated during the preschool and elementary school years when a child's interaction with peers becomes more frequent and intense. As preschool children grow older, demands for socialization cause them to spend less time in nonsocial, individualistic activities. They gradually learn to repress egocentric behaviors in favor of group-approved responses. The sociopsychological processes of interaction through which the individual learns the habits, beliefs, values, and skills for effective group participation are called *socialization*. The stages or periods of socialization are overlapping. The major function of socialization is to transform an untrained human organism into an effective member of a society. The most important elements of socialization take place during childhood, but growth is lifelong.

Growing up is synonymous with developing appropriate skills, knowledge, feelings, and attitudes. As children's physical and psychological capacities develop, they are confronted with new societal expectations and norms. The cultural pressures for conformity are difficult for children without disabilities and almost impossible for those who have them. Common developmental tasks range from learning sex-appropriate behavior to becoming socially responsible.

Havighurst (1953) suggested the following list of developmental tasks:

- *Early childhood*–learning to walk; learning to take solid foods; learning to control the elimination of body wastes; learning sex differences and sexual modesty, learning physiological stability; forming simple concepts of social and physical reality; learning to relate oneself emotionally to parents, siblings, and other people; and learning to distinguish right from wrong
- *Middle childhood* –learning physical skills necessary for ordinary games; building a wholesome self-concept; learning to get along with age-mates; developing fundamental skills in reading, writing, and calculating; developing concepts necessary for everyday living; developing conscience, morality, and a scale of values; achieving personal independence; and developing attitudes toward social groups and institutions
- *Adolescence*–achieving more mature relations with age-mates; achieving a masculine or feminine social identity; accepting one's physique and using the body effectively; achieving independence of parents and other adults; selecting and preparing for an occupation; preparing for marriage and family life; developing intellectual skills and concepts necessary for civic competence; desiring and achieving socially responsible behavior; and acquiring a set of values and an ethical system
- *Early adulthood*–selecting a mate; learning to live with a marriage partner; starting a family; rearing children; managing a home; getting started in an occupation; taking on civic responsibility; and finding a congenial social group
- *Middle age*–achieving adult civic responsibility; establishing and maintaining an economic standard of living; assisting teenage children to become responsible adults; developing adult leisure-time activities; relating oneself to one's spouse as a person; accepting and adjusting to the physiological changes of middle age; and adjusting to aging parents
- *Later maturity*–adjusting to decreasing physical strength and health; adjusting to retirement and reduced income; adjusting to the death of one's spouse; establishing an explicit affiliation with one's age-group; meeting social and civic obligations; and establishing satisfactory physical living arrangements

Erikson (1950) delineated eight stages in the life cycle:

- *Trust versus mistrust (birth to one year)*– If children's basic needs are met, they will think the world is a safe and dependable place. If their basic needs are not met or if they are inconsistently met, they will define the world as a place of fear and suspicion.
- *Autonomy versus doubt (two to three years)*–If children are encouraged to do things they are capable of doing, at their own pace and in their own time, they learn autonomy. If they are encouraged to do too many things–things

they do not want to do or things they can not do–they doubt their ability to deal with the environment.
- *Initiative versus guilt (four to five years)*–If children are allowed to initiate activities and if parents take time to answer their questions, they will not be afraid to tackle new things. If their movements are greatly restricted and they are made to feel that their questions are unimportant, they will feel guilty doing things on their own.
- *Industry versus inferiority (six to eleven years)*–If children are encouraged to make and do things, are allowed to finish what they start, and are praised for the efforts and results, they become industrious. If they are ridiculed or ignored for trying to do things, they feel inferior.
- *Identity versus role confusion (twelve to eighteen years)*–If adolescents succeed in integrating roles in different situations and also experience continuity in their perceptions of self, they develop a positive self-identity. If they are unable to establish a sense of stability in the various roles they play, then confusion results.
- *Intimacy versus isolation (young adulthood)*–This stage is characterized by being pulled to identify with others and, conversely, being repelled by them because of competitive, combative relations.
- *Generalivity versus self-absorption (middle age)*–This is the struggle between establishing and guiding the next generation and being a victim of one's own self-concerns.
- *Integrity versus despair (old age)*–Integrity is acceptance of one's life cycle as something that had to be, while despair is the feeling that time has run out to try alternative roads to integrity.

Piaget (1952) described four stages or periods of intellectual development:

- *Sensorimotor (birth to two years)*–This stage is characterized by learning about properties of things through the senses and motor activity. This leads to new ways of handling situations.
- *Preoperational (two to seven years)*–By learning symbols, children are able to manipulate symbols and objects mentally. This also allows acquisition of language that is egocentric; words have a unique meaning to each child. Gradually, the child learns to think of more than one quality at a time and to understand conversation.
- *Concrete operational (seven to eleven years)*–The child learns to manipulate mentally concrete experiences that earlier had to be manipulated physically; the child develops the ability to deal with operations but not to generalize beyond his or her actual experiences.
- *Formal operational (eleven years and older)*–The child develops the ability to deal with things not present and with abstractions.

Drawing on Piaget's work, Bruner (1962) identified three stages of concept development. During the first stage, *preoperational*, which generally ends at about age five or six, the child is concerned with manipulating objects on a trial-and-error basis. During the second stage, *concrete operations*, which begins after the child enters school, the ability to organize data through contact with concrete objects emerges, and the child learns to use organized data in the solution of problems. During the third stage, *formal operations*, which usually begins between the ages of ten and fourteen, the child acquires the ability to operate on hypothetical propositions without having the concrete objects visible.

Childhood

The average child's physical growth is as rapid from birth to five years of age as it is from six to sixteen. During the first five years, depending on the disability and parental reaction, a child with a disability may grow from a helpless, dependent infant to an active pseudo-independent person. Of course, if parents are overprotective, the child remains helpless and dependent. For most preschool children, the large muscles mature rapidly but are not under complete control.

During childhood, social conflicts tend to decrease and friendly interactions increase. The patterns of friendship change markedly with age changes. For example, between the ages of two and three the number of friends increases; after this time the major change is in the closeness of attachment to a few friends. Varying modes of popularity and leadership emerge. By the time they reach kindergarten, most children have a fairly definite idea of other children with whom they would like to play. Some children with disabilities are constantly sought out by other children for playmates; others are rejected and avoided. A few children with disabilities assume leadership roles; most are content to be followers. On the whole, the interactions of preschool children are characterized by cooperation and friendship.

Unlike preschool friendships, which are casual and transient, elementary school relationships become more intense and lasting. With the exception of their parents and a few teachers, elementary schoolchildren's closest friends are their age-mates.

Middle Childhood (ages six through twelve) is dominated by "gang" activities. The growth of bones, muscles, and nervous tissue is dramatic during this period. The long bones of the legs and arms grow rapidly, and this gives most children a tall, thin look, as contrasted with their previous short, stocky appearance. Along with the rapid development of the large muscles of the legs, back, shoulders, arms, and wrist comes an increase in physical activity. Physically immobile and slow children are left behind. This is especially true for children with impaired muscles and nervous tissue.

The nervous system reaches its maximum rate of development around ten years of age, and at twelve the brain has reached its maximum size. This results in a higher level of intellectual development than of muscular dexterity. Thus, a miniature adult is trapped in a child's body. The quest for redefinition begins. Sexual differences are learned and internalized. So, too, is the need to challenge authority.

Preadolescence or Puberty (ages ten through twelve) is characterized by many conditions, including a growth spurt, awakening sexuality, and an increase in peer group relationships. Except for infancy, the body undergoes the most rapid changes in size and shape during this period. Children aged ten, eleven, and twelve begin to "look down on" little children and underdeveloped age-mates. (Persons with physical disabilities are disproportionately represented in the latter category.) Along with these changes, the reproductive system starts to mature, causing sex-linked physical characteristics to appear: Girls develop obvious breasts and begin to produce female hormones; boys get more muscular and begin to produce male hormones. This is hardly the period of "latency" that early psychologists imagined it to be. Skin blemishes and increased weight add to the awkwardness of this period.

During this period, friends tend to resemble each other in social class, chronological age, physical maturity, and ethnic identity. This, without much doubt, is one of the most difficult periods for socially rejected children with disabilities. Negative attitudes that children have toward disabilities are reinforced, and positive ones are questioned during the pairing off for dates. This also is the time when positive contacts with persons with disabilities can alter prejudicial attitudes. As a group, it is accurate to say, all preadolescents are characterized by prolonged depressed and negativistic states.

The social meanings of their disabilities are learned by most children mainly from interaction with their significant others. Overprotection by parents and siblings provides the child with a disability with his or her first debilitating concept: "I am fragile. I am not expected to do the same things as able-bodied children. I am not responsible for my behavior." This attitude does not prepare children for interacting with age-mates as equals, but it does prepare them for rejection. One of the most devastating realities many children with disabilities experience in childhood is rejection. Consistently being the last person chosen in team sports and being excluded from group conversations and peer activities are demoralizing to young developing egos–and older ones, too.

Children with disabilities tend to develop behaviors to protect their egos from constant rebuffing. Isolation and hostility are only two of the protective behaviors that children with disabilities may exhibit. Sitting in the back of the classroom and not participating in class discussion are early signs of isolation. Becoming a bully and responding defensively to teachers, parents, and other authority figures are not always signs of tough kids. Often these behaviors mask fragile and frustrated lives: Limiting association with people lessens the chances of being rejected by them. The child with a disability may view this behavior as the best way of dealing with his or her frustration. In reality this may be the only way he or she knows to react.

It may be painful for children with disabilities to tell others about the frustration they experience trying to fit in with "normal" people. However, this problem can be effectively handled only by sharing it with caring people and devising appropriate coping mechanisms. Teachers usually are good listeners, and most parents care about the welfare of their children and are interested in such problems. If adults are not acceptable, most children have at least one close friend with whom they can share intimate feelings. Although problems centering on disabilities can be discussed with friends, it is wise to remember that whether or not friends have disabilities they also have problems, and care must be taken not to "dump" a load of problems on them.

Adolescence

The period from puberty to the late teens or early twenties is adolescence. Many of the problems described earlier are carried over into this period, often described as the "impossible period" between childhood and adulthood. Thus, there are fears centering on physical appearance, sex, social status, and vocation. Being denied many of the rights of either children or adults, they are nevertheless expected to fulfill many of the obligations of both groups. That is, they are expected to remain obedient to their parents, to control their sex impulses, to select a vocation, and otherwise to begin to act as adults.

This is a period in which young people need association with the opposite sex; they also need to evolve their own theory of life. Dating becomes a central concern for both sexes. Along with the problem of getting dates come issues centering on the outer limits of heterosexual and homosexual relationships. In general, adolescent girls engage in less premarital sexual intercourse than boys do, but standards of acceptable sexual behavior vary with social class. For example, studies indicate that masturbation is quite widely practiced among middle-class children, whereas sexual intercourse is much more frequent among lower-class children. Because of their more limited opportunities to engage in dating activities, adolescents with physical disabilities, more so than other adolescents, are more likely to masturbate than to engage in sexual intercourse.

Adolescents identify most strongly with their own peers and form cliques. Members of cliques usually come from the same racial and socioeconomic backgrounds and therefore have much the same interests and values. Cliques are dominant forces because they are based on personal compatibility, congeniality, and mutual admiration. If members of cliques are conscious of their physical appearance, youths with obvious physical impairments are excluded.

Most adolescent groups reinforce and strengthen the values that members have acquired from their parents. In other words, peer groups are less originators than reinforcers of values and behaviors developed in the family. This includes values and behaviors pertaining to people with disabilities. However, in some areas, such as dress, music, and slang, peer groups aid adolescents in achieving independence from adults. By sticking together and behaving alike, they are able to insulate themselves from outside pressures to conform to all adult norms and behaviors.

Contrary to some opinions, most adolescents do not view their parents as unnecessary authoritarians. Instead, they consider them as necessary teachers of moral and ethical values. Thus, most adolescents grow up and behave like their parents. Sherif and Sherif (1964) clearly demonstrated the extent to which all adolescents are affected by middle-class values:

> There is one clear and striking generalization about the high school youth which holds in all areas and despite their differing backgrounds: Their values and goals earmark all as youth exposed to the American ideology of success and wanting the tangible symbols of that success. There were no differences between the youth in different areas with respect to desires for material goods. In addition to comfortable housing, the symbols of success for these adolescents include a car in every garage, a telephone, television set, transistor radio, fashionable clothing, time to enjoy them, and money to provide them. (p. 199)

Little has changed since the Sherifs conducted their studies.

This period is especially trying for youths with disabilities who begin seriously to question their future: "Will I get married?" "Will I have children?" "If I have children will they be disabled?" "Will my children be ashamed of me?" "Will I be able to find a job?" These are but a few of the future-oriented questions that nag adolescents with disabilities. All of these are valid questions that must be handled in a caring manner. Failure to do so will only add to the moodiness, confusion, and oversensitivity that characterize adolescents. Unfortunately, most adolescents with disabilities are afraid and ashamed to ask adults these questions. They need to know that some of these questions, particularly those pertaining to marriage, are of concern to children who do not have disabilities.

Adulthood

Depending on the source consulted, adulthood begins at age eighteen, nineteen, twenty, or twenty-one. In some communities, adolescents are physically and psychologically adults but are legally classified as juveniles. Conversely, many persons are adults legally but psychologically less mature than adolescents. Generally, *young adulthood,* up to the age of forty, is a period of great mobility and transition. Most young adults move from economic dependence on parents to self-support, from being at home to starting their own homes. They engage in a variety of jobs and experiment with different lifestyles. These changes are more difficult and less likely for those with disabilities, who frequently are neither encouraged nor allowed to grow up.

The period of *middle age* (from about forty to sixty-five years of age) is characterized by depression, restlessness, irritability, anxiety, and physiological upheaval. Concern about health and physical appearance is increased during the middle years. Consequently, exercise and diets are ritualistically followed. For individuals with disabilities who have been able to secure steady employment during their young adulthood, middle age is a period of economic security and relative comfort. This also is the time when most people realize that they are unlikely to attain many of their childhood dreams of success. For some persons this leads to prolonged disillusionment; for others it leads to contentment with what they have been able to achieve. For persons with permanent disabilities, this is a time to accept their condition or lapse into continual depression.

The period of *old age* starts at about sixty-five years of age. Old age is a great equalizer for individuals who acquired physical disabilities during their younger years. Physical deterioration and chronic disabilities and diseases become prevalent for all people during old age. Physiologically, the body begins to break down, and, psychologically, the mind becomes less proficient. It is during old age that most people become concerned about disabling conditions. Often, their concern is too little, too late. Their fate, like that of many persons with disabilities of all ages, is social disengagement and alienation. Fortunately, conditions are changing for young persons with disabilities and the aged.

Gradually, Americans are beginning to fashion out productive lives during disability and old age.

Although the rest of the authors' comments are directed to people with disabilities, these remarks may be helpful to other persons who find themselves in teaching, counseling, rehabilitation, and other helping roles.

SELF-ACCEPTANCE

No matter what age a person is, it is important that he or she know and accept himself or herself. The person who has a positive self-concept and strong self-acceptance will do more than survive. He or she will flourish as a person (Hahn, 1988). It is difficult to convince other people to accept one, however, if one does not accept oneself. Part of the self-identity of a person with a disability is the disability. The person who has a strong sense of self-acceptance is not afraid to acknowledge his or her disability, nor is he or she afraid to admit strengths and weaknesses or to be rejected by individuals who do not like disabilities. He or she does not waste energies being negative and defensive but instead uses them for positive, creative activities and interactions. The individual who has not learned to accept his or her disability becomes a negative prophecy that fulfills itself.

People with disabilities should accept their disability as a fact of life but not as their whole life. In other words, they should view the disability and its limitations as a reality, but their entire life should not be controlled by it (Kaiser, Freeman & Wingate, 1985; Stuifbergen & Becker, 1994). To be consumed by their disability will not allow the development of their strengths and positive potentials; instead, almost all of their energies—mental, physical, and emotional—will be drained in an attempt to "live with a physical disability." Few people are fortunate enough to learn to accept themselves totally. All people fall short of perfection in almost all matters; all do things that cause them to dislike themselves. This is normal. However, some persons dislike themselves most of the time. That is not normal. They must learn that because they are not able to do some things with the style, grace, or quickness of persons without disabilities, this is not failure. On the contrary, it is *difference*.

People tend to respond to others in ways that reflect how they regard themselves. Self-assured persons do not have to use others to build their own egos. They give freely of themselves and have no need to put others down. Individuals who have low self-acceptance use people to support their own ego but give little to them in return. They are immature and unable to tolerate situations that do not support them. Often they project onto others aspects of themselves that they find despicable. If one is a mature person, one will not have to find scapegoats for one's own inadequacies. Instead, one will seek self-improvement.

The self-assured person who has a disability mixes well with other people and this, in turn, enhances his or her self-esteem. The person who has a low self-concept avoids people or, at the other extreme, displays destructive, competitive, defensive, or dependent behavior. This latter behavior repels friends and irritates enemies. This sets up a no-win situation.

POSITIVE THOUGHTS

An acquaintance of one of the authors decided to establish a business. In the initial planning stage, he talked with many people who had attempted to establish a similar business but had failed. His idea was to learn as many of their mistakes as possible so that he could avoid making them in his own business. Approximately one year after the establishment of his business, the young entrepreneur declared bankruptcy. Part of the reason for his failure was that he had, without realizing what he was doing, programmed himself to think negatively. He became so obsessed with the ways his business could fail that he forgot to think of the many ways to make it succeed.

Several books focusing on positive thinking have been written, and the authors of some of these books make comfortable livings teaching the "power of positive thinking." The main theme running through most discussions of positive thinking is "believe in yourself." Although societal attitudes get in the way of the self-actualization of people with disabilities, the major obstacle often is the people themselves. Too many persons with disabilities allow themselves to think negatively. If a person believes that he or she cannot make a positive contribution to society, it is very likely that he or she will not (LaGreca & Vaughn, 1992).

REALISM

Realistic ideas of one's abilities and limitations are prerequisites to being a successful person. To attempt to accomplish what may seem to be the impossible is not foolish. In fact, many great accomplishments, such as Orville and Wilbur Wright's maiden flight at Kitty Hawk, North Carolina; Henry Ford's horseless carriage; and the development of television, were at one time considered impossible feats. However, continually attempting to accomplish things that have been proven to be beyond one's capabilities is foolish expenditure of one's energies. As has been discussed in previous chapters, everyone has limitations, and the key is to become successful in doing the possible. One must recognize and accept one's limitations as well as identify one's strengths and build on them (Hearne, 1991).

Too often people with disabilities feel that they must become superdisabled in order to be recognized as worthy human beings. In the process of becoming superdisabled they forget to be human. Stated another way, some persons devote so much energy and time to trying to be superstars that they become subnormal failures. They fail to develop into well-rounded individuals who can function in many social and economic settings. They should take inventory of their skills, determining what they do well and also what they do poorly. They should not hesitate to participate in activities in which they are average performers. Most people will have skills similar to theirs; therefore, they will feel comfortable in their presence. If people participate only in activities in which they are the best, friends will avoid them, because no one likes to feel inferior. People should not avoid those things in which they perform poorly; to do so will cause them to miss opportunities to improve their skills. However, they should not subject themselves to humiliation by constantly trying to do things that are virtually impossible for them to accomplish with any degree of skill and success.

restoration, personal adjustment counseling, vocational evaluation, vocational counseling, and job placement create opportunities for independence or dependence. Too much attention and too much care can create a feeling of helplessness. The severity of the limitations imposed by a disability obviously affects the degree of independence one may have. However, dependency should not mean total loss of control over decision making. Individuals with severe disabilities can exercise some control over their lives. Decisions such as what to eat within their diet, what to watch on television, or which book to read can be made by most concerned persons.

It is easy for people to blame others for their own mistakes or problems. In fact, it is psychologically more satisfying to think that others are the cause of a behavior, especially if that behavior is not to their liking. However, personal growth begins when people accept responsibility for their behavior. Becoming a responsible person is not always easy. Being responsible for oneself is a demanding task. Although people have certain basic needs from birth to death that if left unmet will cause them to suffer, especially if they are not naturally endowed with the ability to fulfill them. If the ability to satisfy basic needs were as much a part of people as are the needs themselves, they would not have any psychosocial problems. Being responsible for oneself often is easier said than done.

RESPONSIBILITY

A physical disability is no reason for a person to surrender his or her life to others (Gregory, 1993). Regardless of how caring, empathic, and sincere a helper is, the person with a disability is the best person to control his or her own life. Hospitalization, physical

EFFECTIVE COMMUNICATION

One of the most effective ways of determining one's own destiny is to communicate effectively with others. Effective communication means that one will do the following:

1. **Understand the roles** of each player in the drama of the helping relationship. It usually is quite obvious what the role of the person with the disability is to be: He or she becomes an individual to be helped, to be rehabilitated, to be evaluated. However, in contrast to the role of the client, the role of the helper is not always clear. Questions that a client must ask are "What do you do?" "What kind of help can you provide me?" "What do you expect of me?" "What are your limits?" In other words, "Where does your role end and another helper's role begin?" Once the client has answers to these questions, he or she can effectively interact with helpers. Without answers to these questions, the client will not know what to expect in the helping relationship and should refuse to commit himself or herself to unknown people.

2. **Listen to what others say.** Although total silence is not recommended in the interaction with a helper, neither is nonstop talking recommended. Talking is one way of relieving anxiety, but excessive talking creates anxiety in the person to whom one is speaking. Effective listening requires paying careful attention to not only the spoken words but also the speaker's body language. If a client is sighted, he or she may obtain a great deal of information by observing the helper's facial expressions and body movement. If the client is visually impaired but not hearing impaired, he or she should pay attention to how the helper talks, in other words inflections and pauses.

3. **Organize one's thoughts** and make sense of the many perceptions running through one's mind. Some of these thoughts may be: "I am uncomfortable with what he is saying." "She is asking me to do something I am afraid to do." "That is not what I want to do." "What will my friends think of this?" "I will be embarrassed wearing that thing." "Will my family accept me?" It is imperative that the client learn to sort out and deal with the disquieting feelings of the moment and carefully discuss them with a helper. It is not uncommon when under stress to jump from one subject to another. Therefore, it is helpful to state feelings and make points clearly and coherently.

4. **Wait for a reaction** once something has been presented to the helper. This is more effective than skipping from one concern to another. Waiting for a reaction means more than listening to the words. It also means, where possible, observing the person's body reaction.

5. **Keep an open mind.** This means more than being receptive to the helper's ideas. It means being willing to question the helper's recommendations. Because an individual is a professional does not mean that he or she automatically knows what is best for a client. Besides, it is the client's life.

6. **Make sure of the communication.** Once an agreement has been made regarding the subject under discussion, every attempt should be made to ensure that the client's understanding and the helper's understanding are the same. The best rehabilitation plans will crumble if all parties are not operating from the same reference points.

PRIDE

Many persons without disabilities find it difficult to imagine people with disabilities as being happy. Yet, many of them are happy. Physical wholeness does not bestow virtues, nor does a disability take them away. An individual can, paraphrasing African Americans, have a disability but feel beautiful and proud. By projecting an image of a proud person, the individual projects the image of a person not ashamed of himself or herself.

Of course, there is truth in negative and positive images. Pride is created and projected to others when people with disabilities respect themselves and demand that others do likewise. This demand means that these individuals will not allow others to devalue their abilities by concentrating on their limitations. Pride comes from not devaluing oneself.

SELF-IMPROVEMENT

The self is always in a state of change; it is never a finished product. One will not be, nor should one expect to be, the same person tomorrow as today. People are always, in Allport's (1955) words, in the process of "becoming." However, each individual develops habits and defense mechanisms that slow the process of change. Consequently, it is difficult to make sweeping changes in personality.

Often people with disabilities try to improve their self-esteem through superficial changes such as prostheses, speech, clothing, and cosmetics. These efforts result in real self-improvement only when they accept their disabilities and change their own negative attitudes and behavior. The difficulty inherent in changing some low self-concepts is that they are too deeply rooted in attitudes and defenses that do not give in easily to do-it-yourself approaches. In these instances, professional helpers are needed to facilitate the change process. This help may come in individual or group therapy situations.

Self-help groups for persons with disabilities are springing up all over the world (Haring & Breen, 1992). In many instances they are highly successful in treating individuals who, for various reasons, have turned to lay persons, rather than professionals, for help. The spirit of commitment and fellowship is very high in most of these organizations. Under no circumstances should anyone discount the importance or effectiveness of well-conceived self-help groups. Each individual must determine whether any of them can be helpful to him or her. For many persons and their families, these groups are vital in the rehabilitation process. There is more, not less, cooperation between professionals and self-help groups.

SUMMARY

If a person is to engage successfully in self-improvement, he or she must, as pointed out earlier, first assess strengths and weaknesses to get a clear understanding of what he or she is and would like to become. Being honest about what one sees in the mirror of life can be unnerving. One may see ugliness and weakness in oneself that one deplores. It is seldom painless to view oneself in an objective, detached manner. Most people need help in taking off their rose-colored glasses, and almost all people need help when they try to correct what they do not like about themselves. Self-improvement is a difficult process, but it is achievable. The hallmarks of a person with a disability who is capable of successful self-improvement are honesty, tenacity, and humility.

NOTE TO HELPERS

If helpers are to understand people with disabilities, they must understand people. An individual with a disability is not a alien creature. Torrance (1970) provided an interesting perspective on human behavior. The authors have modified his list of characteristics to fit people with disabilities:

1. *"Wanting to know"*–This is evident in the curiosity of persons with disabilities who ask questions, become absorbed in the search for the truth of their disabilities, try to make sense out of their world, make guesses and test them, and try to discover their limits and the limits of their conditions. *Helpers must help them to know.*

2. *"Digging deeper"*–The genuinely human person with a disability is not satisfied with quick, easy, superficial answers. *Helpers must not give such answers.*

3. *"Looking twice and listening for smells"*–The person with a disability can never be satisfied with his or her situation by looking at it from an intellectual distance or seeing a report or hearing the helper's words or touching equipment. He or she will want to get to know it from different angles, perspectives, and senses. It is not necessarily a sign of distrust when a client tries to learn things on his or her own terms. *Helpers must realize that it is the client's life and let him or her have it.*

4. *"Listening to a cat"*–Too many helpers can neither talk to nor listen with understanding to a cat. Much human communication is nonverbal. In the helping process, words usually are insufficient for communicating the deepest and most genuine concerns of one person for another. *Helpers must learn to communicate nonverbally and to understand nonverbal communication.*

5. *"Crossing out mistakes"*–Persons with disabilities who try to achieve their potentialities inevitably make mistakes. They lose in humanness when they avoid doing difficult and worthwhile things because of the fear of failure. *Helpers must help them not to be afraid to try new things and must not punish or ridicule them if they fail.*

6. *"Getting into and out of deep water"*–Testing the limits of one's skills and abilities, disability, and personal resources means taking calculated risks. It means asking questions for which no ready answers exist. *An effective helper assists clients to sort out possible alternatives.*

7. *"Waving a ball"*–To be truly human is to be able to laugh, play, fantasize, and loaf. *Helpers should encourage their clients to take time out to relax.*

8. *"Cutting a hole to see through"*–This is a tolerance for complexity. By opening up the windows of their lives, persons with disabilities see more of themselves. *An effective helper must be a window through which clients can gain a better understanding of the world beyond themselves.*

9. *"Building sand castles"*–In order to build a sand castle, one must be able to see sand not only as it is but also as it might be. To move from dependency to independence requires persons with disabilities to see their existence as it might be. *Helpers must encourage clients to plan and strive for their dreams but to do so in terms of the materials and resources they can realistically draw upon.*

10. *"Singing in your own key"*–Thoreau stated this idea very poetically: "If a man does not keep pace with his companions, perhaps it is because he hears a different drummer. Let him step to the music he hears, however measured or far away. It is not important that he matures as an apple tree or an oak. Shall he turn his spring into summer . . . ?" *Helpers should let their clients know that it is all right to do things differently, to be out of step with persons who do not have a disability.*

11. *"Plugging in the sun"*–For most persons with disabilities, the source of their energy comes from self-help groups and organizations that focus on the needs of persons with disabilities. *An effective helper learns the names and locations of local or regional organizations that pertain to people with disabilities.*

12. *"Shaking hands with the future"*–Becoming human means growing up or realizing yesterday's dreams and also creating new dreams. *Helpers must be willing to become their client's past, to terminate the helper-client relationship when their client has achieved his or her rehabilitation goals.*

Professional helpers must learn as much as they can about their clients and use this information to help make their rehabilitation as successful as possible. First, however, helpers must be willing to let their clients become whatever they become.

POINTS FOR DISCUSSION AND SUGGESTED ACTIVITIES

1. Ask at least three persons with disabilities to describe some of the most discouraging aspects of having a disability. Also ask them to describe some of the positive experiences they have had.
2. Ask at least three persons with disabilities to describe some of the changes they would like to see in society that they believe would help persons with disabilities.
3. Ask at least three persons with disabilities if they consider themselves to be disabled. If the answer is yes, ask them how they feel about being called a person with a disability.

REFERENCES

Allport, G.W (1955). *Becoming: Basic Considerations for Psychology of Personality.* New Haven, CT: Yale University Press.

Bruner, J.S. (1962). *The Process of Education.* Cambridge, MA: Harvard University Press.

Bruner, J.S. (1966). *Toward a Theory of Instruction.* New York: Belnap.

Erikson, E.H. (1950). *Children and Society.* New York: W. W. Norton.

Gregory, R.J. (1993). A policy by and for people with disability. *Disability & Rehabilitation, 15,* 151–154.

Hahn, H. (1988). Can disability be beautiful? *Social Policy, 18,* 26–32.

Haring, T.G., and Breen, C.G. (1992). A peer-mediated social network intervention to enhance the social integration of persons with moderate and severe disabilities. *Journal of Applied Behavior Analysis, 25,* 319–333.

Havighurst, R. (1953). *Human Development and Education.* New York: Longmans & Green.

Hearne, P.G. (1991). Employment strategies for people with disabilities: A prescription for change. *Milbank Quarterly, 69,* 111–128.

Kaiser, S.B., Freeman, C.M., & Wingate, S.B. (1985). Stigma and negotiated outcomes: Management of appearance by persons with physical disabilities. *Deviant Behavior, 6,* 205–224.

LaGreca, A.M., and Vaughn, S. (1992). Social functioning of individuals with learning disabilities: Annotated bibliography. *School Psychology Review, 21,* 423–426.

Piaget, J. (1952). *The Language and Thought of the Child.* London: Routledge & Kegan Paul.

Piaget, J. (1954). *The Construction of Reality for the Child.* New York: Basic Books.

Sherif, M., & Sherif, C.W. (1964). *Reference Groups.* New York: Harper & Row.

Stuifbergen, A.K., and Becker, H.A. (1994). Predictors of health-promoting lifestyles in persons with disabilities. *Research in Nursing & Health, 17,* 3–13.

Torrance, W.P. (1970). What it means to be human. In M.M. Scobey and G. Graham (Eds.), *To Nurture Humaness: Commitment for the 70's.* Washington, DC: Association for Supervision and Curriculum Development.

SUGGESTED READINGS

Bryan, W.V. (1996). *In Search of Freedom.* Springfield, IL: Charles C Thomas.

Bryan, W. V. (2002). *Sociopolitical Aspects of Disabilities.* Springfield, IL: Charles C Thomas.

Fine, M., and Asch, A. (1988). Disabilities beyond stigma: Social interaction, discrimination and activism. *Journal of Social Issues, 44*:3–21.

Goffman, E. (1963). *Stigma: Notes on the Management of Spoiled Identity.* Englewood Cliffs, NJ: Prentice-Hall.

King, G. et al. (1993). Self-evaluation and self-concept of adolescents with physical disabilities. *American Journal of Occupational Therapy, 47*: 132–140.

Part 2

EMPOWERMENT

Chapters 5 through 8 discuss the importance of persons with disabilities being empowered to handle as much of their daily life activities as they can. There can be no question that many persons with disabilities have limitations that impact some of the things that they may want to do. However, is that not a reality for all humans? Each one of us has limitations that affect the quality of our performance in certain areas. Persons with disabilities must be empowered to control as much of their lives as realistically possible. More importantly, to the extent they are capable, persons with disabilities must empower themselves to be the major decision maker with regard to matters that impact their lives. Chapters 5 through 8 discuss some ways persons with disabilities have been empowered and can be empowered to take charge of their lives.

Chapter 5

EMPOWERMENT

Outline

- Introduction
- Benefits of Empowerment
- Becoming Empowered
- Societal Responsibility
- Persons With Disabilities Empowering Themselves
- Summary
- Points for Discussion and Suggested Activities

Objectives

- To discuss the importance of persons with disabilities becoming empowered
- To discuss persons with disabilities' responsibilities for empowering themselves
- To discuss societal responsibilities with regard to helping empower persons with disabilities

INTRODUCTION

The evolution of social interaction of persons with disabilities with their non-disabled brothers and sisters throughout the world has been, to say the least, an interesting relationship. As extensively discussed in this book, as well as in others, there have been some highpoints that seem to promise rewards of more equal opportunities for persons with disabilities, and there have been a considerable number of devastating low points where persons with disabilities were tolerated and treated as a lesser form of human species. As we have looked backward through the long telescope of history, in many cases, we have judged our reactions to and interaction with persons with disabilities to be less than stellar human relations. Given this historical evaluation, the current question is, 100 years from now, how will social scientists and human relations specialists view our treatment of persons with disabilities? Without question we currently have the opportunity to work with persons with disabilities in assisting them in achieving their goals of being able to contribute and participate in society to their fullest potential. One way to help persons with disabilities to achieve these goals is to work with them in empowering themselves.

There can be numerous definitions of empowerment; the definition depends, to a great extent, on who or what is being empowered and to what the empowerment is being directed. With regard to persons with disabilities, empowerment means having the opportunity to function and achieve to the maximum of their abilities, physical, mental or a combination thereof. In Chapter 1, we discussed concepts of disabilities. In that discussion, we emphasized that the concept of empowerment is one emerging concept for persons with disabilities, and hopefully it will become one of the dominate concepts that will, for a considerable period of time, dominate the human relationships between persons with disabilities and their nondisabled brothers and sisters.

EMPOWERMENT ACTIONS

Empowerment is not a totally new concept for persons with disabilities. In past years, courageous persons with disabilities–with assistance from family, friends, politicians, rehabilitation and human rights persons–have come together, body and spirit, to promote and demand equal rights and access. The Independent Living Center Movement discussed in Chapter 7 is one example of empowerment. We will briefly discuss the following movements of empowerment by persons with disabilities to demonstrate what unity of persons with disabilities and their nondisabled advocates can accomplish: **Wheel of Justice Protest, Deaf President Now Protest, Section 504 Protest, and League of Physically Handicapped Protest**. Bryan (2010) in his book Sociopolitical Aspects of Disabilities discusses these protest movements and with the permission of the author the following information has been extracted.

WHEEL OF JUSTICE PROTEST. The development of the ADA of 1990 occurred as the result of a decade of planning and coalition building, and as the legislation was working its way through Congress, there were some congressmen who felt the act was unnecessary. Because of these feelings and, more important, the fact that some of the congresspersons were powerful enough to either delay, derail or deny passage of the act, disability rights activists felt it necessary to protest, demonstrating their support for passage of the act in its then present state. Thus, the American Disabled for Accessible Public Transit organized Wheels of Justice, which was a series of demonstrations.

> More than 700 people gathered in Washington D.C., where on 12 March, they marched from the White House to the Capitol to listen to speeches by disability rights advocates such as Justin Dart, Jr., Evan Kemp, Jr., James Brady, I. King Jordan, and Mike Auberger. Auberger, at the foot of the capitol steps told the crowd, "We will not permit these steps to continue to be a barrier to prevent us from the equality that is rightfully ours." This was the call to begin "the crawl-up," as people left their wheelchairs to make their way up the 78 steps into the capitol building.
> The next day more than 200 demonstrators occupied the capitol rotunda, meeting with congressional leaders. (Pelka, 1997, p. 322).

In total, more than 150 demonstrators were arrested. However, their arrests were well worth their efforts, for on July 26, 1990, President George H. W. Bush signed into law the Americans with Disabilities Act (pp. 149, 150).

The signing of the ADA legislation was brought about by the efforts of persons with disabilities and their supporters. This is an example that demonstrates that determination can empower a group of people, and empowerment can overcome many obstacles. This is but one example of empowerment of persons with disabilities; another example is the Deaf President Now Protest.

DEAF PRESIDENT NOW PROTEST. In 1998, Gallaudet University, which had been founded as the National College for the Deaf, was searching for a new president. In its more than 120 years of existence, the institution had never had a president who was deaf, and if the board of trustees were to have their way, the next president would also not be deaf. Despite requests by the university's alumni association and several organizations representing people who were hearing impaired that the next president be deaf and the fact that the majority of the finalists for the job were deaf, the board announced they were hiring a nondeaf person as president.

The students of Gallaudet were determined that the Board of Trustees would not get its way in this matter. The organized group of students voted to shut down their campus and keep it closed until the Board reversed its decision and fulfilled their dreams of having a deaf president appointed. The students lived up to their promise of closing the campus and issued what they considered four nonnegotiable demands to the Board of Trustees. The following demands, according to the students, had to be met for the demonstration to end:

1. Resignation of the newly appointed president and the appointment of a deaf president as her replacement
2. Resignation of the Board of Trustee chairperson
3. An increase in deaf representation on the board to a majority (51%)
4. No reprisals against the protesters

The students received considerable support for their demand of hiring a deaf president. The support came from various sources, such as members of the U.S. Congress, civil rights leaders and activists, a labor union, and the faculty of the university. This kind of support undoubtedly boosted their courage and belief in the correctness of their cause.

Three days after the students shut down the campus, the newly appointed president resigned and three days later the Board of Trustees agreed to meet the remaining demands of the students. The Board appointed I. King Jordan president, making him the first deaf president of Gallaudet University (pp. 148, 149).

This protest is an example of persons with disabilities taking charge of their own lives and desires and nondisabled persons seeing their determination and joining to support them. This is the essence of empowerment. The next protest, Section 504 Protest, is yet another example of what empowerment can accomplish.

SECTION 504 PROTEST. Throughout most of the 1970s, the community of persons with disabilities found itself needing to make its plight known to the public. President Richard Nixon vetoed the Rehabilitation Act of 1972; within this legislation were provisions for the establishment of independent living centers. Disability rights activists, advocates, and other empathetic supporters protested President Nixon's action. Unfortunately, the protest did not change the action, and the act died from the lack of presidential support. Despite this setback, the disability rights activists were undaunted in their efforts to ensure that persons with disabilities had available to them the tools to make their lives as independent as possible.

The Rehabilitation Act of 1973 was passed and signed by the President. Although this act did not provide funding for independent living centers (this would not occur until 1978), it did include some very significant provisions that would profoundly affect the lives of persons with disabilities. These provisions were identified in Sections 501, 502, 503, and 504. Although the act was signed in 1973, by 1977 the regulations governing Section 504 had not been issued. Section 504 "prohibited" discrimination against persons with disabilities by any institution receiving federal financial assistance. Stated in other terms, the act prohibited any institution, agency, organization, or program receiving funds from the federal government from denying access, services, or employment to someone solely on the basis of his or her disability. This provision was basically useless without approved regulations. The Department of Health, Education, and Welfare (HEW) was responsible for issuing these regulations. Throughout President Gerald Ford's administration, the Secretary of HEW failed to issue the needed regulations. Therefore, disability rights activists became increasingly concerned because they knew (1) there was virtually no way of enforcing this section until regulations were issued and signed by the Secretary of HEW, and (2) as more time lapsed without the issuance of regulations, the chances of their being issued decreased. In 1977, President Jimmy Carter appointed Joseph Califano as the Secretary of HEW and it became the Carter administration's responsibility to issue the regulations. Califano's stance was similar to his predecessor's. Distressed by this failure to act, the disability rights group American Coalition of Citizens with Disabilities (ACCD) wrote President Carter, informing him that if the regulations were not issued soon there would be protests against his administration. The regulations were not issued, thus protests began at HEW offices in Atlanta, Boston, Denver, San Francisco, and Washington, D.C. Perhaps the most dramatic of the protests was the twenty-five–day sit-in at the San Francisco Health, Education and Welfare office.

These efforts by the disability rights activists resulted in Secretary Califano's signing the regulations on April 28, 1977. In addition, the efforts brought national attention to the needs and desires of persons with disabilities. Moreover, the nation perhaps, for the first time, began to see person with disabilities "in a different light," as strong, capable, and determined people.

The final protest discussed, League of Physically Handicapped, is one that occurred many years ago and is evidence that some persons with disabilities in the United States have had the will and courage to seek their rights and make it known that they are as much American as any other citizen. It also demonstrates that a small number can be empowered to do things that positively affect many.

LEAGUE OF PHYSICALLY HANDICAPPED. Shortly after the October 1929 Wall Street crash, the United States sank deeply into an economic depression that had the effect of making beggars of some previously wealthy individuals. In many cases, not only did some persons who had invested in the stock market lose the most of their financial resources, but also they, along with countless others, were unable to secure adequate employment to support themselves and their families. It was this background that greeted newly elected President Franklin D. Roosevelt. In fact, a major reason he was elected president was that many Americans believed he would be better at getting the United States' economy functioning correctly, as well as returning the masses of unemployed persons to work.

To stabilize the economy and reemploy the legion of unemployed, President Roosevelt established a number of social programs through his "New Deal" policy; one of these programs was the Works Progress Administration (WPA). It was the responsibility of this agency to place unemployed persons in jobs, mostly public-service-type work constructing roads, buildings, and streets to mention three of many projects. During this period, as is currently the case, the unemployment rate of persons with disabilities was much higher than that of the general public; therefore, those who could work were not, in any significant numbers, being referred by the Office of the Emergency Relief Board (ERB) to these jobs. The ERB was the agency designated to screen candidates for this type of employment.

Because of the insensitivity of the ERB toward the needs of persons with disabilities, six persons with disabilities decided to investigate the situation. Having been refused a meeting with the director of ERB, the six decided to conduct a sit-in at the director's office. Initially they were denied entrance to the building; however, a few days later, "three of the six disabled protesters sat in for nine days" (Pelka, 1997, p. 191). Their actions did not change federal policy, but they did gain considerable public support, thus increasing the public's awareness of the needs and mistreatment of persons with disabilities.

Although no policy was changed, some immediate tangible good resulted from their efforts.

> At its height, the league had several hundred members. Among its actions were a three-week picket of the WPA's New York headquarters of the New York Port Authority, pickets and demonstrations at other government offices, and two trips to Washington, D.C. to meet with officials of the Roosevelt administration. Members of the group spoke at labor union meetings, and leftist rallies, trying to raise awareness of the oppression of people with disabilities. The league was able to get WPA jobs for some 500 disabled New Yorkers. (Pelka, 1997, p. 191)

This 1930s movement may have been the genesis of the 1960s disability rights movement. As Pelka stated, one of the original six protesters was involved in disability right efforts into the 1980s.

BENEFITS OF EMPOWERMENT

The four previously discussed actions of protest are good examples of how unity of purpose can lead to action that leads to positive results. The protests led to increased employment in the New York area; passage of a landmark civil rights law; implementation of orders that has benefited thousands, if not millions, of persons with disabilities; and the hiring of a person with a disability in a leadership role that has served as inspiration for other persons with disabilities to be proud of themselves and aspire to leadership positions. The empowerment of persons with disabilities as a result of the previously mentioned actions has inspired thousands of persons with disabilities by demonstrating that they have within themselves the power to help control their own destiny.

Empowerment of persons with disabilities is not only beneficial to persons with disabilities but also beneficial to society. No society can maintain high standards of living and reach even higher levels of functioning when it has a group of people who are willing and capable of making contributions to its society but who are treated as underclass people of the society. The axiom that a chain is only as strong as its weakest link applies to how the lack of empowerment of persons with disabilities can affect the society in which they live. This is not meant to imply that persons with disabilities weaken a society; rather, the implication is that the society could be stronger if many persons with disabilities were given opportunities to function at their maximum level of potential. The paternalistic approach to dealing with persons with disabilities does very little with regard to empowering persons with disabilities. The paternalistic approach, although often well-meaning, results in what we will call a "caretaker society" in which persons with disabilities are too often treated as "wards of society." Wards of society implies that local, state, and/or federal government provides various forms of assistance for the daily living of persons with disabilities.

Providing assistance is beneficial when it is designed to prepare persons to improve their life situation. It is a proven fact that resources provided to educate and/or train persons to become employable and self-sufficient benefits society because the recipients repay the government many times in taxes and spending power.

BECOMING EMPOWERED

Self Acceptance

The journey to empowering ones self begins with believing in ones self, accepting ones self and loving ones self. In part because of societal beliefs and perceptions of persons with disabilities, some persons with disabilities have doubted their own abilities and capabilities. To a significant extent, this self-doubt has caused some persons with disabilities to be ashamed of themselves, feel sorry for themselves, and think of themselves as incapable of being productive members of society. Some psychological counselors emphasize that to effectively accept love and appreciation from another, one has to first love and respect ones self. This means that people have to be realistic and recognize their strengths and weaknesses. They need to be willing to accept the fact that they can be productive using their strengths and are capable of improving upon their weaknesses and—in those cases in which they cannot improve their weaknesses—be willing to accept them as part of their overall life makeup.

Throughout this book we highlight that one of the causes of low self-esteem in some persons with disabilities is the paternalistic attitudes that too often prevail in society. A major problem for persons with disabilities is that people believe that persons with disabilities are weak, defenseless, and dependent. These feelings are certainly not appropriate foundational building blocks for self-empowerment. Therefore, persons with disabilities must first accept the fact that they have a disability. Second, they must realize and project the fact that having a disability is no disgrace and nothing about which to be ashamed. Third, they must recognize the obvious fact about humans: everyone is unique and everyone has both strengths and weaknesses. Persons with disabilities are a representative of this fact. Fourth, from the standpoint of everyone has both strengths and weaknesses, everyone has some limitations and therefore everyone has a disability. Given this reality, disability means limitations and their limitations maybe more visible and/or pronounced than those of some other people. Many persons with limitations are not ashamed of their limitation; thus, a person who has been designated as having a disability should also not be ashamed of his/her limitations. Fifth, persons with disabilities must be cognizant of the fact that most persons without disabilities do not concentrate on their weaknesses, from the standpoint of allowing the weaknesses to keep them from improving upon the weaknesses and utilizing their strengths, thus making their strengths stronger. By increasing the potential of their strengths, they deemphasize their weaknesses. If persons with disabilities would practice these five points they would be well on their way to empowering themselves. Additional means through which persons with disabilities can empower themselves are **education/training** and **meaningful employment**.

Education/Training

Regardless of the type of society—capitalist, socialist, communist or a combination thereof—it cannot sustain itself without its citizens being productive. A precursor of a person becoming productive and a determinant of how productive he or she will become to a large extent depends on the education and training one receives. Likewise, an important factor in persons with disabilities empowering themselves is becoming educated and trained at or close to their maximum level of potential. Unless a person with a disability has a cognitive disability that limits his or her level of educational attainment, most persons with disabilities, if appropriately evaluated, are capable of high levels of educational pursuit and attainment. Persons with cognitive disabilities, if appropriately evaluated and receiving education or training from sensitive, caring educators and trainers, can be educated and trained at levels compatible with their abilities. Too often persons with disabilities are judged by nondisabled persons, either consciously or subconsciously, as not being capable of high levels of education and in some cases as not being able to receive virtually any education. With regard to training, for too many persons with disabilities, they have been judged to be trained in repetitious minimally stimulating areas. The result of poor or inadequate levels of education too frequently has led to many persons with disabilities becoming depressed because they realize they are unable to compete with their nondisabled counterparts. This realization may cause them to develop feelings of self-pity and think of themselves as second-class citizens.

To avoid this devaluation of one's self-esteem requires persons with disabilities and their families to be proactive and demand professional evaluation and appropriate educational and training placement. This requires an understanding of the legal rights of persons with disabilities and, in this case, laws both state and federal, which pertain to education of persons with disabilities. One such law is the federal law, Individual Disability Education Act, which is discussed in Chapter 7. Additional things that should be done to ensure appropriate educational and training opportunities for persons with disabilities are the following:

1. Become aware of issues that come before local school boards and attend meetings to insure that the needs of persons with disabilities are adequately addressed.
2. Become aware of state laws and state legislative committees that are responsible for educational issues. An effective way of dealing with state legislative committees is to become familiar with one's legislative representative and if necessary organize or join organizations that advocate for educational rights of persons with disabilities.
3. For persons who are attending colleges/universities or vocational schools, become familiar with the student affairs offices, because that office is, generally speaking, responsible for assisting persons with disabilities. Most colleges, both public and private, receive some federal monies; therefore, they are required to provide equal opportunities for persons with disabilities. It has been the experience of the authors that most colleges and universities as well as vocational schools welcome persons with disabilities and are eager to assist them so that they can be successful graduates of their educational programs.

Employment

Appropriate education and training prepares persons to be productive citizens. However, regardless of how educated and trained a person may be, her or his chances of making significant contributions to society and contributions to one's self-esteem become limited if she or he is unable to secure gainful employment. It is an unfortunate fact that in the United States, the unemployment rate for persons with disabilities consistently stays in the 30 percent plus range, and when severely disabled persons with disabilities are added the rate can reach into the 70 percent area. The ADA of 1990 and the ADA Amendments of 2008 are major allies to empowering persons with disabilities to secure equal and fair opportunities in the employment arenas.

One of the reasons the unemployment rate for persons with disabilities is extremely high relates to the fact that many employers have misperceptions with regard to the capabilities of persons with disabilities. For- tunately, most employers are willing to be educated with regard to the needs and abilities of persons with disabilities; however, persons with disabilities cannot assume that employers are going to seek information about the population of persons with disabilities. Therefore, it is incumbent for persons with disabilities to make prospective em- ployers aware of their capabilities. This can be done by disability rights groups and other organizations dedicated to working with persons with disabilities who come together to educate employers about the need for employment of persons with disabilities and their abilities to be productive employees.

Persons with disabilities certainly have responsibilities for self-advocacy with regard to removing barriers that are hindering their progress to receiving equal and fair treatment. Additionally, society has equal res- ponsibility to remove various barriers to equal opportunities for persons with disabilities. Two of the major barriers that must be removed are societal perceptions and physical barriers.

SOCIETAL RESPONSIBILITY

The productivity and level of prosperity of any society depends largely on the level and quality of contributions its citizens are able to make. Approximately one fifth of the American population has some type of disability and certainly not every person with a disability is unable to be as productive as he or she would like to be. However, if a conservative figure of 10 percent of the population of persons with disabilities are unable to be as productive as their potentials would allow because of barriers of various kinds, then society is being deprived of desiring and willing talent. Consequently, not only are some persons with disabilities suffering from lack of use of their talents but also society is being deprived of valuable contributions. Therefore, in the United States, it is incumbent upon all persons to help remove barriers that are handicapping anyone including persons with disabilities.

It has been stated that between 30 and 70 percent of the population of persons with disabilities are either unemployed or underemployed. The lack of sufficient employment is a major problem for persons with disabilities who are not being able to be as productive as many would like to be. However, it is not the only problem. Insufficient education for persons with disabilities often contributes to poor employment opportunities. To help empower persons with disabilities, society must help remove the barrier that leads to inadequate education, which leads to unemployment and underemployment, which leads to a significant segment of the American population not being able to be an active part of American society to the extent they would like to be.

Within the United States, especially during the past fifty years, there have been significant improvements with regard to the attitudes of nondisabled persons toward persons with disabilities. It is a rare occurrence for nondisabled persons to speak of persons with disabilities as being inferior. Many nondisabled persons may think of persons with disabilities as being weaker than persons without disabilities are, they may think of persons with disabilities as being unfortunate, and they may think of persons with disabilities as needing to be protected from failure and disappointments, but fortunately, they do not think of persons with disabilities as being inferior. Although these thoughts, to some extent, represent improved attitudes toward persons with disabilities, the protector, paternalistic attitudes that have replaced the second-class citizen attitudes continue to represent a major stumbling block for persons with disabilities. The best way that society can help empower persons with disabilities is to view the result of having a disability as creating a limitation or limitations. Further, the thoughts should be that everyone has limitations, some have more limitations than others. However, similar to limitations with which persons without disabilities are confronted, they learn to either adapt to the limitations or find ways of compensating for the limitations, or both. In most cases, persons without disabilities are not degraded or pitted for not being perfect. Once the nondisabled population stops viewing disabilities as creating a different kind of human being and treats persons with disabilities as equal to any other human being, then as a society we have begun to help empower persons with disabilities.

PERSONS WITH DISABILITIES EMPOWERING THEMSELVES

A change in societal attitudes toward viewing persons with disabilities as capable individuals and equal to persons without disabilities with regard to being members of society will help considerably regarding the empowerment of persons with disabilities. This fact does not relieve persons with disabilities from being the major force in empowering themselves. Stated in other terms, persons without disabilities do not carry all of the responsibilities for the empowerment of persons with disabilities. Persons with disabilities should carry the major responsibility for empowering themselves. When persons with disabilities rely on nondisabled persons to inform and make society aware of their second-class citizenship and other unequal treatments they are receiving, they are reinforcing the conditions that have led to the situations that they are trying to overcome. They are leaving the impression that they are unable to speak for themselves, thus reinforcing the too-often-held belief by society that persons with disabilities are dependent persons.

Counselors, social workers, rehabilitation counselors, and other types of psychological behavioral professionals quite often stress to their clients that they, the clients, are responsible for their behavior and as such they are responsible for managing their behavior. This is advice that persons with disabilities should take to heart. Everybody at various points in their lives need help; however, needing and receiving help does not equate to relinquishing one's responsibilities for determining directions of life to others. Similar to the pioneers of the Independent Living Movement who knew that they had to have help moving from a totally dependent living situation to a living arrangement where they could have more control of their lives, other persons with disabilities must take heed of the example of those pioneers and carry on with the spirit of independence that they projected. By following the previously mentioned example, persons with disabilities will begin breaking the shackles of dependency.

Another thing that some persons with disabilities must do to empower themselves is to disassociate themselves from the **fear of failure**. The fear of failure is not unique to persons with disabilities. When engaging in new and/or unfamiliar activities, most humans have some self-doubt with regard to whether they will be successful in accomplishing the tasks being presented to them. In the process of thinking about the possibilities of either success or failure, the fear of embarrassing themselves if they are unable to accomplish their goals quite often becomes of paramount concern. This is a normal psychological reaction; however, most people accept the risk of failure, realize that if they fail it will not be the end of the world, and further learn, generally speaking, that from failure comes new learning experiences that help them to be successful in other tasks and endeavors. Persons with disabilities who are held back because of fear of failure must learn to accept failure as part of the human growth process. They must recognize that very little self-esteem growth occurs without taking chances, and in the process of taking chances, if they fail, they must learn from the failure and try another approach. In some cases, they also have to learn that what they are trying to accomplish will not succeed. This revelation is also a psychological growth process. Further, persons with disabilities must learn to not be too sensitive and believe that their failures will be judged by nondisabled persons as weakness. Most nondisabled persons like to see persons with disabilities succeed and are willing to assist them in succeeding. Persons with disabilities must accept such help but not depend on the same. This brings us to another point necessary for persons with disabilities to accomplish with regard to self-empowerment: **breaking the act of overdependency**.

As has been implied previously, we need each other to survive and prosper. The problem for some persons with disabilities is that they have become too dependent on assistance from others. In the process of receiving assistance, they have become addicted to the assistance. Psychological growth occurs when we venture beyond our comfort zones and learn new things. As previously stated, this process of venturing beyond our comfort zones sometimes means making mistakes and being unsuccessful. This is not always bad, because in the process of making mistakes we also can learn what not to do and how to do things better. The opposite of moving beyond one's comfort zone is to become psychologically stagnant and dependent on others to meet one's needs.

Other things persons with disabilities can do to empower themselves are to **become engaged in community activities and become knowledgeable with regard to one's civil rights.** Involvement in community activities has the benefit of giving fellow citizens the opportunity to see and interact with persons with disabilities on a level field of human interaction. Stated in other terms, the more nondisabled neighbors and other associates interact with persons with disabilities, the better the chances are they will see persons with disabilities as fellow human beings. This type of interaction will establish persons with disabilities as persons who are interested in similar things in which many others in the community have an interest. The interaction will also establish them as intellectual and capable persons who have things to offer to the well-being of the community. Stated in other terms, many of the mysteries of disabilities will be dispelled by the interaction with community neighbors.

Persons with disabilities must become aware of their civil rights and the laws that protect those rights. There are numerous laws that are designed to assist persons with disabilities to interact with fellow human beings as well as interact successfully within their environment. By not becoming familiar with civil rights laws that protect the rights of persons with disabilities, these laws become ineffective. There are laws that not only empower persons with disabilities with regard to living within society more effectively but also provide educational opportunities that are helpful in increasing chances of upward mobility within society. These laws become ineffective if persons with disabilities do not become aware of them and what they can dom.

SUMMARY

Attitudes toward persons with disabilities with regard to their place in society, what they are capable of doing, and their value to society are improving. Associated with this improvement of attitudes is better access to society's goods and services. Despite the improvement of attitudes, in the United States and some other economically developed countries, all is still not well for many persons with disabilities. A good example of an area that continues to need significant improvement is in employment of persons with disabilities, particularly persons with severe disabilities. In order to overcome some of the current issues that continue to keep persons with disabilities from being adequately included in society, persons with disabilities must practice self-empowerment. Whenever possible, they must avoid being snared in the trap of paternalism, where they become dependent on others to make decisions for them as well as speak for them with regard to their wants, desires, and needs. No one is better at knowing what their wants, desires, and needs are than the people who possess those attributes; therefore, the message is that persons with disabilities must empower themselves by being their own best advocates.

POINTS FOR DISCUSSION AND SUGGESTED ACTIVITIES

1. What does the term empowerment mean to you?
2. How can you help empower persons with disabilities?
3. List some efforts that have occurred in your state and/or community to empower persons with disabilities.

REFERENCES

Bryan, W.V. (2010). *Sociopolitical Aspects of Disabilities* (2nd ed.). Springfield, IL: Charles C Thomas.

Pelka, F. (1997). *The Disability Rights Movement.* Santa Barbara: ABC-CLIO.

SUGGESTED READINGS

Boggs, C. (1986). *Social Movements and Political Power.* Philadelphia: Temple University Press.

Drake, R. (1999). *Understanding Disability Policy.* London: Macmillan.

Hurst, R. (1995). Choice and empowerment–lessons from Europe. *Disability and Society. 10*: 529–534.

Shapiro, J. P. (1993). *No Pity: People With Disabilities Forging a New Civil Rights Movement.* New York: New York Times Books.

Chapter 6

EMPLOYMENT

Outline

- Introduction
- Protestant Work Ethic
- Employment and Self-Esteem
- What About Persons Who Have Disabilities?
- Obstacles to Obtaining a Job
- Preparing for Employment
- Laws That Aid Employment
- Agencies That Aid Employment
- Sheltered Workshops
- Supported Employment
- Maintaining Employment
- Summary
- Points for Discussion and Suggested Activities

Objectives

- To identify and debunk some of the employment myths that hinder the employment of persons with disabilities
- To identify and inform the reader of laws that assist persons with disabilities in preparing for and maintaining employment
- To identify and inform the reader of agencies and organizations that assist persons with disabilities with regard to obtaining employment

INTRODUCTION

As discussed in Chapter 1, many of the negative feelings about and reactions to persons with disabilities are associated with the belief that they are people for whom constant care must be provided. In America, a nation that prides itself on being compassionate toward citizens who are unable to meet their own needs, various forms of social services have been created to help individuals who cannot totally help themselves. Certainly this is preferable to being treated as clowns and court jesters, individuals who fumble and bumble their way through life much like the prototypes of carnivals and circuses. Fortunately, few persons with disabilities have to behave that way before receiving help.

One of the reasons some persons with disabilities accept what many consider to be degrading employment is because this has been the only work available to them. This is especially true for persons with severe or visible disabilities, such as missing limbs, deformed body parts, or bodies that deviate considerably from what the prevailing society considers normal. People who are considered able bodied or whose bodies do not significantly deviate from the norm are sometimes critical of persons with disabilities who work in jobs that cause other persons to view them in amazement—as freaks of nature. If we examine that situation in an objective manner, we may conclude that these persons are not freaks, but people trying to survive. When faced with unemployment, being pitied, being dependent on relatives and friends, being institutionalized or taking employment—albeit distasteful—allows them to have a measure of independence, and independence is precisely what most persons with disabilities want. In his theory of hierarchy of needs, Maslow (1962) stated that there are various needs that humans have, and in ascending order they are: physiological, safety, love, belonging, and self-actualization. Frankl (1965) argued that "meaning" is a higher need than self-actualization is. There is no question that as humans we search for meaning and relevance in our lives; however, this search is an aspect of each of Maslow's needs. Consider a person at Maslow's lowest need level—physiological—who must have food, clothing, and other basic survival things. He is likely to assign some significance or meaning to his current minimal existence life situation. We know that he must have these basic needs met to survive. But even at the lowest level, however, he will seek understanding and try to rationalize why his life situation is what it is. Roe (1956) explains how employment helps to satisfy the basic needs of humans:

> In our society, there is no single situation which is potentially so capable of giving some satisfaction at all levels of basic needs as is the occupation. With respect to the physiological needs, it is clear that in our culture the usual means of allaying hunger and thirst, and to some extent sexual needs and the others is through the job, which provides the money that can be exchanged for food and drink. The same is true for the safety needs. The need to be a member of a group and to give and receive love is also one, which can be satisfied in part by the occupation. To work with a congenial group, to be an extrinsic part of the function to the group to be needed and welcomed by the group are important aspects of the satisfactory job.
>
> Perhaps satisfaction of the need for esteem from self and others is most easily seen as a big part of the occupation. In the first place, entering upon an occupation is generally seen in our culture as a symbol of adulthood, and an indication that a young man or woman has reached a stage of some independence and freedom. Having a job in itself carries a measure of esteem. What importance it has is seen most clearly in the devastating effects upon the individual of being out of work.
>
> Occupations as a source of need satisfaction are of extreme importance in our culture. It may be that occupations have become so important in our culture just because so many needs are so well satisfied by them. (pp. 31–32)

As Roe's comments clearly state, work plays a significant role in our lives. It helps us meet our needs, not only those that are basic to our physical survival, but also our self-esteem needs. Given the fact work is vital to meeting many of our needs as human beings, two questions come to mind: Why is work so important in our lives? How has being employed reached such a lofty position? To answer these questions, let's look at the development of the American work ethic.

PROTESTANT WORK ETHIC

Significant changes have occurred in the concept of work since prehistoric days, when people had to work only enough to meet very basic needs of food, clothing, and shelter. As time passed and human needs became more symbolic, work and work-related activities began to take on meaning that went beyond basic survival. The earliest recorded ideas about work referred to it as a curse, a punishment, an activity not included as part of the good life and, at best, a necessary evil—needed to sustain life (Lofquist & Davis, 1969). People of high status did not work. Only slaves, indentured servants, and peasants worked. The masters or ruling classes did not work; they were preoccupied with intellectual contemplation that could not be sustained through physical labor. Work was considered necessary, but only insofar as to sustain the individual and the group to which he or she belonged.

As Christianity spread, the meaning of work began to change. Martin Luther subscribed to the principle that work is a form of redemption. The religious decree was that all people who are able to work should work, including affluent intellectuals and ascetics. Thus, whether an individual's economic position was high or low, he or she was expected to work in order to serve God. According to Luther, the best way to serve God was by performing work more perfectly. The philosophies of John Calvin and Martin Luther were very similar in regard to work, which they both thought curbed the evil in people. Weber (1930) stated that the belief that work was the highest means of asceticism, and the strongest proof of religious faith had the greatest influences in shaping capitalism. Work became the religious spirit of capitalism and had at least three basic meanings for preindustrial people: (1) it was hard, necessary, and burdensome; (2) it was a means to religious fulfillment; and (3) it was good because it was a creative act.

Noted scholars in the field of occupation and career development (e.g., Chirikos, 1991; Deutscher, 1971; Roe, 1956; Super, 1968; Yelin & Katz, 1994) observed that the meaning of work changed in the twentieth century. Work became valued as a way to get consumer goods and maintain dignity and self-esteem rather than as verification of religious salvation. In the twenty-first century, work continues to be viewed as a way to assert one's independence and bolster one's self-esteem. Obermann (1965) appears to have seen into the future of the twenty-first century when he remarked that the most observable contribution by individuals to their society will be made through their work or occupations. In technological cultures, work or occupation more nearly defines a person's importance. Consequently, job success is likely to help satisfy the need for recognition and status. In today's society, occupation is one of the most important aspects of an individual's life; it helps define our place in our communities. Generally, social status, technical capabilities, and economic level all evolve from occupations (Day & Alon, 1993).

EMPLOYMENT AND SELF-ESTEEM

In simplified terms, the definition of self-esteem is how one values one's self or, stated in another way, what one thinks about oneself. Many factors contribute to the development of self-esteem. Our interaction with the environment, our interaction with significant others, and how we think others view us are a few of the factors. Employment, or lack thereof, plays a major role in how others react to us. To be within the prime employment age of eighteen to sixty-four years and be unemployed quite often causes contemporaries to harbor negative feeling toward you. If an unemployed person is receiving some type of public assistance, additional disdain toward the person is likely. The reality for most unemployed persons, particularly unemployed persons with disabilities, is that they would prefer to have gainful employment. In the second century, Galen, the Greek physician and writer, is reported to have written that employment is nature's best physician, an essential to happiness. Through the centuries, in most societies, work has served as an important force in building and maintaining self-esteem.

With the advent of the Industrial Revolution and the beginning of the Age of Automation, some humans became concerned with the relevance of work to their search for identity. In the 1960s and 1970s, as more jobs became automated, two major concerns began to be voiced by career and occupational development specialists. The first was the fear that automation would place large numbers of persons in the unemployment status, and the second was that workers would have considerably more free time and thus more attention would have to be given to orienting persons to effective use of leisure time. It is true that automation virtually eliminated some jobs such as elevator and telephone switchboard operators; however, as those jobs were eliminated, automation created new jobs. Thus the fear of extreme high unemployment never materialized, and the new jobs helped improve the nation's economy as well as individuals' self-esteem.

Although no society still subscribes to the pre–Industrial Revolution idea of hard work for all, most societies continue to promote the idea that work for the able-bodied is good. Although dated in years, the following comments and results from a 1971 Gallup Poll continue to reflect current public opinion with regard to public assistance.

> If we give people money without working, we will be taking away the individual's incentive to work and his ability to pass this incentive on to his children. To do this would be creating a society of parasites–a something for nothing society.
>
> I don't want my tax money going to someone who is sitting around with his feet up in the air. I feel they should be provided with a job not charity. This gives man confidence by letting him earn the money, thus making him feel like a man. (cited in Wolfbein, 1971, p. 164)

The same Gallup Poll asked, "Would you favor a guaranteed income?" Fifty-eight percent of the respondents disapproved. However, to the question "Do you favor providing enough work for everyone?" 82 percent answered in the affirmative, which reflected an American tradition–the belief that work is good and humans contribute to society through work.

According to Childs (1971), work is more than a means through which goods and services are purchased; it is a means by which an individual purchases his or her dignity. For most Americans, it is through work that their identity and social status are achieved. One of the questions almost always asked of strangers in casual conversation is "What is your job?" The answer to that usually sparks a mental picture that categorizes the individual. Deutscher (1971) offered this cogent analysis of the importance of work in the development of self-esteem:

> Involvement with meaningful work is an adult activity. It helps to establish and maintain adult life. It is not that people work when they become adults, but that they work to become adults, to nourish the adult personality structure with its capacity for intimacy, relatedness, productivity, and participation in community life. Work provides a much-needed link to reality in non-child contexts. Furthermore, it has a fundamental economic reality; most people have to work in order to provide financial support for themselves and their families. Finally, work has a social reality. Through work people earn a place in their community and develop within themselves a sense of accomplishment. (p. 15)

Work status shapes nonjob actions. The U.S. Congress recognized this when it amended the Social Security Act in 1967, stating that doling out funds to unemployed people who were able to work does very little to bolster their self-esteem. The amendments required parents of dependent children to be involved in job training or work. Summarizing various ideas with regard to work, Friedman and Havighurst (1954) listed several common meanings of work:

1. It is a source of self-respect, a way of achieving recognition or respect from others.
2. It defines a person's identity; his/her role in society.
3. It provides the opportunity for association with other persons for building friendships.
4. It allows for self-expression and provides the opportunity for creative and new experiences.
5. It permits people to be of service to others.

Most people want an occupation that will permit them self-expression. The manner in which occupational self-expression is implemented is, to a great extent, determined by external conditions.

WHAT ABOUT PERSONS WHO HAVE DISABILITIES?

Work takes on increased meaning for people who have a disability (Vash, 1981). Such individuals are too often viewed as not being capable persons when so much emphasis is put on physical abilities. Some employers are reluctant to hire persons with disabilities, especially those with visible or severe disabilities. Sadly, they concentrate their thought on the persons' limitation rather than their strengths. To be more succinct, too many employers give more thought to what they think persons with disabilities cannot do rather than what they can do. A result of this kind of thinking is unemployment rates for persons with disabilities being as high as 70 percent. The following facts, extracted from the 1998 National Organization on Disability (NOD)/Louis Harris Survey of American with Disabilities, underscore difficulties persons with disabilities have in securing gainful employment:

> Employment continues to be the area with the widest gulf between people with disabilities and the rest of the population. Only three in ten working-age adults with disabilities are employed full or part-time compared to eight in ten adults without disabilities. Working age adults with disabilities are not more likely to be employed today than they were a decade ago, even though almost three out of four who are not working say that they would prefer to be working. (p. 7)

Other revealing facts from the survey are that among those with disabilities ages sixteen to sixty-four who are not employed, 72 percent said that they would prefer to be working; two out of three adults with disabilities said that their disability prevented or made it more difficult for them to get the kind of job they would like to have.

OBSTACLES TO OBTAINING A JOB

Work is a basic ingredient in modern culture; most people organize their lives around their occupations. Grave psychological disturbance can result when persons with disabilities who are able to work are barred from participating in this most important societal activity. When individuals are unable to find or keep a job because of prejudices about their disabilities, physical disability becomes a handicap. The work capabilities of most persons with physical disabilities have been demonstrated many times. There are several factors more important for the performance of most jobs than physical prowess. This is particularly true given the current state of automation in jobs as well as the ability to handle many tasks through the use of a computer.

Although the following study is quite dated, the results are as accurate today as they were in the 1960s. The staff of the Vocational Rehabilitation Division of the Federal Board of Vocational Education studied 6097 persons who had physical disabilities and were employed after being rehabilitated. The investigation confirmed that (1) rehabilitated persons could perform adequately in a wide range of occupations; (2) persons who have disabilities, even those with similar diagnoses, differed greatly from each other in many occupational factors; and (3) it is not possible to equate disability and occupational capability (Obermann, 1965). In a more current study, the NOD Survey of Americans with Disabilities (1994) found that persons who have disabilities are capable of being employed in essentially the same types of jobs as their nondisabled counterparts. Roe (1956) had the following to say about persons who have disabilities and their ability to work:

> Unlike special abilities which may qualify their holder for desirable, unusual jobs, special disabilities are more likely to function as only limited factors. Blindness, deafness, orthopedic disabilities, chronic illness all have very real effects upon occupational selection. Some of these effects, it is true, are the result of inadequate knowledge on the part of everyone, the disabled, the employers, and society generally as to just what performance limitations are the necessary results of certain disabilities, but some of the effects are genuinely inevitable. A man with one arm cannot perform activities which really require two fully functioning ones, but he can do many more things with one arm and one prosthetic device than might be imagined. Furthermore, there are large numbers of occupations for which a second arm is really unnecessary. (pp. 64–65)

Through the years, individual and group prejudices based on unfounded myths have caused workers who have disabilities to be relegated to dead-end jobs, if any at all (Ondusko, 1991; Satcher & Dooley-Dickey, 1992). This negative attitude is the greatest hurdle that people with disabilities have to overcome, and it is an extremely high hurdle, built on actual disabilities as well as imagined ones (Christman & Slaten, 1991). Most individuals with disabilities strongly desire to live up to societal standards of being economically productive citizens. However, quite often, traditional attitudes toward them do not facilitate this. Even the schools they attend frequently treat them as less capable people. Moreover, some persons who have disabilities themselves may consider their plight as being inevitable.

Although societal understanding of disabilities has improved, there remains a significant lack of understanding of the wants, needs, and capabilities of people with disabilities. Therefore, additional emphasis must be placed on integrating students with mental disabilities into the classrooms with their nondisabled peers. Likewise, employers need to be better educated with regard to the capabilities of persons who have disabilities. In the same vein as "Sunday Christians" who transgress during the week but believe that they have discharged their religious duties by attending church service on Sunday, some educators and employers believe that they fulfill their obligations to persons with disabilities by donating money to charity drives. Despite their awareness of the therapeutic value of education and work, it is still difficult to find effective teachers and gainful employment for individuals who have disabilities.

One of the major obstacles to persons who have disabilities securing gainful employment is the misunderstanding and misinformation that employers and their human resource specialists have with regard to persons who have disabilities. Myths too frequently hamper the chance of persons who have disabilities obtaining gainful employment. Some of these myths are discussed in the next few pages because the authors of this book believe that the reluctance of employers to hire workers who have disabilities stems primarily from false assumptions that are deeply entrenched. Common employment-related myths relate to safety, insurance, liability, productivity, attendance, accommodation, and acceptance in the workforce.

Safety Myth

Myth: Because workers who have disabilities deviate from what employers generally consider normal, in other words, they walk differently, walk with the aid of something, or have a hearing or visual impairment, some employers think they are likely to injure themselves or cause other employees to be injured.

Reality: In studies conducted during the past forty years, comparing safety records of workers who have disabilities and nondisabled persons, the results have shown there were no significant difference in the safety records of the two groups. Many companies such as International Telephone and Telegraph (ITT), IBM, Sears, ConEd, Wal-Mart, and McDonalds, to mention a few, have experienced the same results. In fact, if they did not believe workers who have disabilities were safe and productive, these companies would not hire them.

Insurance Myth

Myth: Insurance companies will not let employers hire workers who have disabilities. "My insurance company will penalize me if I hire a person with a disability. My insurance rates will increase. My worker compensation rates will also increase."

Reality: Insurance companies do not tell employers whom to hire, nor are employers required to get approval from worker compensation insurance before hiring persons who have disabilities (Brantman, 1978). Insurance premiums are based on a company's safety record, not its workers' physiques. As discussed in regard to the safety myth, employees with disabilities are proportionately as safe as employees who do not have disabilities. Worker's compensation insurance rates are determined by several factors, such as the nature of the business, size of payroll, and accident experience. In determining worker compensation insurance rates, occupations are classified so that the cost of accidents can be assessed proportionately to the accident risks involved.

Liability Myth

Myth: An on-the-job accident that, when added to a worker's prior disability, results in permanent total disability will make the company liable for the permanent total disability.

Reality: All fifty states and the District of Columbia now have some type of Second Injury Fund (name may vary by state). The Second Injury Fund assumes the responsibility of compensation to a person with a physical disability who becomes totally disabled through an industrial accident, allocating to the employer's expense only the single injury sustained at work. Because each state develops its own Second Injury Fund, specific provisions and the way they are applied vary by state.

Productivity Myth

Myth: Workers who have disabilities are not capable of performing their jobs; therefore, the other employees have to "take up the slack."

Reality: Mandated by the ADA, all employers with fifteen or more employees must have determined and listed the skill requirements of each job. Even those employers with less than fifteen employees should know the skill level of each of their jobs. If they do not, their employee's poor job performance probably will be the employer's fault in that requirements of the job are not known. If an employer is aware of the skills required for the job and a person with a disability applies and is best qualified, he or she should be hired. Persons who have disabilities should be given an equal opportunity. However, if they do not have the required aptitude or skills, they should not be hired. With regard to productivity, studies by the DuPont Corporation have show that persons who have disabilities are as productive as their nondisabled counterparts.

Myth: Persons who are considered to be mentally retarded cannot be productive in a nonsheltered workshop employment environment.

Reality: Companies such as Pizza Hut and McDonalds, to name only two, are among the leaders in hiring persons considered to have mental disabilities. As a whole, these employees are productive; otherwise, the companies would not hire them.

Myth: It is better not to hire persons who have disabilities because they might fail, thus destroying their self-esteem.

Reality: It is true that some persons who have disabilities will fail at their job; they have the same right to fail or succeed as nondisabled persons. In the attempt to keep them from failing, employers also deny them the opportunity to succeed. With regard to lowering their self-esteem, most persons who have disabilities are not so fragile that a failure will destroy them. Similar to persons without disabilities who fail at a task, if they are properly counseled and encouraged, they have an excellent chance at being successful in tasks compatible with their skills and aptitude levels.

Attendance Myth

Myth: Workers who have disabilities are absent from their jobs a great amount of time because of their physical problems.

Reality: Studies conducted by DuPont and other companies have revealed that the attendance of persons who have disabilities is as good as or, in some cases, better than nondisabled workers. Perhaps the best evidence for their dependability is found in companies such as DuPont, Sears, IBM, Wal-Mart, and McDonalds. Certainly, they would not hire them if they were not dependable.

Accommodation Myth

Myth: Most job sites would have to have extensive renovation to accommodate persons who have disabilities. "Our company will have to spend a fortune to accommodate employee who have a disability. They need a lot of special equipment."

Reality: The ADA does require employers, if requested, to provide reasonable accommodations and if the accommodations do not create an undue hardship. Several points can be made to explode this myth. If the requested accommodation will be too expensive (cause the employer to have financial problems) or change the nature of the business, the employer does not have to honor the request. It should be noted that legal determination of an undue burden is achieved on a case-by-case basis.

The Office of Disability Employment Policy (formerly The President's Committee on Employment of Persons with Disabilities) states that most accommodations cost less than $1000. The Job Accommodation Network's studies document that 15 percent of accommodations cost nothing, whereas 51 percent cost between $1 and $1000, and less than 25 percent cost more than $1000.

There are resources such as the Job Accommodation Network (JAN) available to assist in reviewing a job for reasonable accommodations. Ultimately, making reasonable accommodations is good business; it helps the employee to be more productive. Job accommodations are frequently made for nondisabled persons, all in the name of making them more productive. For example, ergonomic specialists frequently recommend changing the color of walls or playing soft music or using different shaped chairs for office personnel. Relatedly, there should be no difference considered when employees who have disabilities request a reasonable accommodation to make their jobs more comfortable, thus increasing productivity.

Acceptance Myth

Myth: Employees who do not have disabilities will not accept individuals with disabilities. The special accommodations (e.g. designated parking spaces, wheelchair ramps, and elevators) will be resented.

Reality: One of the reasons that nondisabled persons have unrealistic ideas about persons who have disabilities is the fact that there generally is very little one-to-one contact with each other. Once nondisabled persons work with individuals who have disabilities and discover that they are capable of doing their jobs, acceptance or rejection occurs for reasons other than disability. With regard to resentment because of parking spaces, ramps, and other accommodations, depending on the type of company or business, regardless of whether they have workers who have disabilities, they may be required to have a certain number of parking spaces and ramps to accommodate visitors and customers who have disabilities. Therefore, educating the employees on the need and requirements of accommodation should address any concerns.

Elimination of stereotypical thinking and myths about disabilities and persons who have disabilities will be a giant step toward opening employment doors for them. Elimination of stereotypes and myths will make a tremendous difference, but the fact remains that job preparedness is equally important. The next portion of this chapter will deal with preparing persons who have disabilities for employment.

PREPARING FOR EMPLOYMENT

For most persons, the type and amount of education or training one has is in direct relationship to the employability of the person. According to the 2000 NOD/Harris Survey, 78 percent of adults with disabilities had completed high school. This is in comparison to 91 percent for people without disabilities. With regard to college education, approximately 44 percent of adult persons who have disabilities had some college education, with a lesser percentage having completed their college education. These results present a mixed bag of information. On the one hand, this represents a closing of the gap between persons who have disabilities and persons without disabilities with regard to educational attainment. On the other hand, the increase in educational attainment has not translated proportionally into more jobs for persons who have disabilities. The unemployment rate for persons who have disabilities ranges from estimates of 65 percent to 70 percent. The 2000 NOD/Harris Survey found that approximately 32 percent of Americans who had disabilities and were of working age were employed full- or part-time. This is in comparison to 81 percent of Americans who did not have disabilities. There are a number of reasons why with increased education persons who have disabilities continue to have difficulty securing gainful employment, including the following ones:

1. Employers' attitudes are driven by myths and stereotypes. It should be noted that most employers are not opposed to hiring persons who have disabilities; however, many employers continue to maintain false perceptions, such as "persons who have disabilities are unemployable." "There are specific jobs for which persons who have disabilities are suited and their jobs do not fit into these categories." "Persons who have disabilities are economically supported by social service agencies and organizations, thus they are either not interested in work or do not need to work."
2. The attitudes of some persons who have disabilities create barriers to employment. These individuals either give up or do not begin the search for a job because they think they cannot successfully compete with nondisabled persons.
3. With regard to education and training, persons who have disabilities are too often channeled into careers where there are few jobs available. They are frequently steered away from careers where there are a variety of job options, such as medicine, law, engineering, teaching, and architecture.
4. Inadequate transportation is a formidable barrier for some persons who have disabilities. Because of the nature of their disabilities, they have to depend on other people or public transportation to get to and from work.
5. Inadequate vocational evaluation and community assessment also result in being trained for jobs that are not readily available in the local community. Even though the person may have the aptitude for a specific job, it does very little good to train him for something not available in his community. Of course, the individual could move to a location where the jobs for which he is trained are available. In many instances, persons who have disabilities do not have the financial or social resources needed to relocate.
6. Despite laws such as the ADA, which attempts to eliminate environmental barriers, many still exist.

To aid persons with disabilities in their efforts to secure gainful and appropriate employment, there are a number of laws helping professionals should know about, such as the Rehabilitation Act of 1973, the ADA of 1990, the Workforce Investment Act of 1998, and the Ticket to Work and Work Incentives Improvement Act of 1999. They should also be knowledgeable about agencies and organizations such as the Vocational Rehabilitation Agency, the Social Security Administration, the Veterans Administration (VA), sheltered workshop organizations, and job training programs. Each of these will be briefly discussed. It is highly recommended that helping professionals, parents, advocates, and persons who have disabilities become familiar with relevant organizations in their own state and community.

LAWS THAT AID EMPLOYMENT

Rehabilitation Act of 1973

This act will be discussed in more detail in Chapter 7, but Sections 503 and 504 are of particular relevance to persons who have disabilities and are seeking employment. Section 503 requires anyone who does business with the federal government in the amount of $2500 or more to take affirmative action in hiring persons who have disabilities. This does not mean that employers have to set employment quotas but does require them to make positive efforts to recruit, hire, and retain persons who have disabilities. Section 504 requires employers not to discriminate against persons who have disabilities, including not requiring persons who have disabilities to take a physical examination if nondisabled applicants are not required to do so. Individuals who believe they have been victims of discrimination have the right to file grievances through the Equal Employment Opportunity Commission (EEOC).

Americans With Disabilities Act (ADA) of 1990

Whereas the Rehabilitation Act of 1973 applies to federal and state agencies as well as private companies and businesses that receive federal government funds in the amount of $2500 or more, the ADA is a civil rights act that applies to all Americans. In this regard, the ADA strengthens the 1973 Rehabilitation Act. Section 1 of the ADA pertains to employment rights of persons who have disabilities. This act requires employers to provide reasonable accommodations to job applicants; these may include, but certainly are not limited to, providing assistance to persons with hearing impairments or relocating the interview to a location within the building that is accessible to a person who has mobility limitations. Physical examinations can only be required if all applicants are required to take them. An applicant is not required to tell the employer that he or she has a disability; however, it is probably a good idea to do so. Once hired, employees are required to provide reasonable accommodations for the person with a disability, unless the accommodations create a hardship for the business. (*See* Chapter 7 for more details regarding the ADA.)

Workforce Investment Act of 1998

This act restructures existing federal statutes governing programs of job training, adult education and literacy, and vocational rehabilitation, replacing them with streamlined and more flexible components of workforce development systems. Title I of the act provides a clear outline of what is meant by streamlined and flexible components, with the listing of the following elements:

1. Training and employment programs must be designed where the needs of businesses and individuals are best understood.
2. Customers must be able to conveniently access the employment, education, training, and information services they need at a single location in their neighborhood.
3. Customers should have choices in deciding the training program that best fits their needs and the organizations that will provide that service. They should have control over their own career development.
4. Business will provide information and leadership and play an active role in ensuring that the system prepares people for current and future jobs.

An important feature, particularly for persons who have disabilities, is the "one-stop," single location approach. In the one-stop centers, employers have a single point of contact to provide information with regard to employment opportunities. It is intended that employers will benefit from a single system for finding job-ready skilled workers. Equally important, employment seekers will

1. Receive a preliminary assessment of their skill levels, attitudes, attributes, and separate service needs
2. Obtain information on a full array of employment-related services, including information about local education and training service providers
3. Receive help filing claims for unemployment insurance and evaluating eligibility for job training and education programs or student financial aid
4. Obtain job search and placement assistance, and receive career counseling
5. Have access to up-to-date labor market information that identifies job vacancies and skills necessary for in-demand jobs and provides information about local, regional, and national employment trends (U.S. Department of Labor, 1998).

Rehabilitation Act Amendment (Section 508)

This is an amendment to Section 508 of the 1973 Rehabilitation Act. The amendment was included in the Workforce Investment Act of 1998 (P.L. 105-220). The amendment requires federal agencies and departments, including the Postal Service, when procuring, maintaining, or using electronic and information technology to ensure, unless an undue burden is created, that the electronic and information technology allows

1. Individuals who have disabilities who are federal employees to have access to and use of information and data that is comparable to the access and use of the information and data by federal employees who are not disabled
2. Individuals who have disabilities who are members of the public seeking information or services from a federal department or agency to have access to and use of information and data that is comparable to the access to and use of the information and data by such members of the public who are not disabled.

In those instances in which an undue burden is created, the federal department or agency must provide to eligible persons who have a disability alternative means of access and use of the information (U.S. Department of Labor, 1998b).

The Ticket to Work and Work Incentives Improvement Act of 1999

As is true for most acts, there are numerous provisions contained therein; in this act, two of the most significant provisions with respect to the needs of persons who have disabilities are

1. Section 101 of Subtitle A—Ticket to Work and Self-Sufficiency Program. Under this provision, the commissioner of the Social Security Administration is authorized to provide Social Security Disability Insurance (SSDI) and Supplemental Security Income (SSI) recipients who have a disability with a "ticket" that he or she may use to obtain employment services, vocational rehabilitation services, and other support services from an employment network (provider of services) of their choice to enable them to enter the workforce. The employment network could be part of the one-stop delivery system established in the Workforce Investment Act of 1998.
2. Subtitle B—Elimination of Work Disincentive. Under this provision a person with a disability may return to work without that

action triggering a review of his or her impairment to determine whether the conditions is still disabling. This action would determine whether the person continued to receive benefits.

AGENCIES THAT AID EMPLOYMENT

Vocational Rehabilitation

The vocational rehabilitation program is a federal- and state-funded program; its major goal is to assist persons who have disabilities become employed and/or as independent as they are capable of becoming. Each state has a vocational rehabilitation service, and programs offered vary by state. However, some of the most common programs are medical evaluations to determine eligibility, vocational assessment, guidance and counseling, independent living services, training/education, job placement, and post-employment services designed to help the person who has a disability maintain employment. Most vocational rehabilitation agencies provide additional services

When attempting to assist a person who has a disability become gainfully employed, the state vocational rehabilitation agency should be one of the first places to which he or she is referred. Each vocational rehabilitation agency has trained counselors available to assist clients. Counselors can help them to determine eligibility for multiple services; develop a rehabilitation plan, which involves determining the rehabilitation goals and the methods to obtaining those goals; assist with job preparation, which may include training or education as well as job readiness skills, such as learning good work habits; assist with job placement; and, in instances of severe disabilities, assist with supported employment (discussed later in this chapter). Additionally, the counselor may assist the client to receive other supportive services, including psychological tests and family counseling.

Veterans Administration

Similar to state vocational rehabilitation programs, the VA offers myriad services for veterans who have disabilities. Services for veterans are somewhat different from the civilian rehabilitation services. The VA has hospitals and veteran financial services.

State Department of Human Services

Each state has a human services agency that provides a variety of services, some of which target persons who have disabilities. These services vary by state; therefore, helping professionals are advised to consult with the appropriate state agency for services and eligibility standards.

Social Security Administration

When most people think of this agency, they most often think of economic support to older Americans and persons who have become disabled. These are major roles of this agency. Through its SSDI and SSI programs, financial assistance is provided. However, the Social Security Administration is becoming increasingly more engaged in programs that prepare persons for employment, such as the Ticket to Work and Work Incentives Improvement Act of 1999 provisions that provide SSDI and SSI beneficiaries who have disabilities a "ticket" that can be used to obtain employment services.

Now that we have provided brief information about federal laws and federal and state agencies, we will now present information about a few private organizations that help prepare persons who have disabilities for employment.

The previous discussion related information with regard to federal laws and federal and state agencies that are available to assist with preparing a person with a disability for employment. The following will relate information about what generally is a private organization's effort to help prepare persons who have disabilities for employment.

SHELTERED WORKSHOPS

For several decades, sheltered workshops have been leaders in preparing persons who have disabilities, particularly those who have severe disabilities, for employment. Sheltered workshops operated by the Salvation Army and Goodwill Industries often provide both job training and employment for persons with disabilities. These are only two of many sheltered workshops available to assist persons who have disabilities achieve their employment goals. Because types of sheltered workshops vary not only in states but in communities, helping professionals should become familiar with the resources available within their respective communities.

Sheltered workshops were initially established to provide protected employment for some persons with disabilities (Bryan, 1996). Due to the severity or nature of their disability, some persons are unable to secure gainful employment in private industry; therefore, these workshops were established. Initially, they were exempt by the Fair Labor Standard Act from paying minimum wages because the productivity of the persons they employed was considered below industry standards. Also, in past years, some sheltered workshops employed persons who have disabilities to do menial tasks, training them for tasks that were seldom needed in the private sector. Currently, many workshops have changed. They have become progressive with regard to employment and training, continually surveying the job markets to determine job availability and employment opportunities and then structuring their training to the local labor market needs. Additionally, some sheltered workshops aggressively seek and successfully compete with the private sector for employment contracts.

The success of these workshops gives private and public employers proof that persons who have disabilities can perform job tasks as efficiently as their nondisabled counterparts. This success has also improved the economic status of sheltered workshop employees. Their performances have led to at least minimum wages. In some instances, they are paid according to industry standards. In addition to providing meaningful employment, the progressive workshops have begun to provide employment training, commonly called "work adjustment training." This is designed to teach good work habits such as punctuality, cooperation, interpersonal relations skills, and other human relations skills. The ultimate objective of these workshops is to prepare their employees for employment outside the sheltered environment. The success of their graduates is instrumental in helping change attitudes with regard to the employability of persons who have disabilities, especially those who have severe disabilities. Clearly, sheltered workshops are very valuable community resources.

SUPPORTED EMPLOYMENT

As previously stated, the unemployment rate for working-age adult persons who have disabilities has been estimated to be as high as 70 percent. One of the reasons for this is the difficulty many persons in this category have securing employment. Persons with severe mobility, visual, and hearing limitations, as well as those with mental disabilities, have few job opportunities. Their employment is inhibited by factors discussed earlier in this chapter. To counteract obstacles and get them into the employment arena, a very innovative approach called supported employment is used.

What Is Supported Employment?

Supported employment is designed to increase an individual's chances of being employed. This is frequently done by using support services such as a job coach or assistive technology, or both. According to Sinnott-Oswald, Gliner and Spencer (1991), supported employees work full- or part-time for an average of twenty hours per week. They are compensated in accordance with the Fair Labor Standards Act. Through this initiative, a growing number of people who have severe disabilities are able to obtain and maintain meaningful employment. Supported employment has three essential features: (1) employees are paid for doing productive work, (2) ongoing support and training ensure the continued employability of employees, and (3) these workers are socially integrated into their work environments.

According to the Developmental Disability Act of 1984, supported employment

- Supports employment for persons with developmental disabilities for whom competitive employment at or above the minimum wage is unlikely and who, because of their disabilities, need intensive ongoing job support
- Allows supported employment to be conducted in a variety of settings, particularly work sites in which nondisabled people are employed
- Supports activities that persons with disabilities need to sustain paid work, including supervision, training, and transportation.

Purpose of Supported Employment

Supported employment was originally developed to transition individuals who have severe disabilities from segregated workshops to competitive marketplace employment. These individuals traditionally have difficulty getting jobs in places other than segregated or sheltered workshops. The purpose has expanded to include more types of disabilities, such as persons who are substance abusers. Supported employment clients do not have to be in a segregated environment to participate in supported programs.

Philosophy of Supported Employment

All persons who are capable, regardless of the severity of their disability, should be given the opportunity for meaningful, paid work. That is the philosophy of supported employment. The key word is "meaningful." That is, whenever possible, employment is provided in an integrated setting with nondisabled persons. Through this interaction, persons with disabilities are given a chance to be valued, productive citizens.

Models of Supported Employment

Three of the original models were supported competitive employment and enclave and mobile work crews. Supported competitive employment provides "regular" job placement on an individual basis. Enclave employment generally consists of a small group of individuals, usually less than ten, who work as a team. Mobile work crews are similar to enclaves; they consist of a small group of individuals who perform specific jobs. Mobile work crews differ from enclaves in that more than one job coach may work with the group. Additionally, crews generally travel throughout the community in a van or bus, performing contractual jobs such as custodial and grounds keeping.

Job Coach

A key element to the success of any supported employment program is the job coach. The job coach works closely with persons who have disabilities by identifying jobs and helping train them on the job. The job coach usually will adjust his or her services to the needs of the individual. Coaches may initially be involved in helping establish the work environment and assisting with training the individuals to successfully perform their job tasks. Once that is done, coaches leave and may return later if additional instruction and support are needed. In working with a mobile crew, the job coach may be permanent, working daily with crew members. Consequently, the job coach is a key to the success of this form of employment.

The final section of this chapter will deal with maintaining employment.

MAINTAINING EMPLOYMENT

Only a few people would disagree with the assertion that securing employment for many persons who have disabilities is at best difficult. The fact that the unemployment rate for persons with disabilities can be as high as 70 percent is ipso facto proof of the statement. Consequently, the NOD/Harris Surveys (1994, 1998, 2000) have shown that a large percentage of unemployed persons who have disabilities prefer to work but are unable to get or keep a job.

It is also a truism that the most ardent advocates of persons who have disabilities, as well as those persons themselves, do not expect employers to tolerate less productivity from workers with disabilities than they do from nondisabled workers. Getting levels of productivity may mean that reasonable accommodations have to be made for all employees. Such accommodations should be considered as efforts to make employees more productive rather than providing special treatment. As previously mentioned, reasonable accommodations are made routinely for nondisabled persons, including such things as piped-in music, certain colored walls, and ergonomic chairs.

Most fair employers make good faith efforts to help ensure the success of their employees. However, even in those instances, if workers who have disabilities believe they have been denied equal opportunities to succeed, they should consult with the appropriate company official with regard to grievance procedures. Most human resource directors or job supervisors will attempt to resolve a dispute before having it become a formal grievance. If after having gone through the company grievance process the worker still believes she or he has not been treated fairly, the next step may be a consultation with the EEOC, the federal agency charged with the responsibility of hearing and processing complaints of discrimination and unfair treatment. This agency will receive complaints from anyone who believes she or he has been discriminated. Helping professionals should be familiar with this agency's requirement for filing complaints.

Additionally, helping professionals should be aware of the provisions and protection offered by the five titles of the ADA. The ADA is discussed in more detail in Chapter 7. Also, it is helpful to be knowledgeable of the Family Medical Leave Act (FMLA). FMLA applies to all public agencies, including state, local, and federal employees; local education agencies; and private sector employers who employ fifty or more employees in 20-hour or more work weeks in a current or preceding calendar year and who engage in commerce or in any industry or activity affecting commerce. To be eligible for family medical leave benefits, an employee must

- Work for a covered employer
- Have worked for the employer for a total of 12 months
- Have worked at least 1250 hours over the previous 12 months
- Work at a location in the United States or any territory or possession of the United States where the employer within 75 miles employs at least fifty employees.

An eligible employee is entitled to a maximum of 12 work weeks of unpaid leave during any 12-month period for one or more of the following reasons:

- Birth and care of the newborn child of the employee
- Placement with the employee of a son or daughter for adoption or foster care
- Care for an immediate family member (spouse, child, or parent) with a serious health condition
- Medical leave when the employee is unable to work because of a serious health condition.

Finally, upon returning to work from leave, an employee must be restored to his or her original job or to an equivalent one with equivalent pay, benefits, and other terms and conditions of employment. Laws protecting the rights of workers who have disabilities vary by state. Therefore, helping professionals are advised to become familiar with their own state laws.

SUMMARY

Work remains a vital part of most Americans' lives. It provides and contributes to many aspects of one's life. In earlier times, persons who had disabilities were thought to be unable to work in a competitive work environment; thus, sheltered or protective work environments were considered the best, if not the only hope for their employment. Today, sheltered employment, with the addition of supported employment programs, is an option for persons who have severe physical or mental limitations. Additionally, early education efforts, innovative job training programs, and improved employer attitudes concerning the capabilities of people once considered unemployable have altered the life choices of countless Americans who once were written off as being useless. Thus they are empowered to enter mainstream American life.

POINTS FOR DISCUSSION AND SUGGESTED ACTIVITIES

1. Discuss with a representative of your state vocational rehabilitation agency the types of employment preparation services available to persons who have disabilities.

2. Contact at least three employers in your area and discuss whether they hire persons who have disabilities and their work-related experiences with them.
3. Research your state or community's involvement in the Ticket to Work and Work Incentives Improvement Act.
4. Contact a Veterans Administration Office to determine the types of employment or training services they have for veterans who have disabilities.
5. Contact a Social Security Administration office to determine the type of employment or training programs they have for persons who have disabilities.
6. Research the unemployment rate of persons who have disabilities in your community, city, or state; interview at least three unemployed persons who have disabilities to ascertain their experiences trying to secure or keep a job.
7. Contact at least three sheltered workshops to determine the types of services they provide to persons who have disabilities.
8. Locate a job coach and discuss the types of services he or she provides.
9. Locate an employer who is participating in supported employment; ask about his or her experiences in the program.

REFERENCES

Brantman, M. (1978). What happens to insurance rates when handicapped people come to work? *Disabled U.S.A.*, Washington, DC: President's Committee on Employment of the Handicapped, Washington, DC.

Bryan, W.V. (1996). *In Search of Freedom.* Springfield, IL: Charles C Thomas.

Childs, G.B. (1971). Is the work ethic realistic in an age of automation? In H. Peters and J.C. Hansen (Eds), *Vocational Guidance and Career Development.* New York: Macmillan.

Chirikos, T.N. (1991). The economics of employment. *Milbank Quarterly, 69*:150–179.

Christman, L.A., and Slaten, B.L. (1991). Attitudes toward people with disabilities and judgement of employment potential. *Perceptual & Motor Skills, 72*: 467–475.

Day, H., and Alon, E. (1993). Work, leisure and quality of life of vocational rehabilitation consumers. *Canadian Journal of Rehabilitation, 7*: 119–125.

Deutscher, M. (1971). Adult work and development models. In H. Peters and J.C. Hansen, (Eds.), *Vocational Guidance and Career Development.* New York: Macmillan.

Frankl, V. (1965). *The Doctor and the Soul From Psychotherapy to Logotherapy* (2nd ed.). New York: Knopp.

Friedman, E., and Havighurst, R. (1954). *The Meaning of Work and Retirement.* Chicago: University of Chicago Press.

Lofquist, L. H., and Davis, R. V. (1969). *Adjustment to Work.* New York: Appleton-Century-Crofts.

Maslow, A. (1962). *Toward a Psychology of Being.* New York: Van Nostrand.

NOD Survey of Americans With Disabilities. (1994). The new competitive advantage. *Business Week*, May, 1994.

NOD Harris Survey of Americans with Disabilities. (2000). Louis Harris and Associates, Inc.

NOD Harris Survey of Americans with Disabilities. (1998). Louis Harris and Associates, Inc.

Obermann, C. E. (1965). *A History of Vocational Rehabilitation in America.* Minneapolis, MN: T. S. Denison.

Ondusko, D. (1991). Comparison of employees with disabilities and able-bodied workers in janitorial maintenance. *Journal of Applied Rehabilitation Counseling, 22*:19–24.

Roe, A. (1956). *The Psychology of Occupations.* New York: John Wiley & Sons.

Satcher, J., and Dooley-Dickey, K. (1992). Attitudes of human resource management students toward persons with disabilities. *Rehabilitation Counseling Bulletin, 35*: 248–252.

Sinnott-Oswald, M., Gliner, J.A., and Spencer, K.C. (1991). Supported and sheltered employment, quality of life issues among worker with disabilities. *Education and Training in Mental Retardation*, 280–284.

Super, D.A. (1968). Developmental self concept theory of vocational behavior. In S.H. Osipow (Ed.), *Theories of Career Development.* New York: Appleton-CenturyCrofts.

U. S. Department of Labor (1998a). *Workforce Investment Act of 1998* [On-line]. (Plain English Version). www.state.co.us/gov_dir/wdc/wia/plainenglish.htm

U. S. Department of Labor (1998b). Workforce Investment Act of 1998, Sec. 508 Electronic and Information Technology [On-line]. Available: www.usdoj.gov/crt/ 508law.html.

United States Department of Justice. (No Date). Employment Standards Administration Wage and Hour Devision, *Fact sheet No. 028* [On-line]. Available: www.dol.gov/dol/esa/public/regs/compliance/whd/whfs28.htm.

Vash, C.L. (1981). *The Psychology of Disability.* New York: Springer.

Weber, M. (1930). *The Protestant Ethic and the Spirit of Capitalism.* New York: Scribner.

Wolfbein, S. L. (1971). *Work in American Society.* Glenview, IL: Scott, Foresman.

Yelin, E. H., and Katz, P. P. (1994). Making work more central to work disability policy. *Milbank Quarterly, 72*: 593–619.

SUGGESTED READINGS

Christman, L.A., and Slaten, B. L. (1991). Attitudes toward people with disabilities and judgment of employment potential. *Perceptual & Motor Skills, 72*: 4670–4675.

Cimera, R.E. (1998). Are individuals with severe mental retardation and multiple disabilities cost-efficient to serve via supported employment programs? *Mental Retardation, 36*: 280–292.

Johnson, W.G., and Lambrinos, J. (1985). Wage discrimination against handicapped men and women. *Journal of Human Resources, 20*: 264–277.

National Organization on Disability. (1998). *Closing the Gap: Expanding the Participation of Americans With Disabilities.* Washington, DC: Author.

Ravard, J.F. et al. (1992). Discrimination toward disabled people seeking employment. *Social Science Medicine, 35*: 951–958.

Chapter 7

POLITICS OF DISABILITIES

Outline

- Introduction
- Advocacy
- Independent Living Center Movement
- Summary
- Note to Helpers
- Points for Discussion and Suggested Activities

Objectives

- To identify that persons with disabilities have self-advocacy
- To describe why persons with disabilities are capable of determining for themselves what their needs are.
- To identify key legislative acts that protect the rights of persons with disabilities and mandate specific services available to them.

INTRODUCTION

The march toward equal access and equal rights for persons with disabilities' in the United States has been a long and quite often difficult journey. As discussed in this text, the journey is not complete; however, significant progress has been made and hopefully progress will continue to be made. Two actions, advocacy and political action, have helped smooth the way and pave the path to better acceptance and increased access for millions of Americas with disabilities.

The United States commitment to its military personnel who in the course of defending the freedom of all Americans became disabled has been the foundation upon which much of the beginning physical restoration of persons with disabilities began. It is true that much of the beginning concerns for persons with physical disabilities were directed toward military personnel with disabilities; however, the efforts directed toward rehabilitation of injured soldiers and other military men and women had several benefits: (1) national awareness of the needs of persons with disabilities were increased, (2) advancements in psychological and medical treatment of persons with disabilities occurred, and (3) political action in the form of federal legislation was enacted to meet some of the needs of persons with disabilities. As previously stated, a specific population–military personnel with disabilities–initially benefited most from the United States attention to needs of persons with disabilities. Eventually, however, the general population of persons with disabilities began to receive increased attention directed toward their needs.

Perhaps one of the lessons the nonmilitary population of persons with disabilities learned from the previously mentioned experiences was the fact that, although significant issues exist, it does not mean timely attention will be forthcoming. In an open democracy in which there are numerous issues that need attention, or at least some of its citizens strongly believe there is a need for attention, the reality, generally speaking, is that issues which are persistently and sometime articulately promoted get the first and most attention. Therefore, advocacy became a vehicle for those representing the needs of persons with disabilities to bring to the attention of the general population that all persons with disabilities were being treated as second-class citizens. As a result of this advocacy, many pieces of federal legislation were enacted to help meet some of the needs of persons with disabilities. There can be no question that most of the initial advocacy agencies and organizations acting on behalf of persons with disabilities produced some very good and useful results. However, as is discussed in this chapter as well as other chapters, there was a downside to the early advocacy: too often persons without disabilities were both determining the needs of persons with disabilities and introducing those needs to the public, rather than persons with disabilities taking the lead on their own behalf. The result of persons with disabilities being in the background while nondisabled persons spoke for them and represented them was that this became their media identity. There were two major problems with this approach to advocacy: (1) an impression was given that persons with disabilities were incapable of determining their own needs and (2) the image of persons with disabilities as being dependent on persons without disabilities became a major perception of the nondisabled. Funk (1987) pointed out that this approach has left society with a persisting image of persons with disabilities as being deviant, incompetent, unhealthy objects of fear who are perpetually dependent on the welfare and charity of others. In opposition to Funk's proclamation, some researchers have concluded that the advocacy of others on the behalf of persons with disabilities has had some positive effects. The truth of that statement cannot be denied, but it is also true that persons with disabilities have begun to advocate for themselves and have had some significant results, such as the Section 504 protest, the Deaf President Now Protest, the Wheel of Justice Protest, the passage of the ADA of 1990 and its amendment of 2008, and the Independent Living Center Movement, all of which are discussed in this text. In addition to the previously mentioned discussion, significant legislative action is discussed, some of which occurred as a result of advocacy by persons with disabilities and others not specifically as a result of action by persons with disabilities, but as a result of meeting needs of various disability groups. The discussion in this chapter begins with advocacy followed by what some have referred to as the beginning of the disability rights movement and continuing with early legislative action and some of the more recent legislative action designed to improve the lives of persons with disabilities.

ADVOCACY

Visions of telethons generally come to mind when one thinks of advocacy for persons with disabilities. Most telethons have been conducted by national organizations that raise money for disability-related research and other relevant services. In previous years, some of the techniques used in telethons, such as displaying persons with disabilities as helpless persons, have been criticized. Currently, most telethons have developed more sensitive approaches to assisting persons with disabilities.

Despite millions of dollars that have been raised through telethons and other advocacy efforts, the impression that frequently remains is that others, particularly the nondisabled, have to be advocates for persons with disabilities. Stone (1984) noted that few people expect to see persons with disabilities as advocates for themselves. Because professional associations have been so visible in their advocacy efforts, the fact that persons with disabilities have a long history of advocating for themselves is not well-known. Pelka (1997) states that as early as the 1850s, persons who were hearing impaired had established a local organization to advocate for their interests.

There have been other advocacy organizations and efforts led by persons with disabilities, such as the League of Physically Handicapped Protest, Section 504 Protest, Deaf President Now Protest, and the Wheels of Justice Protest.

The League of Physically Handicapped Protest was organized during the Great Depression of the 1930s to protest the ERB's reluctance to refer persons with disabilities for jobs provided through President Franklin Roosevelt's WPA program. The ERB was the agency designated to screen candidates for employment. Although the protest did not change federal policy, it gained public support and made society in general aware of the desires and employment needs of persons with disabilities.

The *Section 504 Protest* occurred in 1977 as a reaction to the failure of the federal government to issue regulations governing Section 504 of the Rehabilitation Act of 1973. Specifically, Section 504 prohibits discrimination of persons with disabilities by any institution receiving federal financial assistance; the organized protest was by the ACCD. Their 25-day sit-in at the San Francisco HEW offices was duplicated in Atlanta, Boston, Denver, and Washington, D.C. The sit-ins forced the Secretary of Health, Education and Welfare (now the Department of Health and Human Services) to sign the regulations on April 28, 1977. Then the provisions of Section 504 became enforceable.

The *Deaf President Now Protest* occurred in 1988, when the Board of Trustees of Gallaudet University failed to hire a deaf person as president. Gallaudet University was founded to educate persons who are deaf. Students of the university shut down the campus and vowed to keep the campus closed until the following demands were met:

1. Resignation of the newly appointed president and the appointment of a deaf president as her replacement
2. Resignation of the Board of Trustee Chairperson
3. An increase in deaf representation on the Board to a majority
4. No reprisals against the protesters.

Three days after the students shut down the campus, the newly appointed president resigned. Within three days, the Board of Trustees agreed to meet the remaining demands of the students. I. King Jordan was appointed, and he became the first deaf president of the university.

In the late 1980s, the American Disabled for Accessible Public Transit Organization organized the *Wheel of Justice Protest* to make known their support of the then pending legislation entitled the Americans with Disabilities Act. Several powerful members of Congress and the Senate believed the act was unnecessary, thus the strength of the act was being threatened. The protesters, some 200 strong, gathered on the steps of the nation's capitol and made their feelings known and their voices heard. In part because of their efforts, the ADA was signed into law by President George H. Bush on July 26, 1990.

INDEPENDENT LIVING CENTER MOVEMENT

Spencer (1990) reminds us that prior to the independent living movement, which began in the early 1970s, many persons with severe disabilities either lived in an institution or were cared for by family members. There is little doubt that the majority of the care received was helpful; however, in most instances it did not provide many opportunities for persons with disabilities to develop independent living skills. Reflecting on this experience, some persons with disabilities began to realize that to be truly free they must take and maintain control of their lives. This belief resulted in the development of independent living centers (ILCs).

Dejong (1982) provides a brief history of the genesis of ILCs: a small group of persons with disabilities at the University of Illinois and the University of California at Berkeley moved out of residential hospitals into the community and organized their own survival services systems. The centers created by these students became the blueprint from which future centers would be established. Following each center's success, the scope of ILC services expanded. Even with new services, the basic principle of persons with disabilities taking greater control of their lives did not change. Perhaps Dejong best summarized the independent living philosophy when he said the dignity of risk is what the ILC movement is all about. Without the possibility of failure, a person with a disability lacks true independence, the mark of one's humanity: the right to self-actualize.

The Uncertainty of Choice

When one considers that the independent living movement was initiated by persons with disabilities, many of whom were persons with severe disabilities such as spinal cord injuries, it becomes quite apparent that those individuals exhibited courage of the highest magnitude. Prior to the movement, they lived in conditions that made them almost totally dependent on others. Even so, for the most part, they lived in safe environments. Therefore, abandoning the status quo involved confronting many uncertainties, namely physical and social barriers designed to restrict the space of free movement of persons with disabilities. The founders of the movement were cognizant that the challenge would be great. They believed the reward of becoming more independent was worth the risks they would encounter.

Similar to the civil rights movement, the founders of the independent living movement had well-conceived ideas and goals. Frieden and Cole (1985) provide insight into some of the founders' thinking. First, they believed that supportive programs could be established to meet their emotional needs as well as to provide environmental accommodations that would allow them to have opportunities previously available only to people without disabilities. Second, they refused to accept the popular notion that they should be confined to an institution. Third, they rejected the assumption that persons with disabilities had fewer rights than the nondisabled had. Likewise, they did not accept the idea that the federal government's obligations to them were limited to abating physical disabilities (Lozano, 1993).

Toward a Definition

There are many definitions of independent living. According to Eisenberg, Giggins, and Duval (1982), independent living means persons with disabilities have opportunities for gainful employment, living in a wholesome family, and having the rights and responsibilities of community life. To achieve these goals, most ILCs have three guiding principles: (1) individuals with disabilities know best how to meet their own needs, (2) the needs of persons with disabilities can be met most effectively through comprehensive programs that provide a variety of services, and (3) persons with disabilities should be integrated as fully as possible into their communities. The hallmark of successful ILCs is evident: They evolve around freedom of choice, the right to live where and how one chooses and can afford (Laurie, 1982). The centers allow for living alone or with a roommate of one's choice. Consequently, independent living is deciding one's own pattern of life–selecting one's own food, entertainment, leisure, and friends. In essence, this is to take risks and freedom to make mistakes.

Frieden and Cole (1985) defined the independent living concept as control over one's life based on the choice of acceptable options that minimize reliance on others in making decisions and in performing everyday activities. This includes managing one's affairs, participating in day-to-day community activities, and fulfilling a range of familial roles. Indeed, this is making decisions that lead to self-determination and the minimization of physical or psychological dependence on other persons.

Sustaining the Initiative

Frieden, Richards, Cole, and Bailey (1979) were among the first writers to note that the independent living movement can be sustained only with support services that help adults with disabilities to effectively manage their own affairs. Anything less is a distortion of the movement. Central to the philosophy of the independent living movement initiative is full participation in community life by as many participants as possible. Relatedly, both short-term and long-term community support is central to ILCs. Gradually, ILCs are changing American attitudes and beliefs with regard to the needs and abilities of persons with disabilities. Spencer's (1990) research documents the positive changes the centers spawned through agencies in California, Massachusetts, Michigan, and Texas that provided state-level support for independent living programs prior to passage of federal legislation.

Although it is very important to note that the independent living movement was initiated by persons with disabilities, it must also be noted that federal support, especially funding, was needed to strengthen and stabilize ILCs. Funding was needed to expand and improve the delivery of services as well as to expand the number of centers throughout the United States. The Rehabilitation Act of 1973 was passed by Congress and amended in 1978 to add Title VII, Comprehensive Services for Independent Living. With the amendment, Congress authorized support for community-based ILC that in turn had the effect of establishing a major change in federal disability policy.

To date, more than 200 ILCs have been developed in the United States'–each state has at least one center. The concept has spread to become international. For example, in the United Kingdom there are more than 30 disabled living centers (DLCs). In addition to ILCs in Canada, there are hundreds of centers scattered throughout the world, mainly in Europe. There are many types of ILCs and related programs. In fact, they have become somewhat specialized. Some centers exist for developmentally disabled youth and adults, other centers have been established for the elderly, still other centers are for persons with mental and emotional problems, and many are for persons with physical disabilities. Therefore, the services provided vary depending on the needs of the population served. Examples of some of the types of services provided are housing, attendant care, readers, interpreters, information with regard to goods and services relevant to the population served, information regarding transportation, peer counseling, professional counseling, independent living skills training, advocacy regarding political action, equipment maintenance and repair, social-recreational services, financial counseling, vocational assistance, and meal preparation (Frieden & Cole, 1985; Futter, Rossi, Gerken, Nosek & Richards, 1990; Lozano, 1993).

Because occupational therapists teach independent living skills, they have become very active as ILCs service providers. Bowen (1993) described occupational therapists as a group involved in the centers as primary caregivers. Neistadt and Marques (1984) researched an independent living skills training program for adults with multiple handicaps. Other researchers have critiqued independent skills transition programs for adolescents with development disabilities (Jackson, Rankin, Sheifkin & Clark, 1986). Nochajski and Gordon (1987) and Neistadt (1987) described community living skills training programs for adults with developmental disabilities. Independent living initiatives can be subsumed under two programs: transitional and cluster.

A transitional program was defined by Frieden and Cole (1985) as an independent living program that facilitates the movement of persons with severe disabilities from comparatively dependent living situations to comparatively independent living situations. They further point out that transitional programs are usually goal-oriented and time specific. These programs generally provide instruction in areas of mobility, medical self-care, financial management, attendant care, housing, personality, and social skills, to mention a few. Transitional programs have the same goal as most other independent living programs: to encourage the participants to make decisions that affect their lives, thus taking responsibility for the direction of their lives.

According to Spencer (1990), the cluster model of independent living focuses on situations in which support services are shared by a group of persons with disabilities who live in close proximity. In contrast to individual-oriented programs, clusters of persons pool their resources in order to find housing or attendants or transportation. Although services vary according to the population served, most ILCs and their programs reflect a common goal, which, according to Townsend and Ryan (1991), is to advocate for "independence" in making decisions about one's life. This does not mean all persons with disabilities must physically perform all daily living tasks. Instead, independent living means the ability to direct, manage, or control the accomplishment of community living through one's own actions or through directing the action of others. Bowen (1993) emphasized that the independent living model focuses on changing the community (e.g. eliminating architectural and attitudinal barriers) rather than the person with the disability. That is, consumers choose the services and the service providers they need.

Townsend and Ryan (1991) listed four major roles of ILCs: (1) to control and direct personal and community services, including planning and organizing transportation, finances, paid work, cooking, laundry, housekeeping, and general assistance; (2) to facilitate participation in leisure and recreational activities, including social skills, emotional stability, motivation, attitudes and interaction support needed to participate at home or outside the home; (3) to assist with the development and use of each individual's education, employment, and social potential and talents; and (4) to contribute to the well-being and betterment of society, including each individual's ability to give as well as to receive help. In the end, this is not independent living. It is interdependent living under conditions that are mutually gratifying (DeLoach, Wilkins & Walker, 1983). The independent living initiative has occurred as a result of a history of stepping stone legislative actions designed to make persons with disabilities as independent as possible.

Legislative Action

In 1917, Congress passed the Smith-Hughes Act, a landmark education act that set the precedent for subsequent federal funding of educational programs, not only for people with disabilities but also for other people (Cull & Hardy, 1973). In addition, the act called for a Board of Vocational Education to spearhead the drive for vocational education. This board was to become the foundation for vocational rehabilitation in the United States. The first Board of Vocational Education was funded in 1918 under the Soldier Rehabilitation Act to operate a program of vocational rehabilitation for World War I veterans. Better known as the Smith-Sears Veterans' Rehabilitation Act of 1918, it provided the following general purview for federal vocational rehabilitation services: "An act to provide for the vocational rehabilitation and return to employment of disabled persons discharged from the military or naval forces of the United States and for other purposes." After this seed had been planted, state and federal vocational rehabilitation programs developed. However, before these programs evolved to their present status, they progressed through several stages.

Smith-Fess Act (1920)

President Woodrow Wilson's signature on PL-236 (the Smith-Fess Act) in 1920 made public rehabilitation programs a long-awaited reality. This act established federal and state rehabilitation programs and provided for an equal sharing of expenditures for them. The act was not without limitations, however. Funds were provided only for vocational guidance, training, occupational adjustment, prostheses, and placement services. In short, rehabilitation services for persons with physical disabilities were to be vocational in nature; physical restoration and sociopsychological services were excluded.

Actually, the Smith-Fess Act was an extension of earlier vocational education legislation. It added the provision making rehabilitation services available to people with physical disabilities. Also, this was temporary legislation and remained operative only by additional legislation. In 1924, federal legislation was passed that extended the life of state and federal vocational rehabilitation programs for an additional six years. It was not until the 1935 Federal Social Security Act that state and federal vocational rehabilitation programs became permanent. The long and tedious battle to institutionalize vocational rehabilitation for persons with disabilities was finally won.

Barden-LaFollette Act (1943)

More commonly known as the Vocational Rehabilitation Act of 1943, the Barden-LaFollette Act strengthened vocational rehabilitation programs by providing physical restoration services to people with disabilities. In addition, it extended vocational rehabilitation services to persons with mental disabilities. In 1954, this act was again amended, and the following significant changes were made:

1. More funds and additional program options were provided to state agencies.
2. Federal-funded research programs were established.
3. Training funds were added for physicians, nurses, rehabilitation counselors, physical therapists, occupational therapists, social workers, psychologists, and other specialists in the field of rehabilitation.

Vocational Rehabilitation Act Amendment (1965)

These amendments further strengthened vocational rehabilitation programs by (1) providing monies to states for innovative projects that developed new methods of providing services and otherwise serving persons with severe disabilities; (2) creating a broader base of services to persons with disabilities, including individuals with socially handicapping conditions; and (3) eliminating economic need as a requisite for rehabilitation services. Slowly, the related pieces to comprehensive care were coming together to form a meaningful whole.

Rehabilitation Act of 1973

PL-112 of the Ninety-third Congress replaced the Vocational Rehabilitation Act as amended in 1968 with this new act, which maintained the major provisions of the 1968 amended act and added the provision that before receiving funds a state must conduct a thorough study to determine the needs of its handicapped citizens. Other significant provisions of the act were the inclusion in Title V of Sections 501, 502, 503, and 504.

SECTION 501. This section established the Interagency Committee on Handicapped Employees. The Committee consists of federal agency heads, who have the responsibility to review annually the adequacy of federal hiring, placement, and job advancement of persons with disabilities. Based on each review, the Committee can recommend further legislation and administrative changes.

SECTION 502. This section established the Architectural and Transportation Barriers Compliance Board, which has the responsibility of monitoring the construction of new federal buildings and the remodeling of old ones to ensure that they are accessible to persons with physical disabilities. Existing federal buildings that are not being remodeled do not have to be made accessible.

SECTION 503. The words *affirmative action* were introduced into the vocabulary of rehabilitation in Section 503, which requires that every employer doing business with the federal government under a contract for more than $2500 take affirmative action in hiring persons with disabilities. Throughout the various stages of employment (recruiting, hiring, upgrading, transferring, advertising for recruitment, establishing rates of pay, and selecting persons for apprenticeships), affirmative action must be taken.

SECTION 504. If the laws contained within Section 504 were followed to the letter, at least 80 percent of the employment problems of persons with physical disabilities would vanish. This section calls for nondiscrimination in employment. Every United States institution that receives federal financial assistance must take steps to ensure that people with disabilities are not discriminated against in employment.

It is important to note that the enactment of Sections 503 and 504 began a major change in America's national commitment to citizens with disabilities. In the 1990s, equality under the law became a reality for persons with disabilities. The Disability Rights Education and Defense Fund (DREDF) correctly assessed the situation when it stated,

"Never before had the exclusion and segregation of people with disabilities been viewed as discrimination." Few people other than social scientists, rehabilitation workers, and, of course, those with disabilities recognized the impact society's perceptions and attitudes had on the well-being of persons with disabilities. Certainly no previous legislation had addressed this issue.

The enactment of Section 504 signaled Congress' realization that the inferior social and economic status of persons with disabilities was not the result of disabilities per se; it was a manifestation of societal barriers and prejudices. Another important aspect of Section 504 is the fact that this was the first federal legislation that viewed people with disabilities as a class. Previously, federal legislation and policies separated disabilities by diagnosis. By viewing people with disabilities as a minority group, they were all defined as being potential victims of discrimination in employment and education.

The Rehabilitation Act of 1973 was amended in 1974 and 1978. The 1974 amendments significantly strengthened programs for persons who are blind that were first authorized in 1936 by the Randolph-Shepard Act. (This act had authorized states to license qualified persons who were blind to operate vending stands in federal buildings.) In addition to providing increased funding to states, some provisions of the amendments to the Rehabilitation Act of 1973 focused on employment opportunities and independent living for people with disabilities. Specifically, the provisions provided for (1) community service employment pilot programs, (2) projects with industry and business to accelerate the training and employment of persons with disabilities, (3) grants and contracts with individuals with disabilities to start or operate business enterprises, (4) loans from the Small Business Administration to persons with disabilities when other financial assistance is unavailable, (5) funds for comprehensive services for independent living for individuals with severe disabilities, and (6) grants to states for the establishment and operation of ILC.

Education of All Handicapped Children Act of 1975

Perhaps the most significant of all legislation for children with disabilities is the Education of All Handicapped Children Act, later renamed the Individuals with Disabilities Education Act. In some respects, particularly for children, this legislation can be compared in importance to the Americans with Disabilities Act.

Individuals with Disabilities Education Act

The Individuals with Disabilities Education Act (IDEA) is a federal law that supports special education and related services for children and youth with disabilities. The law was originally enacted in 1975 as the Education of All Handicapped Children Act to establish grants to states for the education of children with disabilities. A major component of the law is the requirement that all eligible school-age children with disabilities are to be provided a free, appropriate, public school education, particularly services that

1. are provided to children and youth with disabilities at public expense, under public supervision and direction, and without charges
2. meet the standards of the appropriate state education agency that must include the requirements of the Individuals with Disabilities Act
3. include preschool, elementary school, or secondary education in the state involved

4. are provided in keeping with an individualized education plan (IEP) that meets the requirements of the law

In 1986, the Education of All Handicapped Children Act was amended to provide special funding incentives for states that would make a free appropriate education available to all eligible preschool-aged children with disabilities, three to five years of age. Additional provisions include financial help to states to develop early intervention programs for infants and toddlers with disabilities. The act was amended in 1992 and 1997.

The Act requires schools to hold an annual meeting with the parents to discuss their children's progress with respect to IEP goals, which are to be developed by a team whose members review the assessment information available on each child who has a disability. The team must consist of the following: one or both parents; at least one of the child's regular education teachers; if appropriate, at least one of the child's special education teachers; if appropriate, a representative of the public agency who is qualified to provide the appropriate services; and the child, if appropriate. The IEP should include

1. a statement of the child's present level of educational performance
2. a statement of measurable annual goals, including short-term objectives
3. a statement of various services to be provided to the child
4. an explanation of the extent, if any, to which the child will not participate with nondisabled children in a regular class
5. a statement of any modifications that will occur for the child to participate in the state or district-wide assessments
6. a timetable of when services will be provided
7. a statement of how goals will be measured
8. a statement of how services will be transitional at various ages, such as at ages 14 and 16
9. a statement about the transfer of the child's rights when he/she reaches the age of adulthood

Americans with Disabilities Act of 1990

Most writers acknowledge that the ADA is the farthest reaching and most influential bill of its kind to date. By passing this law, Congress made several important acknowledgments that persons with disabilities, their families, friends, and rehabilitation workers have known for many years:

1. American society had isolated and segregated individuals with disabilities
2. Persons with disabilities were victims of serious discrimination
3. Discrimination against persons with disabilities was a pervasive social problem
4. The result of discrimination against persons with disabilities was problematic in the critical areas of employment, housing, public accommodation, education, transportation, communication, recreation, institutionalization, health services, voting and access to public services
5. There was no legal recourse for persons with disabilities who were victims of discrimination
6. Many of the acts of discrimination encountered by persons with disabilities were blatant and intentionally exclusionary
7. Persons with disabilities occupied an inferior status in the American society
8. Persons with disabilities are a minority group that was relegated to a position of political powerlessness

Because the act is extensive, the authors of this book chose not to attempt a detailed analysis. Instead, the reader is encouraged to obtain a copy of the *Americans With Disabilities Act: An Implementation Guide* published by the Disability Rights Education and Defense Fund, Inc. We also recommend the reader to contact the Equal Employment Opportunity Commission, the United States Departments of Justice and Transportation, or the Federal Communication Commission in order to obtain specific interpretations of relevant regulations. For the purposes of this text, highlights of the law are presented below.

PERSONS WITH DISABILITIES DEFINED. The ADA defines a person with a disability as (1) a person with a physical or mental impairment that substantially limits one or more major life activities, (2) a person with a record of such a physical or mental impairment, or (3) a person who is regarded as having an impairment. A closer analysis of this definition provides the following observations:

1. A person is considered disabled if her or his condition creates limitations in performing any major life activity such as walking, seeing, hearing, speaking, breathing, learning, working, or caring for one's self.
2. A person is considered disabled if he or she has a history of a disability. A major consideration is whether employers and others discriminate against him or her because of a past record of disability.
3. A person is considered disabled if others regard him or her as disabled and he or she meets one of the following criteria: (a) does not have a substantial limitation of a major life activity but is treated by an employer or others as though the impairment creates such a limitation; (b) has a physical or mental impairment that substantially limits major life activities only as a result of the attitudes of others, in other words, an individual who has epilepsy seizures that are controlled by medication, but he or she has difficulties due to employers' or others' negative attitude about epilepsy; (c) has no impairment but is treated by employers or others as if he or she has a substantially limiting impairment, in other words, someone who is mistreated because of a disfiguring birthmark.

EXCLUSIONS. The definition of a disability is quite broad, but there are some exclusions, such as addiction to and use of illegal drugs, homosexuality and bisexuality, transsexualism, transvestism, pedophilia, exhibitionism, gender identity disorder not resulting from a physical impairment, voyeurism, other sexual behavior disorders, kleptomania, pyromania, psychoactive substance use disorder from current illegal use of drugs.

There are specific circumstances that determine whether or not someone addicted to drugs is considered a person with a disability. For instance, individuals addicted to and using *illegal* drugs are not protected by the ADA; however, individuals addicted to and using *controlled* drugs are protected by the ADA. Individuals addicted to but *not using* either controlled or illegal drugs are protected by the ADA. The ADA defines a person as being disabled if his or her disability "substantially limits" the performance of major life activities. According to the EEOC, substantially limits means:

> Unable to perform a major life activity that the average person in the general population can perform or significantly restricted as to the condition, manner or duration which an individual can perform major life activity as compared to the condition, manner, or duration

under which the average person in the general population can perform the same major life activities.

According to the DREDF, the following factors should be considered when determining whether an individual is substantially limited in a major life activity:

- The nature and severity of the impairment
- The duration or expected duration of the impairment
- The permanent or long term impact
- The expected permanent or long-term impact of, or result from impairment.

Although the act is entitled "Americans With Disabilities," any individual with a disability in the United States, regardless of citizenship is covered. The act consists of five titles: Title I, Employment; Title II, Public Services, Title III, Public Accommodations and Services Operated by Private Entities, Title IV, Telecommunications Relay Services; and Title V, Miscellaneous Provisions.

TITLE I. The "Employment" title was phased in, effective July 26, 1992, and all private employers who had twenty-five or more employees were subject to the ADA. Effective July 26, 1994, all private employers who have fifteen or more employees were subject to the ADA. It should be noted that employers that have less than fifteen employees, although they are not subject to the employment provisions, may be subject to the public accommodation provisions. As an example, a barber shop that employs seven barbers is required to provide public accommodations accessible to persons with disabilities. State and local government employers have no size limitation; they are subject to the ADA regardless of the total number of employees.

The ADA requires an employer to identify job positions in a manner that clearly identifies required job skills, experience, education, and any other job-related requirements. In other words, the essential functions of jobs must be clearly outlined. The ADA does not force employers to hire persons with disabilities over equally qualified persons without disabilities. However, if two applicants are equally qualified, an employer is prohibited from selecting the person without a disability if hiring the other person would require some kind of special accommodations. Unless they can prove that making the accommodation would create an "undue hardship," employers must provide reasonable accommodations for persons with disabilities. Reasonable accommodations mean (1) modifications or adjustments to the work environment or to the manner or circumstances under which positions are held or customarily performed that enable qualified individuals with disabilities to perform the essential functions of the positions (2) or modifications or adjustments that enable employees with disabilities to receive the same benefits and privileges as their coworkers who do not have a disability.

TITLE II. This title prohibits discrimination of persons with disabilities in all services, programs, and activities provided by or made available by state and local governments. Title II consists of two subtitles: Subtitle A covers state and local governments' activities other than public transit and Subtitle B covers the provision of publicly funded transit. Title II extends the nondiscrimination requirements set forth by Section 504 of the 1973 Rehabilitation Act to the activities of all state and local governments, regardless of whether they received federal financial assistance.

The ADA defines "public transportation" as transportation by bus or rail or by any other conveyance (other than air travel) that provides the general public with general or specific services (including charter service) on a regular and continuing basis. This title requires public entities to make public transportation vehicles accessible to persons with disabilities, including those using wheelchairs. It sets forth regulations with regard to the accessibility of new, used, and remanufactured vehicles.

The title established a provision whereby if the public entity can prove that providing the service creates an undue burden, it does not have to provide the requested accommodation. The entity, however, is required to provide services to the extent that doing so would not impose an undue financial burden. "Public entity" is defined as any department, agency, special-purpose district or other instrumentality of a state or local government, as well as Amtrak and certain commuter rail agencies. Regardless of the number of employees they have, public entities such as state and local governments are subject to the ADA through Title II.

TITLE III. The essence of this title, "Public Accommodations and Services Operated by Private Entities," is stated in the General Rule: No individual shall be discriminated against on the basis of disability in the full and equal enjoyment of the goods, services, facilities, privileges, advantages, and accommodations of any place of public accommodation. A "private entity" is defined by this title as an individual as well as a company, business, or other entity.

An important difference exists between Title I and Title III with regard to who is subject to the ADA. Specifically, companies with less than fifteen employees are not subject to the employment provisions; however, such a company may be subject under the public accommodation provisions. For example, an owner of a bed and breakfast establishment who employs seven people is not subject to Title I; however, the owner is subject to Title III because the business is open to the public. In other words, all public accommodations are covered by the ADA.

Religious organizations and some private clubs are exempt. Private clubs that are exempt under Title II of the Civil Rights Act of 1964 are exempt under the ADA. Public accommodation cannot restrict "service animals," even if they have a policy against allowing "pets" into their establishments. The public accommodation cannot separate the person with a disability from his or her service animal. Public accommodations cannot be refused to persons with disabilities on the grounds that the organization's insurance coverage is based on the absence of persons with disabilities. Similarly, insurance companies must justify with sound actuarial data any differential treatment of persons with disabilities. Title III of the ADA considers it an act of discrimination if the public accommodation fails to provide a person with a disability with an auxiliary aid or service that if by providing it a person with a disability will not be excluded or segregated and/or denied goods or services. The ADA provides some latitude for public accommodations in that organizations need not provide an auxiliary aid or service if it would fundamentally alter the nature of the service provided, or it would be an undue burden on the organization. "Undue burden" means significant difficulty or expense.

TITLE IV. This title, "Telecommunications Relay Services," attempts to minimize isolation of persons with disabilities. There are two major provisions of this title. Telecommunication relay services and closed captioning of all federally funded television public service announcements are included. In 1934, Congress passed the Communication Act, which directed the Federal Communication Commission (FCC) to make available, as much as possible, a rapid, efficient, nationwide and worldwide wire and radio communication service with adequate facilities at reasonable charges to all the people of the United States. Title IV amended the 1934 Act by adding a section mandating the FCC to ensure that interstate and intrastate telecommunication relay services are available, to the extent possible and in the most efficient manner, to hearing-impaired and speech-impaired individuals (Jones, 1991). The statutory requirements for relay services are the following:

1. Continuous services: All relay services must operate twenty-four hours per day, seven days a week.
2. No content restrictions: Relay operators are prohibited from failing to fulfill the obligations of common carriers by refusing calls or limiting the length of calls.
3. Confidentiality: Relay operators are prohibited from disclosing the content of any relayed conversation and from keeping records of the content of any such conversation beyond the duration of the call.
4. Unaltered messages: The ADA prohibits relay operators from intentionally altering a relay conversation. The only exception to this rule applies to hearing-impaired individuals who use American Sign Language (ASL), a language that differs in grammar and syntax from English. These individuals may want their messages interpreted into English for hearing people and may want English messages from those persons interpreted into ASL.
5. Charges billed to relay users: Users of relay services cannot be required to pay rates greater than rates paid for functionally equivalent voice communication services with respect to such factors as the duration of the call, the time of day, and the distance from point of origin to point of termination.
6. Closed caption: Title IV states that any television public service announcement produced or funded in whole or part by an agency or instrumentality of the federal government shall include closed captioning of the verbal content of the announcement.

TITLE V. "Miscellaneous Provisions" make a clear statement that nothing in this act shall be construed to reduce the scope of coverage or apply a lesser standard than the coverage required or the standards applied under Title V of the Rehabilitation Act of 1973 or the regulations issued by federal agencies pursuant to such title. Stated in other terms, the ADA's goal is to strengthen existing laws, both state and federal, as they relate to providing equal access for persons with disabilities. For example, if a state or a federal law provides more protection to a person with a disability than the ADA does, that law supersedes the ADA. Conversely, if the ADA provides better protection to the person with a disability, then the ADA supersedes the weaker law.

States can be sued under the ADA. The act states that no individual shall discriminate against any other individual because such other individual made a charge, testified, assisted, or participated in any manner in any investigation, proceeding, or hearing under this act. Title V authorizes various federal agencies, commissions, and so on, to provide technical assistance with the intent of assisting entities covered under the act to understand their responsibilities under the act. The National Council on Disability must conduct studies and produce reports on the effect of the practices of wilderness land management and the ability of persons with disabilities to use and enjoy these areas. This section of Title V identifies what is not considered a disability primarily related to sexual preference and illegal drug or substance use.

The One hundred first Congress passed the legislation and President George Bush signed into law the ADA, but the real forces behind the establishment of the act were persons with disabilities. Most writers agree that the ADA is a step in the right direction as the United States moves toward equal rights for all people. However, it is a truism that attitudes cannot be legislated. Therefore, persons with disabilities will only be able to cast away the bonds of isolation and neglect when other people accept and cherish them (Eisenberg et al., 1982).

Americans with Disabilities Act Amendments of 2008

It could be considered ironic that President George Herbert Walker Bush signed the Americans with Disabilities Act into law and his son President George W. Bush in 2008 signed into law the amendments to the act his father signed.

As has been mentioned previously the ADA is a civil rights law that protect persons with disabilities from discrimination because of their disability. The Act was designed to increase the possibilities of persons with disabilities accessing and utilizing the goods and services of America. One of the things that have made the United States a prosperous and free country is open access, for most of its citizens, to employment opportunities, recreational facilities, as well as, myriad other services. Despite the attempts to provide Americans significant opportunities, some of America's citizens have not had as free and open access and opportunities as others have. Many persons with disabilities can be included within this category. When the ADA was implemented, the vision was that the provisions within the law would help remove some of the obstacles persons with disabilities faced in seeking equality. One can imagine that neither the persons who fought for the development of the legislation nor the framers of the legislation were so euphoric that they believed that the law would solve all of the problems persons with disabilities faced and would continue to face in their attempts to become first-class citizens of America. Rather the advocates and sponsors of the 1990 ADA knew there would be challenges to some provisions of the law and that the law would eventually need some revisions. This belief of the framers of the ADA was indeed correct. The United States Supreme Court in some of its rulings with regard to some aspects of Title I (employment) began to, in the opinion of disability advocates, narrow and restrict some of the positive impacts the law could have for persons with disabilities. The following statement by the Congress of the United States in Public Law 110-325 Americans with Disabilities Amendments Act of 2008 clearly explains some of Congress' concerns: "as a result of these Supreme Court cases, lower courts have incorrectly found in individual cases that people with a range of substantially limiting impairments are not people with disabilities." "Congress finds that the current Equal Employment Opportunity Commission ADA regulations defining the term 'substantially limits' as 'significantly restricted' are inconsistent with congressional intent, by expressing too high a standard."

The amendments to the ADA became effective January 1, 2009, and are designed to restore some of the intent of the original law. It was the opinion of persons with disabilities, disability advocates, and people in the United States Congress that some Supreme Court rulings had taken away a part of the power of the 1990 Act to make inclusion of some persons with disabilities into the mainstream of American society. The amendments among other things had at least seven major points that restored some of the strength of the ADA. One major point is the fact that mitigating measures are no longer to be used to disqualify a person for reasonable accommodations. With regard to mitigating measures, some courts had ruled that if certain aids had helped the person with a disability significantly lessen his or her limitation or when using the aids the limitations associated with the disability were eliminated, then the person with the disability no longer qualified for reasonable accommodations. The ADA amendments proclaim that with the exception of regular eyeglasses and contact lens, mitigating and corrective measures are not to be considered in determining whether services are to be provided. The Americans with Disabilities Act Amendments of 2008 state the following: "the determination of whether an impairment substantially limits a major life activity shall be made without regard to the ameliorative effects of mitigating measures such as medication, medical supplies, equipment, or appliances, low-vision devices (which do not include ordinary eyeglasses or contact lenses), prosthetics including limbs and devices, hearing aids and cochlear implants or other implantable hearing devices, mobility devices, or oxygen therapy equipment and supplies; use of assistive technology; reasonable accommodations or auxiliary aids or services; or learned behavioral or adaptive neurological modifications." This is a significant change because without this change, persons with disabilities would be penalized for taking measures to improve their life situations by limiting the impact of the limitations caused by their disabilities. This is an important and significant change that will benefit many persons with disabilities. However, one can envision some future ethical issues to be raised. To be more specific, as science develops improved prosthetics and other disability aids, as well as scientific and medical advances producing medicines that can effectively control some disabilities, will they be added to the list of mitigating and corrective measures similar to regular eyeglasses and contact lens? The ethical issue is whether the use of these devices and/or medicines eliminate the disability or are simply masking the disability?

A second change relates to reasonable accommodations. The amendments attempt to clarify reasonable accommodation by pointing out that employers do not have to provide reasonable accommodations to a person who is not actually disabled but is regarded as disabled by the employer. The ADA Amendments Act of 2008 identifies a person regarded as having an impairment with the following statement: "(A) An individual meets the requirement of being regarded as having such an impairment if the individual establishes that he or she has been subjected to an action prohibited under this Act because of an actual or perceived physical or mental impairment whether or not the impairment limits or is perceived to limit a major life activity." With regard to not providing reasonable accommodations to persons who are regarded as having a disability, the Act states the following: "A covered entity under Title I, a public entity under Title II, and any person who owns, leases (or leases to), or operates a place of public accommodation under Title III, need not provide a reasonable accommodation or a reasonable modification to policies, practices, or procedures to an individual who meets the definition of disability in Section 3 (1) solely under subparagraph (C) of such section." The persons identified in Section 3 are persons who do not have a disability but are regarded as having a disability.

A third change relates to the type of life activities that are restricted and bodily functions that may be restricted and are to be considered in qualifying a person for protection of the ADA. The amendments kept the major life activities that are in the 1990 Act and added major life activities not identified in the ADA, including reading, bending, and communication. Additionally, the following major bodily functions were also included: functions of the immune system; normal cell growth; and digestive system, bowel, bladder, neurological, brain, respiratory, circulatory, endocrine, and reproductive functions.

A fourth change produced by the amendments that strengthens the act deals with the concept of substantially limited. The amendments lessen the proof needed to prove substantially limited.

A fifth impact of the amendments is the clarification of what is meant by transitory impairment and how it is to be treated with regard to the ADA. The amendment excludes transitory impairments receiving protection under the ADA. Transitory impairments are considered to last six months or less.

A sixth improvement of the act involves who cannot claim reverse discrimination. The amendments do not allow recognition of claims regarding reverse discrimination by nondisabled persons.

The seventh major change relates to the overall intent of the amendments. The amendments emphasize that the definition of a disability should be interpreted broadly.

Rehabilitation Act Amendments of 1992

The purpose of these amendments is to (1) empower persons with disabilities in the areas of employment, economic self-sufficiency, independence, and inclusion and integration into society and (2) ensure that the federal government plays a leadership role in promoting the employment of individuals with disabilities, especially individuals with severe disabilities. The amendment provides for expansion of independent living of persons with disabilities. It provides training opportunities to persons with disabilities through vocational rehabilitation. The amendment also provides for research and demonstration projects with the intention of using relevant discoveries to the benefit of persons with disabilities.

Efforts by persons with disabilities to sensitize the nondisabled public and policymakers have paid dividends as indicated by the data that Congress used to support the Rehabilitation Act Amendments of 1992:

1. Millions of Americans have one or more physical or mental disability, and the number is increasing.
2. Individuals with disabilities constitute one of the most disadvantaged groups in society.
3. Disability is a natural part of human experience and in no way diminishes the right of individuals to: (a) live independently, (b) enjoy self-determination, (c) make choices, (d) contribute to society, (e) pursue meaningful careers, and (f) enjoy full inclusion and integration in the economic, political, social, cultural, and educational mainstream of American society.
4. Increased employment of individuals with disabilities can be achieved through the provision of individualized training, independent living services, educational and support services, and meaningful opportunities for employment in integrated work settings through provision of reasonable accommodations.
5. Individuals with disabilities continually encounter various forms of discrimination in such critical areas of employment, housing, public accommodations, education, transportation, recreation, institutionalization, health services, voting, and public service.
6. The well-being of the nation includes the goal of providing individuals with disabilities with the tools necessary to (a) make informed choices and decisions and (b) achieve equality of oppor-

tunity, full inclusion and integration in society, employment, independent living, and economic and social self-sufficiency for such individuals.

Rehabilitation Act Amendments of 1993

The Rehabilitation Act Amendments of 1993 amended the Rehabilitation Act of 1973 and the Education of the Deaf Act of 1986. Some noteworthy aspects of the amendments are the provisions for separate independent state commissions to operate or oversee the vocational rehabilitation programs for the individuals who are blind or who have other disabilities. Specifically, provision was made to establish state rehabilitation advisory councils to include at least one representative from the statewide independent living council, at least one representative from a parent training and information center, at least one representative from the client assistance program, as well as representatives of disability advocacy groups to represent a cross-section of disabilities, family members/guardians, and advocates.

Rehabilitation Act Amendments of 1998

Workforce Investment Act among other provisions contained within the Rehabilitation Act, enhanced consumer choice, and the State Rehabilitation Advisory Council is renamed the State Rehabilitation Council and given expanded responsibilities. In addition, the Rehabilitation Act Amendments of 1998, which were included within this act, strengthened Section 508 of the 1973 Rehabilitation Act and the Rehabilitation Act of 1986. Section 508 requires federal agencies that purchase, develop, and/or maintain electronic and information technology to be accessible to persons with disabilities. (*See* Chapter 5 for more details.)

Ticket to Work and Work Incentives Improvement Act of 1999 established a Ticket to Work and Self-Sufficiency Program to provide SSDI and SSI beneficiaries with a ticket they can use to obtain vocational rehabilitation services, employment services, and other support services from an employment network of their choice. (*See* Chapter 5 for more details.)

SUMMARY

Structures must be devised to provide opportunities for continual feedback and evaluation in the change process. Without open channels of communication, people with disabilities and their supporters cannot know the outcome of their efforts; they are neither confronted with failure nor rewarded for success. Criteria that measure success in achieving self-determination should be part of the annual evaluation of all relevant organizations.

NOTE TO HELPERS

All groups and individuals should be treated equitably. Nothing should be done to create or perpetuate race, color, nationality, religion, sex, age, or disability stereotypes. Effective helpers show personal concern for all their helpers. They budget time to talk with and listen to them. Trust and respect are the essential characteristics of successful helpers. In summary, they teach acceptance by living it.

POINTS FOR DISCUSSION AND SUGGESTED ACTIVITIES

1. Research your state's laws that either protect rights of or ensure services to persons with disabilities.
2. Determine if there have been any protests in your state led by or for persons with disabilities.
3. Determine what kind of independent living facilities are available in your community for persons with disabilities.
4. Describe the types of disability advocacy organizations that exist in your community.
5. Survey some local employers to determine the extent of their knowledge of the Americans with Disabilities Act.
6. Survey parents of school children with disabilities to determine the extent of their knowledge of the Individuals with Disabilities Education Act.
7. Describe your local school-to-work program.

REFERENCES

Bowen, R.C. (1993). The use of occupational therapists in independent living programs. *American Journal of Occupational Therapy, 48*, 105–112.

Cull, J.G., and Hardy, R.E. (1973). *Adjustment to Work.* Springfield, IL: Charles C Thomas.

Dejong, G. (1982). Independent living. In M. Eisenberg, C. Giggins, and R. Duval (Eds.), *Disabled People as Second-Class Citizens.* New York: Springer.

DeLoach, C., Wilkins, R., and Walker, G. (1983). *Independent Living: Philosophy, Process and Services.* Baltimore: University Park Press.

Eisenberg, M., Giggins, C., and Duval, R. (Eds.). (1982). *Disabled People as Second-Class Citizens.* New York: Springer.

Frieden, L., and Cole, J. (1985). Independence: The ultimate goal of rehabilitation for spinal cord-injured persons. *American Journal of Occupational Therapies, 39*, 734–739.

Frieden, L., Richards, L., Cole, J., and Bailey, D. (1979). *ILRU Source Book.* Houston, TX: Independent Living Research Utilization Project.

Funk, R. (1987). From caste to class in the context of civil rights. In A. Gartner and T. Joe (Eds.), *Images of the Disabled.* New York: Praeger.

Futter, M.J., Rossi, M.S., Gerken, L., Nosek, M.A., and Richards, L. (1990). Relationships between independent living centers and mental rehabilitation programs. *Archives of Physical Medicine & Rehabilitation, 71*, 519–522.

Gartner, A., and Joe, T. (Eds.). (1987). *Images of the Disabled.* New York: Praeger.

Jackson, J., Rankin, A., Sheifkin, S., and Clark, R. (1986). Options: An occupational therapy transition program for adolescents with developmental disabilities. *Occupational Therapy in Health Care, 6*, 33–51.

Jones, N. L. (1991). Essential requirements of the act: A short history and overview. *The Milbank Quarterly, 69*, 20–25.

Laurie, G. (1982). Independent living programs. In M.G. Eisenberg, C. Giggins, and R.J. Duval (Eds.), *Disabled People are Second-Class Citizens.* New York: Springer.

Lofquist, L.H., and Davis, R.V. (1969). *Adjustment to Work.* New York: Appleton-Century-Crofts.

Lozano, B. (1993). Independent living: Relation among training, skills and success. *American Journal on Mental Retardation, 98*, 249–262.

Neistadt, M.D. (1987). An occupational therapy program for adults with developmental disabilities. *American Journal of Occupational Therapy, 41*, 433–438.

Neistadt, M.D., and Marques, K. (1984). An independent living skills training program. *American Journal of Occupational Therapy, 38*, 671–676.

Nochajski, S.B., and Gordon, C.Y. (1987). The use of Trivial Pursuit in teaching community living skills to adults with developmental disabilities. *American Journal of Occupational Therapy, 41*, 10–15.

Pelka, F. (1997). *The Disability Rights Movement.* Santa Barbara, CA: ABC-CLIO.

Spencer, J.C. (1990). An ethnographic study of independent living alternatives. *American Journal of Occupational Therapy, 45*, 243–251.

Stone, D.A. (1984). *The Disabled State.* Philadelphia: Temple University Press.

Townsend, E., and Ryan, B. (1991). Assessing independence in community living. *Canadian Journal of Public Health, 82,* 52–52.

SUGGESTED READINGS

Bryan, W.V. (2006). *In Search of Freedom.* Springfield, IL: Charles C Thomas.

Bryan, W.V. (2010). *Sociopolitical Aspects of Disabilities.* Springfield, IL: Charles C Thomas.

Dell Orto, A.E., and Marinelli, R.P. (Eds.). (1995). *Encyclopedia of Disability and Rehabilitation.* New York: Simon & Schuster Macmillian.

Funk, R. (Ed.). (1987). *Disability Rights: From Caste to Class in the Context of Civil Rights.* New York: Praeger.

Pardeck, J.T., and Chung, W. S. (1992). An analysis of the Americans with Disabilities Act of 1990. *Journal of Health & Social Policy, 17*:100–112.

Pelka, F. (1997). *The Disability Rights Movement.* Santa Barbara, CA: ABC-CLIO.

Reed, K.L. (1992). History of federal legislation for persons with disabilities. *The American Journal of Occupational Therapy, 46*: 397–408.

Schneid, T. (1992). *The Americans With Disabilities Act.* New York: Van Nostrand Reinhold.

Stone, D.A. (1984). *The Disabled State.* Philadelphia: Temple University Press.

Verville, R.E. (1979). Federal legislative history of independent living programs. *Archives of Physical Medicine & Rehabilitation, 60*: 447–451.

Chapter 8

FAMILY

Outline

- Introduction
- Members of the Family Drama
- Normal Feelings and Behaviors
- Self-Directed Children
- Relieving Pressures
- Marital Problems
- On Caring
- Burnout
- Summary
- Note to Helpers
- Points for Discussion and Suggested Readings

Objectives

- To identify the impact the family has on the maturation of children with disabilities
- To provide information with regard to how parents can care for themselves as they care for their child with a disability
- To provide suggestions with regard to things parents of children with disabilities can do in their quest to assist their children

INTRODUCTION

Each person with a disability must live with his or her disability and adjust to the disability. Perhaps the most difficult aspect of this process is learning to accept the responses of nondisabled people to the disability. This is especially difficult because there is no foolproof way to predict whether onlookers will display acceptance or rejection. When decoded, a large number of public responses convey rejection, pity, and overprotectiveness. Although caring persons wish that none of these things would happen, realistic persons know that they can and often do happen.

Ross (1981); Perske (1981); Featherstone (1980); and Innocenti, Huh, and Boyce (1992) pointed out that the emotions surrounding a physical disability go up and down as if on a roller coaster, moving through remorse, relief, and resolution. In reality a disability is a family condition; it is never a problem of just the person with the disability (Padrone, 1994). Of all the family member, parents are the most affected. In this chapter, the authors will use the term child and children to mean a person or persons of any age from birth to death, because a child–whatever his or her age–is a child to his or her parents.

MEMBERS OF THE FAMILY DRAMA

All members of the family are important. However, depending on the situation, some are treated as if they are more important at a given moment than others. Rehabilitation is easier when persons with disabilities and their relatives accept the disabilities without guilt or hostility. Frequently this requires relatives to leave the physical care to others while they provide emotional care. Kvaraceus and Hayes (1969) observed that when parents learn of their child's permanent disability they usually pass through three stages. It does not matter if the disability occurs at birth or during late adulthood; most parents do some fairly predictable things.

Stage 1 is the period of trying to find proof that the child is not permanently disabled. This consists of taking the child to see several physicians in order to get "the good news" that the disability is temporary and does not permanently impair the individual's functioning. This stage also includes voracious reading about the disability and seeking out other persons who have experienced disabilities. During this stage, there is a frantic search to find someone or something to make the disability go away. While searching for a positive diagnosis, finances are drained in middle-income families and depleted in low-income families.

Stage 2 is the period in which parents are determined to prove that the experts are wrong. This could be called the "pray for miracles" stage. Usually, one parent becomes obsessed with taking care of the child. Gradually, the interaction between spouses changes as the child becomes a wedge between them. It is not uncommon for one spouse to lose interest in sexual intercourse, refuse to associate with other people, neglect her or his duties within and outside the home, and spend an inordinate amount of time with the child trying to help him or her to be like a "normal" person. It is typical for the consumed parent to convince herself or himself that the child is a misunderstood genius. If there are other children in the family, they begin to feel neglected, and the other relatives begin to feel estranged from the situation. This then, is the most crucial period in family interpersonal relationships.

Stage 3, if it occurs, is characterized by both parents accepting the child's disability as being permanent but not a disaster. Often, parental separation or divorce precedes this stage. Only by accepting the disability are parents able fully to accept the child and, relatedly, themselves. It need not be, but it often is, a personally painful and financially costly journey from Stage 1 to Stage 3. Nor is it necessary to go through all three stages. Throughout the entire drama, it becomes clear that family member and the child are persons first and social role players second. Parents in particular tend to forget or not learn this basic fact. Buscaglia (1975) wrote; "only in rare instances does becoming a parent drastically change the person one is. Most generally, a thoughtful person will make a thoughtful parent. A loving person will be a loving parent. On the other hand, a confused or neurotic person will also make a confused and neurotic parent" (p. 84). There are good and bad actors playing parent roles.

The Mother Role

A woman's concept of the mother role is shaped by the culture and social class in which she lives. Initially, she is likely to respond to maternal cues in the same way her mother or mother surrogate responded to similar cues. The mother role is learned; it is not in the genes. Motherly love can be the strongest emotional tie between two human beings, or it can be the weakest. Most societies ascribe the nurturing role to the mother. Thus, it is expected that mothers will have the responsibility for taking care of their children's emotional needs. Fathers are not unable to do this, but they seldom are conditioned or expected to take on this responsibility. Fortunately, with regard to family roles, in many countries men are beginning to engage themselves in roles that previously were assigned to women.

In most societies, it is expected that two of the primary female roles in marriage are wife and mother; the corresponding male roles are husband and father. The father and mother roles are concerned mainly with providing love and discipline to their children. To do this effectively, some mothers delegate to the father, and some fathers delegate love sharing to the mother. In a balanced marriage, however, mothers and fathers share these responsibilities. There is no valid reason to attribute nurturing behavior to women in their wife and mother roles and discipline behavior to men in their husband and father roles. What is more important in terms of effective parenthood is that there is teamwork in caring for children, especially children with disabilities.

The Father Role

There has been considerably less attention given to father roles. This is the case even though there is a difference between fatherhood and being a father. Like the mother role, the father role is learned. The image of the virile male is believed by many people to be incompatible with tender feelings. To deny fathers their social or individual right to express tenderness and gentleness is to deny them emotions they naturally feel for their children. Some fathers voluntarily deny these feelings, however. In an attempt to wall out "feminine" and tender feelings, some fathers go to great lengths not to show their love. C. S. Lewis (Rosewell, 1972) cautioned these persons: "if you want to make sure of keeping your heart intact, you must give it to no one. Avoid all entanglements, lock it up safe in the coffin of selfishness. But in that coffin–safe, dark, motionless, airless–it will change. It will not be broken; it will become unbreakable, and irredeemable..." (p. 112).

Because the bonding between most mothers and their children is very strong, the father's role is likely to seem secondary, and he may feel left out. If the child with a disability is male, a father is likely to have conflicting feelings–anger and pity. Females with disabilities are less difficult to accept as dependents. After all, there is little shame in a father taking care of a daughter, whatever her age. However, sons are expected to take care of not only themselves but also their own families when they grow up.

The Other Family Members' Roles

In most cases, the concerns parents have for a child with a disability are family concerns and must be treated as such. It is counterproductive to define a child with a disability as a responsibility only of his or her parents. All members of the family, including extended family members, should be involved in the rehabilitation process. To do this, they must have an accurate understanding of the child's disability and be in touch with their own feelings about the disability and the child. The family members' role in the helping process first begins in handling their own negative feelings of shame, anger, self-pity, hurt, and frustration. Second, they need to learn helpful ways to relate to the child. Throughout this process, care must be taken to not neglect the other family members.

In the end, it is not so much what medical, rehabilitation, and educational personnel do that brings about a satisfactory adjustment to a disability but, instead, what the family does. This is not to say that the family members alone can bring about an effective adjustment. They certainly need the help of friends, professionals, and self-help groups, nor are family members ever neutral in the rehabilitation process. On the contrary, they are positive or negative catalysts for adjustment.

NORMAL FEELINGS AND BEHAVIORS

Tucked securely somewhere in the minds of most people is the belief that they should not display behavior that indicates feelings of weakness or culpability. Yet, it is the denial of these feelings that renders would-be helpers ineffective when dealing with people who have a disability. Parents are particularly sensitive to what they believe is the need of their child who had a disability to not be upset by the negative feelings of others. Katz (1961), Spock and Lerrigo (1965), Featherstone (1980), and McCallion and Toseland (1993) provide informative, sensitive views of being parents of a child with a disability. Feelings are neither logical or predictable; they just are. Some parents make the mistake of singling out other parents whom they admire and then try to emulate them. Each parent of a child with a disability usually learns how to deal helpfully with his or her feelings, not by example but by trial and error experiences. Behaviors that fit one parent may not fit another. Like the helpers described in other chapters of this book, parents must be congruent in their feelings and behaviors, which should be positive toward their children.

Each member of the family, including the person with the disability, will feel different about the disability at different times. Whatever their feelings, it is important to discuss them openly and honestly. Admit-tedly, this is easier said than done. There is a danger in open dialogues of this kind. They should not be discouraged if a family member expresses negative feelings. An open, honest dialogue is just that; It is the way people feel at the time of the discussion. Some parents scold siblings for expressing jealousy or hatred of a brother or sister with a disability. Rather than scolding, it is more helpful to try to determine why they feel the way they do about their sibling. Little is accomplished when parents try to sqelch expression of these feelings. Besides, with or without approval, they will surface.

It is difficult for most persons to state their negative feelings about a loved one, and it is exceptionally difficult to share negative feelings about a family member who has a disability. Few families openly and honestly deal with any interpersonal problem. Generally speaking, there is a conspiracy of silence when the members are together and secret character assassination when they are apart. The more productive sharing session also includes positive feelings. If a family convenes to talk about problems but seldom about feelings of happiness, pride, and positive growth, they will split into pieces that can not be put back together.

Self-Pity

Anything that diminishes the social worth of children also damages the ego of their parents, siblings, and other relatives. Pity expressed for the person with a disability often is displacement of deeply felt self-pity. For example, in their solitude, parents may ask; "Why did this terrible thing happen to us? What have we done to be punished this way? What will the neighbors think?" Parental self-pity is heightened by the realization that some of the dreams they had for the child with the disability will not be realized. The young child will not become a candidate for the prettiest baby contest, the teenage child is not likely to become a superstar in sports, and the adult may not be able to have children. (Interestingly, few nondisabled children can make most of their parents' dreams come true either.) Exaggerated self-pity can cause parents to view the child as their personal "cross to bear." They become God's self-appointed martyrs.

To a certain extent and depending upon the circumstances it is normal to engage in some self-pity and to grieve. Most parents wish the best for their children. In many ways, children who have spina bifida, cerebral palsy, loss of hearing or vision, or some other disability to some extent are different. It is important to remember that these children are not dead; most have plenty of life and potentials. However, some parents tend to refer to them as though they are dead, for example "Jonny was so full of life" or "Sue was a joy to be around." Unfortunately, persons with disabilities who hear their parents making these statements may give up on some of their dreams and ambitions. In their minds they may be thinking "if mom and dad are thinking of me in that way, perhaps I can't accomplish my dreams.

Magic Cures

The desire to cure the child that has a disability leads some parents down several false trails, and they run faster when they see children approximately the same age as their child doing things they would like their child to do. There are nagging "what if" thoughts that may even drive parents to seek miracle or magical cures from known charlatans. Dreams of success are not easily abandoned and are seldom forgotten. The quest for cure is accelerated when a child begins to lose control of muscles or limbs or body functions. Also, congenital disabilities are often easier for parents to accept than those resulting from accidents.

It is normal to be shocked and to disbelieve the diagnosis of permanent disability. There are no good ways to prepare oneself or others to accept a disability. However, some ways are less traumatic than others are. Understanding the medical aspects of a disability does not lessen the anguish, but it allows one to act from intelligence instead of ignorance. When "what if" is asked, the answer is always the same: no amount of conjecture will alter the fact of the disability. By dwelling on idle speculation, parents and others often overlook an important fact: most people with permanent disabilities cannot be cured, but they can still be productive. A permanent disability does not ipso facto mean a permanent handicap. Indeed, most people with disabilities can be, and usually are, happy and well-adjusted.

Guilt and Shame

Sometimes parents feel guilty when they wish the child with a disability had not been born or wish that he or she were dead. These are not always evil wishes, but they are always developed from feelings of helplessness. These feelings may also be developed from a feeling of wanting to protect the loved one from hurt and harm; thus they wish the person had not been born so he does not have to go through what they think will be difficulties in life. Feelings of guilt are not the same as feelings of shame. Guilt is self-centered and shame is other-centered. Parents who feel guilty are likely to ask what they have done to cause the disability. Parents who feel ashamed worry about what other people–friends, neighbors, and other relatives–will think about the child who has a disability. Excessive shame can lead people to think that they are sinful and unworthy of love, whereas excessive guilt causes them to know that they are sinful and unworthy of love.

It is normal to have feelings of guilt and even some feelings of shame. However, it is not normal to have excessive feelings of this nature. Parents of a child with a disability must accept themselves and their child if their home is to be a good environment for all members. If parents can publicly present their child to others without feelings of excessive guilt or shame, then the child can more easily take pleasure in being himself as well as take pleasure in public activities.

Overprotection

Often guilt gives way to overprotection. "This is my child and nobody is going to abuse him. He may have a disability but he's my baby," a mother said. Her baby was thirty years old, and she treated him like a ten year old. Under most conditions, it is difficult for parents not to overprotect a child. It is even more difficult when the child has a disability. Overprotection weakens parents and their children. It is an act of love to give children room to grow and learn.

It is normal for parents to want to protect their children from physical and emotional pain. How much hurt can parents spare their children? Obviously, parents cannot wish away or stop their children's pain, but they can minimize the pain. In reality, parents cannot spare children the hurt others will inflict on them, so some parents try to prepare their children for a variety of societal reactions. Thus, instead of focusing on what a child cannot do, the more helpful parents focus on what he or she can do. The goal of parenting is to prepare children for lives away from their parents. This requires a realistic assessment of each child's skills, abilities, and potential.

Resentment

Caring for any child is a chore, and caring for a child with a disability can add extra dimensions in the child-caring process. Overprotection can give way to resentment. Feeling trapped in a series of activities that seem to have no end, parents of a child with a permanent disability often become entombed in their own altruism. This feeling is heightened when friends and funds begin to wane. Sibling problems are likely to become acute when most of the family's time and financial resources are spent taking care of one of its members (Stoneman, Brody, Davis & Crapps, 1991). Well-intentioned relatives only add to the resentment when they, too, treat the child with a disability as a special person. They forget that all children (and adults) should be treated as special persons.

It is normal for parents who spend an inordinate amount of time with their children to sometimes feel resentful. It is also normal to complain and even cry when they feel overworked and locked into an activity. This feeling is often related to overprotection. The child with a disability should be fitted into the family schedule instead of vice versa. Much of the resentment parents feel could be avoided if the child were allowed to be a regular member of the family. Care must be taken not to cause the child with a disability to be physically in but socially out of the family.

It is parental love that allows a child to cope with his or her disability as a member of the family. Some parents do not realize that their children need time away from them, too. In order to stay in the family, persons with disabilities must respect themselves and other people and their spaces. Any change in one family member affects the other members, and it is within the family that the child with a disability learns whether it is okay to be himself or herself. Much of the time that family members spend with the child is not helpful because it is spent treating him or her like an invalid and not like a person of equal value. The key is to encourage people with disabilities to be independent in most activities and able to ask for help in those situations requiring assistance.

SELF-DIRECTED CHILDREN

Parents who do not produce self-directed children fail everyone—their children and the society they will serve. The older children become, the more difficult it is for them to learn to be self-directing. The question is, "How can parents produce self-directed children with disabilities?"

First, parents must believe that self-direction is important. Each parent must be willing to put it to practice in the home and must not simply give lip service to the concept. Self-direction should be a living concept; it must be given as much practice as subject matter recitals in school. All children learn by doing, and they learn best by assisting in planning and carrying out their own activities.

Second, parents must trust their children to learn. As noted, too many parents try to protect their children from failure and, consequently, do not give them difficult chores. Responsibility and self-direction are learned. If children with disabilities are going to learn self-direction, then it must be through being given opportunities to succeed and fail in family-related activities. Along this line of thought, if a child believes in his or her own inadequacy or lack of power when confronted with new situations, failure is certain. As a child falls further and further behind his or her peers in skill development, there is a diminishing of his or her self-concept (Mayberry, 1990). Parents cannot do a task for a child and develop his or her task mastery. A sense of success comes only from an individual's own task mastery.

Third, parents of a child with a disability need to maintain an experimental attitude. When their child is given the opportunity to try new (or old) behaviors, parents should not be alarmed or disappointed when he or she makes mistakes. Letting children make mistakes is not easy, for most formal education is built on correct answers. Wrong answers are regarded as failures and are to be avoided. Parents conditioned to think this way are fostering an attitude that stands squarely in the way of encouraging children's self-direction and independence. People fearful of making mistakes will not risk trying. Without trying, self-direction, creativity, and independence cannot be discovered. One of the nice things about self-direction is that it does not have to be taught. It needs only to be encouraged.

Fourth, children with disabilities must learn the meaning of responsibility. The implications of decision-making experiences must be understood by them. Parenting should be thought of not as providing children with the correct answers but rather as providing them with opportunities to learn many ways of solving problems—not imaginary, make-believe problems but real ones in which decisions count.

RELIEVING PRESSURES

Wherever one goes in the world, one hears talk about external pressures that affect adults who do not have disabilities. At the same time that these people complain about the pressures that bother them, they do not seem to be fully aware of the pressures on people with disabilities. Individuals with disabilities are pressured to behave in a socialized way: to be popular, belong to a group, achieve in school, hold their own in a competitive world, take advantage of all opportunities, and be happy in a world that even people without disabilities do not believe is safe and secure. In short, people with disabilities frequently are expected to be better citizens than people without disabilities are.

Children—with or without disabilities—cannot escape from all pressures, and it is not desirable that they do. A certain amount of pressure acts as a driving force, kindling the desire to finish a job or task, to go on to the next step. However, there are differences between constructive and destructive pressure. Constructive pressure is closely tied to two other parts of learning: motivation and the reward or satisfaction obtained through achievement. When conditions are not favorable for success and achievement, increased pressure is likely to result only in attitudes of distress and defeat. If parents are to aid their children in learning to live successfully with external pressures, they must know when to exert pressure.

Pressure applied for its own sake or a perverted reason to make them tough will almost always fail, and parents who nag children to do better—without understanding why they are not making progress—will produce even greater underachievers. Pressure is positive only when it is combined with cues that arouse curiosity and interest and cause a person to exert pressure from within himself or herself to succeed. Parental pressure is of little value when the inner drive is missing in a child. Furthermore, success related to inner pressure is much more effective and infinitely more rewarding. Here, again, parents must be sure that pressure is applied toward a goal that is possible for a child to achieve. Negative pressure is often used carelessly by parents. A look of disappointment, sarcastic and undermining remarks, and comparing low-achieving children with siblings and peers are examples of negative pressures applied to shame a child into doing better. Such pressure tends to destroy children's faith in themselves as well as in their parents.

Obviously, if parents want their children to be optimally creative, external pressure is not the answer. Creativity develops from internal pressure. It comes from the reservoir of ideas that flow out of the mind and demand recognition. Parents can create an atmosphere or a safe place in which this can happen, but they cannot create the ideas. Children who feel comfortable at home—who find it safe to ask questions, express ideas, and try new behavior—respond to pressure within themselves through self-expression. They become well-balanced persons.

MARITAL PROBLEMS

When there is conflict centered on children, it is not helpful for parents to pretend that no conflict exists. Only by acknowledging that they have problems are they able to resolve them. Setting aside time to discuss points of distress is a good beginning, but it is only a beginning. Problem resolution must follow. Most parents forget that they were husbands and wives or lovers before they were parents. They will need to build on all of these previous foundations to keep their marriage together. If the marriage is to survive, the neglected person must be brought back into the relationship.

Problem solving or adjusting to conflicts centered on a child with a disability can be one of the most trying aspects of a marriage. Running away from the issue by leaving home is not helpful. Another counterproductive approach is anger. However, productive anger is not the same as outbursts of hostility used exploitatively to get a spouse or a child to yield because of fear. Aristotle observed, "Anyone can become angry–that is easy; but to be angry with the right person, and to the right degree, and at the right time, and for the right purpose and in the right way–that is not within everybody's power and is not easy."

When conflicts arise and anger is one of the resulting emotions, the partner who is not angry should realize that the anger is an indication of how strongly the other person feels about the situation. In this respect, feelings are emotional barometers that should be carefully read in order to predict the human relations climate. Often, there is a calm period before an outburst of anger. Silent suffering is seldom productive, particularly when the issue is a child who has a disability. If grievances are held in, tension will build up and eventually explode outward against the other partner or the child, or it will explode inward against the angry person and cause considerable psychological damage.

An important role for both partners in a marriage is listener. If one partner is troubled, the other needs to understand, and this requires listening. However, the listener should heed the words of the prophet Kahlil Gibran (1961): "The reality of the other person is not in what he reveals to you, but in what he cannot reveal to you. Therefore, if you would understand him, listen not to what he says but rather to what he does not say" (p. 14). A major aspect of listening is being able to understand nonverbal messages: frowns, sighs, closed body positions.

Mothers in particular should make an attempt to include fathers in the care of children. Fathers can feel abandoned, too. Most fathers want very much to be parents in nurturing and caring for their children. Love that grows in a family is best maintained by attachment and release. Attachment is in the form of closeness, companionship, and caring for each other; release is in the form of trusting, respecting, and allowing the other person enough private space. In the center of this matrix are the children. If parents cannot let go of their children, the family becomes an unhealthy place. These families should have the following sign, like the warning on cigarettes, posted on their doors: "Beware, this family is dangerous to the health of its members."

Not all marriages that have a child with a disability turn sour, but many become emotionally colder. The disability is but another factor added to already strained interpersonal relations. As most marriages progress, disengagement tends to be the rule rather than the exception. Couples begin to pay less attention to each other; they frequently become bored with each other. The child with a disability is seldom the reason for the drifting apart, but he or she is often cited as the reason. Effective ways of coping can seldom be taught. At best, general guides can be offered, but each person must learn the coping styles that work in his or her situation. Drawing on the experiences of others gives parents a much-needed awareness that they are not the only ones with a particular problem but that, if they are not careful, they may be the only ones unable to resolve the problem. Help for children with disabilities must necessarily come from a network of persons: the children themselves, their parents, relatives, and friends, and professional and paraprofessional helpers.

ON CARING

Parents who care about their children view them as being part of themselves and also separate entities. They do not try to dominate or posses their children. Rather, they recognize their own and their children's need to grow. In order to do this, parents must feel good about themselves and their children. Self-honesty will allow parents to evaluate accurately their behavior and that of their children. No one would try to teach a turtle to fly or an elephant to bake a cake, but there are many things that turtles and elephants can do. Children are like turtles and elephants. Why try to teach children who have severe visual problems to pole vault or children who are have hearing impairments to judge a musical contest? There are many other things they can do. Caring parents have a true appreciation of their own potential abilities as well as their children.

Caring is not a spectator sport; it requires active participation by all the parties involved (Moxley, Raider & Cohen 1989). Parents who care learn from their mistakes and try not to repeat them. By modeling this behavior, they teach their children to learn from their mistakes, and in the process of learning, they develop humility. Parents learn from children, children learn from parents, and parents and children learn from themselves about themselves. They are not humiliated by having others see their weaknesses, nor are they vain when others see their strengths, for what they show is neither good nor bad. It is merely a condition that can be accepted or rejected. That is, they are never ashamed of themselves—of their negative behavior, perhaps—but never of themselves. Also, parents who care do not ask, "Aren't you ashamed of yourself?"

Parents who care about their children have a sense of humor. They are able to laugh at themselves and with their children. Christenson and Miller (1980) show how this is done. Humor is the lubricant that gets most parents over difficult spots, but they do not use humor to put down their children or to keep them dependent.

Parents who care about their child with a disability have a large amount of empathy and little sympathy. They do not hold out false hope to themselves or their child. Quick-fix solutions are not their style, and pity is buried in the past. The parents are realists. They talk with professionals who can help them to understand their child's diagnosis, treatment, and prognosis. They leave little to their fantasies and fears as they seek a clear prognosis and a clear understanding of the rehabilitation regimen. This is supplemented by current information about disabilities that are found in professional journals, textbooks, novels, autobiographies, and other library data. Caring parents tend to be well-read.

Parents who care do not treat their children like the other-directed people Reisman (1950) wrote about. Other-directed people are unable to distinguish thoughts from feelings and are unable to express feelings even when recognizing them. Indeed, overprotected and overindulged children are unable to distinguish between what they want and what they ought to want. They become, generally speaking, helpless, passive, and indecisive and have low self-esteem. Sadly, they defer to "normal" people when decisions about them are being made. It takes a lot of negative conditioning to produce other-directed people.

Parents who care meet their own physical and emotional needs. Individuals who give almost everything to others and little to themselves burn out as parents. Thus, they contribute to their own demise and that of their family. A truly caring relationship is mutually beneficial and, therefore, mutually growth producing and freeing. It is this freeing process that cements the bond that binds family members to one another. The binding is not in titles or ranks or physical condition but in human beings caught up in each others' lives and yet free to let go if that will enrich them.

BURNOUT

The longer parents are together, the less they tend to do together. Slowly a light seems to go out in their eyes, and they have difficulty seeing each other. The deadening effect of routine role conformity by parents of a child with a disability and the draining effects of trying to hide their feelings of frustration, loneliness, anger, and inadequacy should not be minimized. The inability of many individuals to find a way to relieve the incipient stress of parenting leads to burnout, the syndrome of emotional exhaustion and cynicism that occurs after long hours of physical and psychological strain.

In some cases, to burn out means that a parent will become an alcoholic, a drug addict, or mentally ill or even commit suicide. Freudenberger (1980) poetically and cogently summarized this decline: "Under the strain of living in our complex world, people's inner resources are consumed as if by fire, leaving a great emptiness inside, although the outer shells may be more or less unchanged" (p. xv). Contrary to many of their wishes or fantasies, parents are but mortal beings. Yet, there are numerous examples of parents who believe that they must be in control of themselves and their children at all times. Their children, they concede, can be out of control, but not them.

Some parents even believe that assisting their children to self-actualize is enough reward to keep themselves going. These martyrs get a kind of vicarious gratification from the successes of their children. Obviously this places a tremendous strain on their children to be socially successful. The self-denial of parents who push their own needs into the background is the volatile fuel that, when ignited, burns up their energies and dreams. There is a tendency for most parents to minimize the importance of self-love. Only if they have strong positive feelings for themselves are parents able to have these feelings for their children. However, parents who gratify their own appetite and emotions in self-destructive ways lack the qualities necessary to show their children restraint. It is a delicate balance that must be kept between self-love and self-indulgence.

It is erroneous to assume that burnout will disappear if it is ignored. This is a tragic belief because burnout does not get better by being ignored. The person burning out may be irritable, angry, resistant to change, or listless. Fatigue is a frequent symptom that many parents of a child with a disability experience because of the erosion of their ability to cope with their child's condition. Social symptoms include (1) high resistance to going home, (2) a feeling of failure, (3) guilt and blame, (4) avoiding contact with friends, (5) reverting to strict rules and regulations, and (6) looking forward to the child with a disability going to sleep or away from home. Physical reactions to psychological stress centering on children with disabilities include (1) migraine headaches, (2) backaches, (3) colds, (4) diarrhea, (5) excessive salivation or dryness of the mouth, (6) heartburn, (7) ulcers, (8) asthma, and (9) rhinitis. Sometimes parents can indeed acquire disabilities while trying to take care of their children. Moreover, burnout affects not just the isolated individual but the whole family.

Parents who burn out imagine themselves as somehow being responsible for the decisions and behaviors of their children. Thus, anguish, abandonment, and despair are natural responses to this unrealistic responsibility.

Most parents who accept this type of responsibility cannot help but feel a profound sense of guilt, even anxiety, when they choose destinies for their children. "Who can then prove that I am the proper person to impose, by my own choice, my conception of man upon mankind?" Sartre asked, "if a voice speaks to me, it is still I myself who must decide whether the voice is or is not that of an angel" (Kaufman, p. 293). Burnout is sometimes the result of parents discovering that they hear neither angels nor devils, only human voices telling them what to do.

There are several ways parents can avoid burnout. Most parents do not do enough for themselves. Prolonged stress centering on a child with a disability can affect the parents' personal lives away from home. It can make them unhappy with their loved ones and unable to be happy during "free" times and leave them generally listless and angry. Parents must learn to pay attention to physical symptoms, to put parenting goals in proper perspective, and to understand the nature of burnout. Only then can they control parenting activities rather than allowing the activities to control them. When parenting becomes a job, those who work at it must learn to vary the activities, avoid involvement in the activities for a time, and share the activities with other.

There are two reliable cures for burnout: closeness and being inner directed. Closeness is anywhere and with anyone a person chooses. Before a person can achieve closeness with another, however, he or she has to achieve closeness with self. Parents who burn out seldom spend enough time with themselves in a constructive manner; thus they do not adequately take care of their personal needs. Inner directedness is not being selfish; rather, it is taking time out for oneself. The purpose, of course, is to do things that are good for one's renewal.

Parents should watch for tiredness and pay attention to physical symptoms such as colds or nagging pains in the back. Also, they should monitor themselves for shifts in attitude, especially toward self-doubt or self-pity. There are many other things parents can do to prevent burnout. Parents should (1) learn to ask for help, (2) be aware of their strengths and weaknesses, (3) take time out to do things they want to do, (4) learn to say no, (5) not feel guilty because they have not lived up to their ideal of a perfect parent, (6) exercise, and (7) set realistic goals for themselves. To help their children, parents must be good to themselves.

SUMMARY

The home is the key institution in personality formation. Children with disabilities have close ties with their parents in particular and other family members in general. Even in homes in which parents love and respect their children, there will be conflicts. Reacting to pressures in their own lives, some parents become demanding or overindulgent or overprotective. At the other end of the continuum, some parents abuse and neglect their children. Most parents manage to do a good job caring for themselves and their children. They would do a better job if they learn basic coping skills.

NOTE TO HELPERS

Parents and other family members vary in their ability to cope with disabilities. Professional helpers can assist them by providing them with needed information and, when appropriate, assurance that their feelings and emotions are part of the rehabilitation process. Kaplan and Mearig (1977) suggested that informal problem solving is the most effective way professionals can help. This is not inconsistent with the goals of counseling, which include helping clients to become independent as soon as possible. Helpers should not expect instant coping or independence, however.

It is important that helpers not try to rescue the family and make decisions for them, nor should they compete with parents and other family members for the affection of the child with a disability. Admittedly, it is difficult to care for the family instead of just the child, but this is exactly what the helper must do. The most effective treatment plans change to reflect changing family relationships. Failure to integrate rehabilitation goals and family members is likely to result in additional family stress and conflicts.

Most families have feelings of grief, hostility, guilt, and shame. They should not be made to feel guilty about their real and imagined inadequacies. It is unrealistic to expect them to handle their emotions and problems without help. Above all else, they need help understanding their feelings, the disability, and the treatment plan. Versluys (1980) offered a practical approach to helping the family adjust to the disability. The following are some of her suggestions.

- Be available and therapeutic with the family.
- Identify and appreciate the feelings of family members.
- Encourage and unconditionally accept ventilation of "hidden" feelings.
- Help family members see that their feelings are normal and acceptable.
- Keep the focus on real issues or crises.
- Provide praise for small accomplishments.
- Provide programs and services that are responsive to family and client needs.
- Discuss meaningful alternatives to rehabilitation problems.
- Provide information concerning procedures, simple facts about the disability, and purpose of treatment methods.
- Listen without offering false hope.

The helper must be able to project to the family an image of genuine concern, empathy, and technical skill. Even this may not be sufficient to dissolve family members' fears and anxieties, but it is a good place to begin. Most frequently, family members take their cues from professional helpers. They need time to understand the disability and to learn how to cope with the situation.

POINTS FOR DISCUSSION AND SUGGESTED ACTIVITIES

1. Interview at least three parents of children with a disability to determine the following: (a) What are the most rewarding things encountered while rearing the child? (b) What are the most difficult things encountered while rearing the child? (c) How independent is the child? (d) What are their recommendations to parents of children with disabilities?
2. Interview at least three parents of children with a disability to determine their reactions to discovering that their child has a disability.
3. Interview a sibling of a person with a disability to determine his or her feelings about having a brother or sister with a disability. Also ask how the sibling has reacted to his or her disability.
4. Interview at least three persons with a disability to determine how they perceive their parents and siblings reactions to the disability.

REFERENCES

Buscaglia, L.C. (1975). *The Disabled and Their Parents: A Counseling Challenge.* Thorofare, NJ: Charles B. Slack.

Christenson, K., and Miller, K. (1980). *Tributes to Courage.* Golden Valley, MN: Courage Center.

Featherstone, H. (1980). A *Difference in the Family: Life with a Disabled Child.* New York: Basic Books.

Freudenberger, H.J. (1980). *Burn-out: The High Cost of Achievement.* New York: Doubleday.

Gibran, K. (1961). *Sand and Foam.* New York: Alfred A. Knopf.

Innocenti, M.S., Huh, K., and Boyce, G.C. (1992). Families of children with disabilities: Normative data and other considerations on parenting stress. *Early Childhood Education, 12,* 403–427.

Kaplan, D., & Mearig, J.S. (1977). A community support system for a family coping with chronic illness. *Rehabilitation Literature, 38,* 79–82, 96.

Katz, A.H. (1961). *Parents of the Handicapped: Self-Organized Parents' and Relatives' Group Treatment of Ill and Handicapped Children.* Springfield, IL: Charles C Thomas.

Kaufman, W.A. (Ed.). (1965). *Existentialism from Dosteovsky to Satre.* New York: Meridian Books.

Kvaraceus, W.C., and Hayes, E.N. (Eds.). (1969). *If Your Child is Handicapped.* Boston: Porter Sargent.

Mayberry, W. (1990). Self-esteem in children: Considerations for measurement and intervention. *Journal of Occupational Therapy, 44,* 729–734.

McCallion, P., and Toseland, R.W. (1993). Empowering families of adolescents and adults with development disabilities. *Families in Society, 74,* 579–587.

Moxley, D.P., Raider, M.C., and Cohen, S.N. (1989). Specifying and facilitating family involvement in services to persons with developmental disabilities. *Child & Adolescent Social Work Journal, 6,* 301–312.

Padrone, R.J. (1994). Psychotherapeutic issues with family members of persons with disabilities. *American Journal of Psychotherapy, 48,* 195–207.

Perske, R. (1981). *Hope for the Families.* Nashville, TN: Abingdon.

Reisman, D. (1950). *The Lonely Crowd: A Study of the Changing American Character.* New Haven, CT: Yale University Press.

Rosewell, N. *Successful Living Day by Day.* New York: Macmillan.

Ross, B.M. (1981). *Our Special Child: A Guide to Successful Parenting of Handicapped Children.* New York: Walker.

Spock, B., and Lerrigo, M.O. (1965). *Caring for Your Disabled Child.* New York: Macmillan.

Stoneman, Z., Brody, G.H., Davis, C.H., and Crapps, J.M. (1991). Ascribed role relations between children with mental retardation and their younger sibling. *American Journal of Mental Retardation, 95,* 537–550.

Versluys, H.P. (1980). Physical rehabilitation and family dynamics. *Rehabilitation Literature, 41,* 58–65.

SUGGESTED READINGS

Bryan, W.V. (2006). In Search of freedom (2nd. ed.). Springfield, IL: Charles C Thomas.

Bryan, W.V. (2009). T*he Professional Helper: The Fundamentals of Being a Professional Helper.* Springfield IL: Charles C Thomas.

Bryan, W.V. (2010). *Sociopolitical Aspects of Disabilities.* Springfield, IL: Charles C Thomas.

Dyson, L.L. (1993). Response to the presence of a child with disabilities: parental stress and family functioning over time. *American Journal on Mental Retardation 98*: 207–218.

Singhi, P.D. et al. (1990). Psychosocial problems in families of disabled children. *British Journal of Medical Psychology, 63*: 173–182.

Tunali, B., & Power, T.G. (1993). Creating satisfaction: A psychological perspective on stress and coping in families of handicapped children. *Journal of Child Psychology & Psychiatry & Allied Disciplines, 34*: 945–957.

Part 3

PSYCHOSOCIAL INTERVENTION

Chapters 9 through 12 to a major extent continue with the theme of Part 2 with the emphasis on how helping professionals can assist in empowering persons with disabilities. As stated in some of the chapters in Part 2, no one is capable of meeting all of her or his needs; therefore, dedicated trained helpers can be important assets to persons with disabilities. Chapters 9 through 12 emphasize how professional helpers can effectively support persons with disabilities.

Chapter 9

HUMAN SERVICES PERSONNEL

Outline

- Introduction
- Purpose of the Interview
- A Delicate Balance
- People Who Care
- Establishing Rapport
- Beyond Telling
- Conference Etiquette
- Optimally Effective Helpers
- Self-Actualization
- Summary
- Note to Helpers
- Points for Discussion and Suggested Activities

Objectives

- To identify things that human service personnel can do to be effective helpers of persons with disabilities
- To provide suggestions for effective approaches to assist persons with disabilities

INTRODUCTION

All people with disabilities are in simultaneous states of *being* and *becoming* something. Whatever they are, they are not stagnant. Even dying is an active process. Those who are socioeconomic failures would like to become successes, and those who are successful try to be even more successful. A major aspect of the upward quest for adjustment centers on social acceptance by peers. A typical change in status involves shedding the stigma attached to a disability. The most obvious status changes are economic ones, whether upward or downward. It is short-sighted to ignore upwardly and downwardly mobile people and focus attention only on individuals and families that are well-established in the middle and upper classes.

It is true that there is less social risk working with economically well-established people with disabilities, but it is also true that they are not the largest group. There are more marginal-income than stable-income Americans with disabilities. Moreover, contrary to popular opinion, it is not too late to alter the employment and living conditions of lower-class adults with disabilities. Concerned human services personnel can and do make a difference. This chapter will use adult clients as the treatment group, build on points made in the earlier chapters, and add a few new tips.

PURPOSE OF THE INTERVIEW

Interviews with clients with disabilities serve many purposes, but the major ones are to obtain and give information, to provide clients an opportunity to ventilate their feelings and relieve tension, and to assist clients in understanding and resolving their problems. In order for helpers to be optimally effective, they must have respect for people with disabilities as human beings, not as disabled people. This includes taking into account the clients' needs, problems, fears, and cultural backgrounds. It is important to give clients credit at the outset for having the capacity to select their own solutions or answers. Thus, the job of the helper is not to solve clients' problems but instead to strengthen their ability to do so.

The success of any interview depends primarily on the helper's ability to establish and maintain a healthy interpersonal relationship with the client. The attainment of such a relationship is to a great extent based on intangibles such as warmth, sensitivity, and interest. Speech alone is seldom adequate to convey these traits. To all but the visually impaired client, the helper's physical appearance, movement, facial expressions, and demeanor all convey acceptance or rejection. Touch is also an important aspect of the helping relationship.

The major task of human services personnel is to help clients adjust to their problems (Ippoliti, Peppey & Depoy, 1994). This means guiding them to information pertaining to their disabilities and attitudes about themselves and other people. Effectively listening as the client speaks is one of the most valuable tools available to a helper. What at first glance appears to be a natural process is in fact a deceptively difficult art that must be learned. It seems easy, but effective listening requires helpers to put aside their own personal needs to talk, explore things, and solve personal problems in order to assist someone else. Most conversations are barely listened to. For most people, hearing is natural, but listening is not. Attending to the verbal and nonverbal communications of clients with disabilities is an art and a skill that most helpers learn on the job, if they learn it at all. The sensitive helper knows that clients with physical disabilities need more than physical rehabilitation. A successful interview can provide the client with a rare opportunity to be heard in a noncritical setting.

A DELICATE BALANCE

Physical disability is a social, mental, and physiological condition. Much of the job of the helper is to assist or accompany clients as they deal with discrimination, rejection, and low social status. Sometimes these problems are overt, but most often they are covert. Specific goals of helping include

1. Reaffirming to clients the fact that they are people first and people with disabilities second
2. Assisting clients to understand the physiological facts and social issues involved in their disabling conditions
3. Encouraging clients to deal with their feelings centering on having a disability
4. Aiding clients to accept their disabilities emotionally and intellectually without devaluing themselves

Clients with disabilities are people, not things to be manipulated. Sometimes they are fragile people–frightened, confused, and defensive–but they are seldom "sick" people. Helpers should not be impatient or insensitive to their hurts, fears, and hostility. In previous chapters we have talked about empathy, congruence, and unconditional positive regard. These concepts apply here, too. Like teachers, other helpers should be guides, not gods. The more effective helpers acknowledge their own humanity, but too often professional helpers forget that people with disabilities are, as Menninger (1942) pointed out, people: "The world is made up of people, but the people of the world forget this. It is hard to believe that, like ourselves, other people are born of women, reared by parents, teased by brothers, . . . consoled by wives, . . . flattered by grandchildren, and buried by parsons and priests with the blessings of the church and the tears of those left behind" (p. 114).

The words inscribed on a plaque hanging in the office of a professional helper are also instructive: "I feel so much better, less helpless and guilty since I found out I was not chosen to be God." All humans fail from time to time. This is not the worst that can happen to helpers or their clients, if they admit their failures and, where appropriate, refer clients they cannot help to someone they think can. Throughout the helping process the identity of the helper and that of the client with a disability must not be destroyed.

> To incorporate another person is to swallow him up, to overwhelm him; and thus to treat him ultimately as less than a whole person. To identify with another person is to lose oneself, to submerge one's own identity in that of the other, to be overwhelmed, and hence to treat oneself ultimately as less than a whole person. To pass judgment . . . is to place oneself in an attitude of superiority; to agree offhandedly is to place oneself in an attitude of inferiority. . . . The personality can cease to exist in two ways—either by destroying the other, or being absorbed by the other—and maturity in interpersonal relationships demands that neither oneself nor the other shall disappear, but that each shall contribute to the affirmation and realization of the other's personality. (Storr, 1961, pp. 41–43)

It is crucial that those involved in the helping relationship avoid labeling, stereotyping, and rationalizing away the unique person who defies reduction and simplification (Huitt & Elston, 1991; Carney & Cobia, 1994). Behavioral sciences theories certainly have their place and have provided invaluable heuristic tools for helpers to use. Even so, helpers must be willing to discard these theoretical devices when they do not fit the situation or when they cease to provide understanding of individuals or groups of persons with disabilities. Harding (1965) is correct: "We cannot change anyone else; we can change only ourselves, and then usually only when the elements that are in need of reform have become conscious through their reflection in someone else" (p. 75).

Helpers must be in touch with and have grasp of what is going on within their own selves before they can help their clients to make choices. Whether they are involved in a helping relationship as professionals, paraprofessionals, or friends and confidantes, it is inevitable that at some point in the relationship the problem of making choices will arise. Helping relationships in which choosing is being continually delayed or postponed by the helper and avoided or procrastinated by the client should be seriously questioned. All too often the helper is meeting his or her own needs by being too protective and not allowing the client to experience the pain and discomfort that generally accompany choosing between alternatives.

Kiekegaard (1962), the father of contemporary existentialist philosophy, described the task of the helping person in this manner: "The highest one human being can do for another is to make the other free, to help him to stand on his own feet—alone. . . .

When a person has overcome all, precisely then is he perhaps closest to losing everything . . . no longer can he fight against something or someone else . . . now he must stand alone" (p. 22).

In summary, there is a delicate balance between helping and doing. Clients with disabilities must be allowed to do all that they can for themselves with the assistance of the helper. The work of the professional includes helping them to fill a need, receive a service, and otherwise solve or resolve a problem. The core material of the helping relationship is interaction of the basic attitudes and emotions of the helper and client. All clients need to be treated as individuals, to be allowed to express their feelings, to receive empathic responses, to be allowed to make choices and decisions, and to have their secrets kept.

In order to help their clients, human services personnel must be willing to learn from them, to discover not only their weaknesses but also their strengths. First, helpers must learn what a client knows and would like to know and what he or she can do, cannot do, and would like to do. Second, helpers must be astute observers of role behaviors. This means analyzing the actions and reactions among people; sorting out their attitudes, values, and beliefs; and understanding the emotions underlying human behavior. Roles are never static, not even the role of "cripple."

PEOPLE WHO CARE

The various styles of helping that professionals and paraprofessionals use when interacting with clients have been described in many ways, including *authoritarian, democratic,* and *laissez-faire.* Authoritarian helpers unilaterally set goals for their clients. Furthermore, they collect all the information and make all the arrangements without permitting their clients to assist in planning. Authoritarian helpers produce a great deal of work-oriented behavior but a low degree of personal involvement. Furthermore, clients who have authoritarian helpers tend to be easily discouraged.

Democratic helpers attempt to identify their clients' goals and needs and allow them to assist actively in the initial planning as well as subsequent action. As would be expected, client morale is high with democratic helpers. Laissez-faire helpers assume no active participation and allow clients to do whatever they want; most or all of the initiative is left to the clients. As might be expected, the laissez-faire helper is the least effective of the three.

Effective helpers assist clients to succeed in achieving their goals while minimizing their failures. The *authority role* of the helper need not be synonymous with *domination.* Some clients are not cooperative merely because they do not like authority in any form. Needless to say, helpers determined to "show these people who's boss" are likely to discover obstinate and recalcitrant individuals who would rather fail than be treated in this manner. For this reason, a helper's behavior should say to the client, "I am here to understand you so that I can help you." This type of authority extends beyond finding fault and prescribing cures. Clients with disabilities need to feel that their helpers understand and accept them as unique individuals with value beyond a promotion or a day's work. In the end, the respect clients have for a helper will be determined by how successful the helper is in assisting them to adjust to their unique situations.

Individuals who do not feel accepted and wanted will find it extremely difficult to relate to helpers in a positive manner. They may withdraw, not pay attention in conferences, complain easily, not provide needed information, miss appointments, and, finally, terminate the relationship. When this happens, clients appear to have no interest in completing the helping process. In reality, they have little or no interest in completing the process *with their current helpers.* Their uncooperative behavior is a not too subtle way of breaking off a relationship so that they can try to find more suitable helpers. Thus, it should be evident that rejection works two ways. Not only do human services personnel reject people with disabilities, but people with disabilities reject insensitive would-be helpers, too.

Successful helpers are able to give of themselves and unconditionally receive their clients. The act of unconditional acceptance communicates to individuals with disabilities: "I acknowledge your physical differences. I am here to help meet your needs, but I will not cause you to lose your self-esteem." Acceptance does not, however, mean feeling *like* individuals with disabilities or anyone else, but it does mean feeling *with* them. No individual can feel like another because no two persons live in the same cognitive world. However, by trying, human services personnel can understand the environmental forces having an impact on the lives of persons with disabilities. The best way to get a feeling for clients' living conditions is to visit their homes, walk around their neighborhoods, visit their friends, talk with neighborhood merchants, and read current books and journals focusing on disabilities.

An optimum helper–helpee relationship involves two people freely responding to each other. This does not mean that the relationship will always be pleasant or comfortable. Rather, it is a relationship in which both parties feel free to say, "I agree" or "I disagree." There are two important ways this open, honest interaction can be beneficial to persons with disabilities who live as second-class citizens in their respective communities. First, helpers can assist them to differentiate between opportunities available in their neighborhoods and those available in the larger community. Second, helpers can assist individuals with disabilities to acquire needed skills and resources. This, then, is an action-oriented approach to helping. To be successful, it requires open, honest communication.

Channels of communication are open only when helpers uncritically accept each client's efforts to communicate. This means learning to "hear" nonverbal communication such as sighs, frowns, and smiles. Obviously, this kind of understanding comes from being familiar with each client's background and disability. Although the negative effects of a person's physical or environmental restrictions cannot be completely erased, they can be ameliorated by offering hope in the place of despair and confidence instead of insecurity. It is important to remember that most people with disabilities are very sensitive to what helpers do not say as well as what they do say. The key is not to give up on persons before trying to understand and help them.

Nonverbal communication should never be considered an acceptable substitute for words unless the client has a hearing impairment. Nonverbal communication is commonly called *body language.* Technically, it is the science of *kinesics.* This science includes the study of reflexive and nonreflexive movements of a part or all of the body used by a person to communicate a message. There are several kinds of body language that helpers use, including the following.

GESTURES AND CLUSTERS OF GESTURES. There are approximately 1 million distinct gestures that have meaning to people around the world. They are produced by facial expressions; postures; and movements of the arms, hands, legs, and so forth. Gestures are essential face-to-face communication.

MANNER OF SPEAKING. The tone of a helper's voice and the placing of oral emphasis are closely related to gestures. Specifically, the manner of speaking includes the quality, volume, pitch, and duration of speech. Indeed, how a message is delivered greatly influences clients.

ZONES OF TERRITORY. Hall (1959) coined the term *proxemics* to describe human zones of spatial territory and how they are used. Zones of movement increase as intimacy decreases. That is, the more space available without other persons present, the more movement is likely to occur. In informal gatherings, a distance of six to eighteen inches is considered too close for the average white American male without a disability, whereas this distance does not cause discomfort for the average person with a disability or for white females without disabilities.

EYE CONTACT. Most Americans are taught not to stare at other people. Instead, they learn to acknowledge another person's presence through deliberate and polite inattention. That is, they look long enough to make it clear that they see the other person and then look away. Most professional helpers are taught to stare at clients—even if it embarrasses them.

TOUCHING. The sense of touch conveys acceptance or rejection, warmth or coldness, positive or negative feelings. This is the singlemost difficult aspect of nonverbal communication for helpers dealing with clients who have disabilities. Most helpers devise ingenious ways to occupy their hands so as to avoid touching persons with physical disabilities.

LISTENING. Effective helping does not occur unless effective listening also occurs. Agency interviews are designed to get and give information. It is during the interview that listening skills become crucial to diagnosis.

Caring about clients is based on the premise that the primary emphasis within the helping process should be on cooperation rather than on control. Helpers who become preoccupied with filling out forms, improving their pep talks, and maintaining rigid time schedules are not likely to be flexible enough to help people with disabilities. Successful helpers are able to provide both *structure* and *freedom* during the helping process. In short, they are able to stay loose and still provide adequate guidance. It is one thing to know what someone needs to do; it is something else to devise a way to help him or her to do it.

The helper who understands people is better able to win their confidence and perceive alternatives for meeting their needs. This kind of helper does not join the local Quitter's Club, whose members look forward to and devise unhelpful methods for terminating relationships with persons who have severe physical limitations. The major goal of quitters is to get these clients into the first activity or situation available, even if it is not what they want or need. Caring primarily about their own discomfort, these helpers are basically negative about interacting with people with disabilities, whom they believe to be ugly and of low status. Individuals who are obsessed with sorting out physical abilities, colors, races, and social classes are not likely to treat all people fairly. They cannot assure rejected clients that they care about them, because they do not. Helpers who really care about people are not uncomfortable around individuals because of their physical conditions, color, or ethnic identity.

Because most people enter the helping relationship wanting to be accepted, to be accepted by human services personnel is a sign of their social worth, and to be accepted by a helper they like and respect causes them to feel very special. Clients who feel the need to move away from helpers are frightened, and those who believe they must move against them are angry. Both types of behavior are easily triggered by human services personnel who do not care. There are obvious risks in caring about clients, however. The temporary nature of most helper–helpee relationships is stressful for both parties. This is compounded by the fact that some persons have physical and psychological limitations that no helper can alter. To care under these conditions is to become frustrated by an inability to succeed.

Some minority-group helpers are afraid to care about persons with disabilities because they believe they will lose their newly achieved middle-class status. For example, some African American helpers with disabilities are unwilling to work with lower-class blacks with disabilities. These reluctant helpers do not want to be identified with poor people, especially poor black people with disabilities. Their self-hatred becomes intensified when community norms force them to live in neighborhoods with lower-class black people. Minority-group helpers who reject their own ethnic identity are not likely to be cultural bridges between themselves and other people.

ESTABLISHING RAPPORT

Anger about their perceived low status causes some persons with disabilities to view every professional worker who does not have a disability with deep suspicion, for example, the hearing impaired are constantly on their guard around professionals who are not hearing impaired. In addition, the rise in consciousness of minority-group people involved in the disability rights movement initially heightens their feelings of distrust of the nonmembers. Extreme cases of distrust result in the erroneous belief that only helpers with the same disability as the clients' are qualified to work with them, in other words, helpers with visual impairments with clients who have visual impairments, hearing-impaired helpers with hearing-impaired people, and so forth. Such an elitist, exclusionary view is not one that the authors of this book support.

The challenge to the human services worker is to demonstrate that competence and empathy are not traits unique to persons with a particular disability. For example, a competent helper can be, when judged by his or her deeds, a kindred soul to all clients. A disability is more than a clinical condition. It is thinking, behaving, and accepting the disability. When this happens, people with disabilities admit that some helpers without disabilities have "soul." Relatedly, competent helpers with disabilities have been able to prove to clients who do not have disabilities that they have soul too. Physical disability is neither a guarantee of, nor an automatic deterrent to, establishing rapport with clients. Attitudes and human relations skills are more important factors.

The first step in establishing rapport with clients is to help them relax. In order to do this, the helper must be relaxed. When helpers do not know how to communicate with clients, neither party will relax. Instead, helpers will hide behind their desks and academic degrees, and clients will hide behind their disabilities. Both helpers and clients who behave this way believe the media stereotypes of persons with disabilities being inferior or strange people. Thus, the discomfort of helpers can produce feelings of discomfort in their clients. During these stressful periods, conversation related to educational or technical subjects may panic the clients. Yet, it is precisely these subjects that the helper is likely to feel most comfortable discussing. A few minutes of informal talk can often reduce the stress. A warm, informal, down-to-earth approach to each person is a prerequisite to establishing rapport (Marini, 1992). The message to helpers is: "Don't fake it. Be yourself–that is, be your warm, caring self, if you have one."

Some clients approach professional helpers in ways that are outright defensive. Those using defensive mechanisms usually do not have faulty personalities. Instead, it is their environment that is faulty. Protection of the ego is normal, but a disproportionate use of defenses indicates a lack of security. Clients with disabilities who imagine that they are objects of rejection or ridicule develop rigid, persistent, and chronic ego-protection devices. Continued feelings of rejection result in behavior inappropriate to reality. This behavior was demonstrated by a client who imagined that his rehabilitation counselor disliked him. To protect himself, he withdrew from all voluntary contact with her. One day the counselor asked him, "Why do you avoid me?" The client answered, "Because you don't like me. You smile at the nondisabled people and joke with them, but you never do these things with me."

Issues that center on disabilities cause many helpers to overreact. Often it is difficult to sift out fact from fiction, objectivity from subjectivity, but it must be done. The development of excessive ego defenses by the client is disturbing to helpers who are unaware of having done anything to elicit such behavior. A smile or an approving nod are small but often effective ways to communicate acceptance and break down the defensive barriers. Asking individuals what is bothering them provides them with an opportunity to get some things out in the open. The key is to try to establish rapport. Sometimes clients need love and acceptance most when they are most unloving and unaccepting of others.

The willingness of clients to continue interacting with professionals and paraprofessionals who want to help them is affected in part by the attractiveness of the arrangement (What is in it for them?) and in part by the belief that only through a cooperative effort can they achieve certain goals. In short, there must be some real or imagined payoff when they cooperate with helpers. The old "do as I tell you because I am the expert" approach works only if clients are intimidated by the helper's status. Open, honest expressions of feelings obviate the necessity for hidden anger. Indeed, freedom of expression should be not only allowed but also encouraged.

An *open dialogue* is not synonymous with *automatic approval*, however. Helpers should make it clear that encouraging candid expressions of feelings does not mean that they necessarily agree with the feelings verbalized. Such conversations or dialogues will probably be a new experience for many persons with physical disabilities. People without disabilities seldom ask people with disabilities what they think; they usually tell them what they should be thinking. Thus, when asked to participate in uncritical discussions, many clients with disabilities will be unprepared and even hesitant. However, once they start talking, the danger is not that they will be silent again but that they may not stop talking. Good helpers are good listeners. They learn to listen with all their senses, not merely their ears.

The first concerns expressed by clients may not be the ones they really want to discuss. That is, they may want to talk about sex or school or a job rather than physical disabilities per se. In the end, whatever pressing problems a person brings to a helper are the ones he or she will discuss, one way or the other. It is not enough to encourage an open discussion; helpers must also accept the client's views. The attention of a reticent client has been compared to a wild animal that must be lured, caught, and held. Along with honest dialogue, the helper must show interest and involvement. Nods and blank stares from the helper are not always interpreted by clients as understanding. It is important for the helper to communicate what he or she understands and what the client needs to do.

People with disabilities cannot respond with conforming behavior if they do not know what is expected of them. Helpers should not be like the near-hysterical beginning teacher who rushed into the principal's office and cried, "This is the last straw. I quit. Those kids are sleeping and running all over the room. I can't control them." The principal thought for a minute, then asked, "Have you told them to sit up, sit down, and be quiet?" As if struck by a bolt of insight, the teacher ran out of the office and back to the classroom. She had been so eager to begin the lesson that she had forgotten to call the class to order. Similar to students in a class, some clients are apathetic, low in energy output, and passive in behavior. Others are impulsive, hyperactive, and diffuse in behavior. It is this wide range of behaviors that makes it impossible to characterize people with disabilities and illustrates why helpers should refrain from stereotyping them.

BEYOND TELLING

Many individuals grieve when a permanent disability is diagnosed. Helpers should be aware of their stages of grief, which are similar to those of terminally ill patients:

1. **Denial and isolation**—refusal to accept the permanence of their disabilities and desire to be alone
2. **Anger** at professionals and friends for giving up on them
3. **Bargaining**—trying to strike a deal with God or some other supernatural force by stating that they will do something good in exchange for restoration of the body function or limbs
4. **Depression**—a sense of loss and realization that they are permanently disabled and, finally, for most persons,
5. **Acceptance** of their disabilities.

It is important to know what stage the client is in.

During the early stages of grieving, a client's attitudes and behavior may change from day to day. Yesterday they wanted to talk about their disability; today they deny that they have a disability. It is therapeutic for helpers to elicit emotional expression rather than emotional repression. A free exchange of thoughts is the beginning of the rehabilitation process. It is of utmost importance to know what the client is feeling. Physicians usually can relieve the physiological symptoms of a disability, but other helpers are needed to relieve the psychological pain from the loss of body image and self-esteem. Family members and friends can help in this process. Effective helping occurs within the context of environment, culture, social roles, and power.

ENVIRONMENT. It is only necessary to look around in order to see how the physical environment affects the quality of the helper–helpee interaction, considering the differences between inner-city slums and affluent suburbs, mountains and seashores, chemically polluted and nonpolluted communities. Environments are equivalent to nonverbal statements about health care. They cause clients and their helpers to feel fearful or relaxed, cheerful or sad, open or closed.

CULTURE. Culture preference is a major problem in most helper–helpee interactions. Members of different cultures live in different worlds. Inability to understand and communicate with culturally different persons renders would-be helpers therapeutically impotent. It is culture more than disability that stands between helpers and clients.

SOCIAL ROLES. Shakespeare said it well in *As You Like It*: "All the world's a stage, and all the men and women merely players. They have their exits and their entrances, and one man in his time plays many parts...." Some helpers forget that "professional" is a role and not themselves. Conversely, "handicapped" is a role and not the essence of the individual so labeled. Inflexible role players are unable to change when solutions require role adaptation.

POWER. It is clear that most helpers have a degree of power over clients. As noted earlier, helpers who are authoritarian and dominating tend to be less helpful than their colleagues who are democratic and encourage client initiative. Part of the helpers' dilemma is that they must be sufficiently detached from clients to exercise sound judgment and at the same time have enough concern to provide sensitive, empathic care. It is possible for professional helpers to suppress emotional responses on a conscious level while counseling and assisting clients, but this detachment does not remove the stress and concern hidden in the unconscious domain of their minds. The pathological process of detachment that tends to produce mature helpers also tends to produce cynical clinicians.

Helping clients with disabilities to tell what they feel requires more than a receptive listener, and it is more than collecting predetermined data. Helpers who believe that the predetermined interview schedule is the only effective method of eliciting pertinent data should learn from the experiences of social workers. Perlman (1957) wrote,

> It has long been said in casework, reiterated against the sometime practice of subjecting the client to a barrage of ready-made questions, that the client "should be allowed to tell his story in his own way." Particularly at the beginning this is true, because the client may feel an urgency to do just that, to pour out what *he* sees and thinks and feels because it is his problem and because he has lived with it and mulled it within himself for days or perhaps months. Moreover, it is "his own way" that gives both caseworker and client not just the objective facts of the problem, but the grasp of its significance. To the client who is ready and able to "give out" with what troubles him, the caseworker's nods and murmurs of understanding–any of those nonverbal ways by which we indicate response–may be all the client needs in his first experience of telling and being heard out.

Not all clients can easily talk about their disabilities. Comments such as "I imagine that this is not easy for you to talk about" and "Go on, I'm listening" may be enough encouragement for some reticent persons. Others will need direct questions to help them focus their conversation. Accurate information is not the result of passive listening; it is the by-product of interpretive talking and active listening. Effective listening is demanding; most people have to work hard at listening to hear what others are trying to say.

Few people know exactly how they feel about their disabilities until they have communicated sufficient data to another person. To tell someone what and how they feel is in itself a relief for many clients, but telling is not enough. Problem resolution must follow if the helping relationship is to be complete. This is likely to occur when the client's questions pertaining to his or her problem are amply discussed. The words of Tournier (1957) sum up the process of helping persons with disabilities to communicate: "Through information I can understand a case, only through communication shall I be able to understand a person" (p. 25).

The dynamics of problem solving are threefold. First, the facts that surround the disability must be understood. Facts frequently consist of objective reality and subjective reactions to it. Second, the facts must be thought through. They must be probed into, reorganized, and turned over in order for the client to grasp as much of the total configuration as possible. Third, a plan must be devised that will result in some type of adjustment.

Fact finding is more complex than many authors suggest. Seldom are professional helpers taught to elicit information–how to talk, to listen, and to provide feedback. However, this does not mean that there are only a few professionals who can communicate effectively with people with disabilities. There are many who do so, but most of them are self-taught. Something as important as communication should not be left to intuition or chance. It should be a part of all college curricula and in-service training programs.

Numerous studies have concluded that a large number of persons with disabilities receive insufficient information about their conditions and coping skills. For example, many persons terminate agency relationships without ever having understood what their helpers decided were their needs, why certain procedures were followed, what, if anything, their failures consisted of, and what the reasons for them were. The rights of clients include the right to courteous, prompt, and the best treatment. They also include the right to know what is wrong, why, and what can be done about it. A case could be built that this ignorance is a by-product of the helping mystique. That is, professional and lay helpers typically are perceived as being men and women whose training and predilections place them in a special service category. To put it even more bluntly, there is a tendency for clients to be in awe of individuals who help them. This intangible dimension of the helping process is one reason, but attention must be given to other reasons communication breaks down.

There are many reasons for an individual's failure to communicate pertinent information. Some persons with disabilities make no effort to communicate information about their situation. In other instances, helpers fail to request needed information, particularly that which would give them basic understanding of the individual with a disability. Since human communication is a two-way process, both helpers and clients distort messages. Some individuals forget information that had been clearly communicated to them.

Furthermore, research demonstrating that people who understand their illness adjust more quickly than those who do not is sparse. From this narrow perspective one could conclude that clients' understanding of their disabilities is unimportant. However, if a goal of helping is educating or informing people, then it is important for clients to understand what is happening to them. In the end, the quality of the information helpers are able to give is directly proportional to the quality of information they solicit. Additional tips for facilitating the communication process are as follows:

1. Respect the family. In most instances, the family is very much involved in decisions made by a member who has a disability. The final decision may be made by the client, but only after considering the feelings of other family members.
2. Call people by their right names. In Spanish, for example, each person has two last names. The first last name is the father's family name, and the second last name is the mother's family name. Use both last names so as not to insult the client. Also, use the correct pronunciation of names.
3. Try to understand local customs.
4. Analyze your feelings about various physical disabilities.

5. Avoid patronizing or condescending approaches.
6. When giving information, do not merely ask if clients understand what you have said. Ask them to tell you what they think you have said.

In the end, the most successful helpers are linguistically compatible with their clients, empathic, and well-trained. This means that the initial edge held by a helper with the same disability or from the same ethnic group as the client will be lost if he or she cannot go beyond physical identity and ethnicity. A helper does not have to have a disability in order to assist people with disabilities effectively.

CONFERENCE ETIQUETTE

Human services workers should not jump to false conclusions when some clients arrive late to their appointments. It is possible that because of their disabilities they have seldom been asked to be on time by their parents or friends. Thus, the term *C.P. (crippled people) time* connotes being chronically late. Interestingly, there are many people without disabilities who are chronically late to meetings, too. This does not mean that they cannot be punctual if asked to be. When clients do arrive on time, human services workers should not show surprise by commending them for being punctual, and certainly they should not be like the teacher who began a school program by announcing, "This is truly an historic occasion. You parents have proven that Indians can be on time."

Agency personnel also should not be surprised if individuals with physical disabilities do not exhibit psychopathic or sociopathic personalities. Most people with disabilities are quite normal. Many of them have adapted to the realities of their limited physical abilities and restricted social and employment opportunities.

The first impressions a client forms of a helper are frequently lasting impressions. During the first meeting, the professional helper should welcome clients, shake their hands, call them by their names, and introduce himself or herself. Whether or not to shake hands with females (if they have hands) is not so much an issue as is the type of handshake. A limp, spongy handshake is hardly the way to communicate acceptance to males or females. Helpers must treat all clients with respect and speak to them with words they can understand. Talking over someone's head or in a patronizing manner, for example "Honey, you'll like this" or "Sweetie, the depreciation of this property can be enough to capitalize a bond investment," is not an effective way to build rapport. The more effective helpers keep the conversation simple and to the point, and they get technical only when necessary or the client asks technical questions.

Each conference should begin with a topic that is pleasant. However, caution should be taken not to delay too long before beginning to discuss the matter at hand. In any case, the helper should begin the discussion by focusing on the client's assets. In addition to being reassuring, this approach is likely to evoke minimum stress and less defensiveness. In order to be successful, helpers should clearly delineate information that is needed and steps to be followed in trying to achieve rehabilitation goals. Communication based on concrete problems or issues generally is productive; conversation that is abstract and vague tends to be anxiety producing. Once rapport is established, the client may volunteer personal and embarrassing data. This information must be kept in the utmost confidence.

When helpers visit clients' homes, they should arrange for the visit well in advance. Most people tend to resent individuals "popping in" just to be friendly. Unannounced visits may disrupt the household routine as well as embarrass or anger people. Although not an absolute necessity, it is best if helpers who go to homes in which English is the second language are able to speak the client's first language, for example, Spanish. Also, before making home visits, helpers should learn the social codes of the community. This will prevent gossip and needless errors in judgment. In some communities, it is taboo for males to visit a married couple's home if the husband is absent. In other communities, it is considered bad manners to refuse to drink or eat food that is offered, no matter how unattractive the refreshments may look. The helper who refuses to sit down or play with young children is frowned upon in most communities. Visiting clients requires adhering to their norms. Emerson was correct in saying that "good manners are made up of petty sacrifices."

There are many valid reasons helpers may visit clients' homes, including (1) to inquire about their health, (2) to obtain additional information needed to complete the analysis, (3) to see what their current needs are, and (4) to tell them about new opportunities for economic or physical improvement. It is essential that family members and helpers know the purpose of the visit. In all instances, helpers should behave as guests. This does not mean being solicitous, but it does mean being polite.

OPTIMALLY EFFECTIVE HELPERS

Optimally effective helpers are able to manage their negative feelings. This is not to say that they are completely objective and treat all clients as equals but that they minimize unfair treatment and maximize fair treatment. Getting to know persons with disabilities may not alter negative attitudes toward them, but it will enable one to respond better to them. Although it would be ideal, a helper need not like persons with disabilities in order to be of assistance to them. Understanding and empathy can occur without condoning or liking.

There are no truly homogeneous groups of persons with disabilities. Within each ethnic group there are rich and poor, cooperative and uncooperative, dependent and independent. Poverty or affluence per se are not absolute determinants of cultural disadvantages or advantages. It is true that poverty-stricken people with disabilities are usually denied adequate socioeconomic opportunities. It is also true that some affluent people do not take advantage of available opportunities. Differences in physical abilities, race, color, or national origin do not in themselves result in a particular condition. For example, African Americans are not as a group subjected to the same kinds of socialization as middle-class, "White, Anglo-Saxon Protestants" (WASPs), but neither are other groups. Puerto Ricans, Mexican Americans, American Indian, Asian Americans, and poor whites who do not speak "correct" English are also disadvantaged when competing with WASPs. However, cultural *difference* should not be equated with cultural *deprivation*. These groups are not deprived of culture.

The quality of human relations within the helper–helpee relationship can be measured by many variables, including how well helpers get along with each other and their clients. One of the first prerequisites for a smoothly functioning helping situation is that persons with disabilities feel welcome and accepted. Without a doubt, the helper is the key person in establishing this atmosphere. People with disabilities should be given the same courteous treatment as all other people. Usually, it is their bodies that are impaired, not their minds or sense of equity. Helpers can find almost anything they want in their clients: Mr. Smith, the loudmouth, is merely the other side of Mr. Smith, the insecure person. When looking at a client, some helpers see only dirty or clean clothes, neat or unkempt hair, straight or twisted bodies. They do not see people. Even worse, they do not accept clients for what they are: people in need of the best help available. Rejection of this kind causes clients to feel like inferior beings who somehow must emerge as "normal" people. Only a body transplant can bring about this feat!

Clients with disabilities in a therapeutically helpful agency environment see themselves as important. What magic will allow helpers to cause this to happen? None! It does not require magic, only common sense, human relations skills, and patience. These are the hallmarks of optimally effective helpers. They are able to accept people with disabilities as they are. They are not shocked by what they see or what their clients say. Relatedly, they are able to reject the inappropriate *behavior* but not the *persons*. Dual standards are not used, and all clients know what is expected of them. Because they know that identical behavior can come from diverse causes, optimally effective helpers avoid making snap judgments. In short, their ethics are situational.

There are many ways clients may respond in crises situations. Some withdraw, shutting out the world around them; for them the only reality is their imagination, the world within themselves. They may think about the "good old days" when they were younger and there seemed to be fewer problems associated with their disabilities. Others ignore the crisis, refusing to acknowledge that they have problems. Some clients even believe that the only problems people with disabilities have are in the minds of other persons who are trying to stir up trouble (the radicals). The majority of clients with disabilities seek constructive solutions to their problems. They are not immobilized by self-pity, despair, euphoria, or anger.

The human relations problems confronting professional helpers and paraprofessionals are varied and awesome. A quick summary of the seemingly insurmountable and rapidly worsening problems that persons with disabilities face can all but immobilize the best-meaning helpers. Yet, even though they have been shocked awake by the world's imperfections, effective helpers know that standing wide-eyed in horror is an inadequate stance to assume. If human services personnel and their clients are to find solutions, they must forsake the posture of untrained, traumatized innocents. The options are clear: They can either hire out as mourners or try to become actively involved in abating and preventing social problems associated with physical disabilities. Professional and lay helpers must become the realists about whom Boyd (1971) wrote:

> Shallow activism must . . . be changed into a considerably deeper and more sophisticated sense of involvement. This calls for listening to people outside one's own ingrown and myopic clique as well as sober examination of self-righteousness in one's motives and actions. . . . A realist throws away rose-colored glasses, straightens his shoulder and looks freely about him in all directions. He wants to see whatever there is to see, in relation to other people and things as well as to himself. A realist alone comprehends hope. Optimism is as antithetical to authentic hope as pessimism. Hope is rooted in realism. (p. 128)

Commitment to social change means not disorder but a new order. Human services personnel do not remain detached, objective, and neutral—far from it—for they are first of all human beings, with their own sets of values, attitudes, beliefs, fears, and dreams, not supermen and superwomen. They are individuals who are superperceptive and untiring in their efforts to eradicate discriminatory behaviors. They do not do this because it will get them a letter of commendation or a promotion. They do it because it is morally, socially, and legally right. They could no more cease trying to bridge cultural gaps than cease being themselves.

There is a bit of the skeptic in the more effective helpers. They do not believe that time will take care of things or that most people would not be prejudiced against people with disabilities if they lived with them. Time, they know, is a neutral concept and takes care of nothing. People take care of things. They also know that human services workers do not have to be college trained in order to understand and help people with disabilities. They merely need to care about them and seek out relevant information and experiences. There seems to be some intangible feature that separates effective helpers from ineffective ones. Words such as *understanding, acceptance,* and *caring* do not adequately describe the inner stuff of this characteristic. One thing seems certain: Optimally effective helpers are not gods and goddesses; they are human beings who somehow manage to climb above the inhumanity surrounding them and help their neighbors with disabilities to do the same.

SELF-ACTUALIZATION

The only way to help ourselves is by helping others, for as Buber (1957) surmised: "He who calls forth the helping word in himself experiences the world. He who offers support strengthens the support to himself. He who effects salvation to him salvation is disclosed" (p. 110). From this perspective, there is a godlike quality in helping other people, especially people with disabilities. Buber defined God as one who gives meaning to personal life, the being who makes persons capable of meeting, associating with, and helping one another. It is clear that, whether or not they acknowledge it, some agency personnel behave like malevolent gods when determining who shall not be helped. By assisting clients who have disabilities to get an adequate education, housing, jobs, and self-esteem, helpers help themselves and other persons to self-actualize.

Maslow (1970) described what he called a *hierarchy of needs* peculiar to human beings. The most basic needs are the physiological ones that sustain the body, such as food and sleep. When they are satisfied, the human organism begins to concentrate on fulfilling a need for safety, which usually is accomplished best in an environment that is structured in an orderly and secure fashion. Not until the basic physiological and safety needs are satisfied do people turn their attention to fulfilling their needs for affection, love, and belonging. For helpers to self-actualize, they must do what only they as unique persons can do to help other people. What are the characteristics of these rare people? How can they be recognized? What kind of behavior do they manifest? Maslow gave an almost poetic description of them:

> Self-actualizing people are, without one single exception, involved in a cause outside their skin, in something which fate has called them to somehow and which they work at and which they love, so that the work joy dichotomy in them disappears. One devoted his life to the laws, another to justice, another to beauty or truth. All, in one way or another, devote their lives to what I have called the "being values" ("B" for short), the ultimate values which are intrinsic, which cannot be reduced to anything more ultimate. There are about fourteen

of these B-values, including truth and beauty, and goodness of the ancients and perfection, simplicity, comprehensiveness, and several more. (p. 43)

SUMMARY

In order to help clients achieve their goals, optimally effective helpers are first able to take care of themselves. The people being helped can comprehend the "wholeness" or "togetherness" in these persons. Each success for a client is a personal success for the helper. In the words of Carkhuff (1969): "In a real sense then, the helping process is a process of personal emergence and/or reemergence. It is a process in which each barrier looms higher than the last, but one in which the rewarding experiences of surmounting previous hurdles increases the probability of future successes. If the helper is not committed to his own physical, emotional, and intellectual development, he cannot enable another to find fulfillment in any or all of these realms of functioning" (p. 31). The authors of this book do not agree with Carkhuff's last assertion. Human services personnel can effectively help clients without taking care of their own needs. However, the price is quite high: Burnout usually occurs. Although no one wishes burnout for everyone, there is something ennobling about burning out while trying to help other people.

NOTE TO HELPERS

Problem solving consists of three operations: fact-finding, analysis of facts, and implementation of action steps. To achieve greater effectiveness, persons with disabilities must be fully involved in efforts to solve their problems. It is possible for professionals to define the problems and prescribe the solutions, but this weakens their clients' self-responsibility. After all, clients own the problems; their helpers do not. The following principles are crucial to problem solving:

1. **A problem can be solved only if the necessary resources are available.** A helper may want to understand people with disabilities but be unable to do so because he or she does not have adequate resources–reading materials, for example. Most helpers are unable to learn about people with disabilities because of missing or inadequate resources. In any puzzle, if pieces are missing, one cannot see the whole picture.

2. **Many clients do not know how they feel about their disability until they communicate their feelings to someone**. They may be vaguely aware of internal discomforts but totally unaware of their implications. Providing clients an opportunity to tell how they feel is usually the first step to isolating negative feelings. Some clients will communicate internal discomforts in a childlike manner by striking, laughing at, or ignoring others. Allowing clients to "tell it like it is" is not the end of the process, however. The helping relationship should have purpose beyond relating unpleasant feelings. If solutions are not sought, talking will serve only to frustrate clients further.

A distinction should be made between thinking *about* a problem and thinking *through* a problem. In the first instance, little more than free association of ideas takes place. In the second instance, more purposeful things occur. A problem is acknowledged, its implications are examined, and solutions are contemplated. Thinking through a problem is physically as well as mentally stimulating. The heart beats faster, and perspiration may break out. The whole person gets caught up in thinking through a problem. Helpers must not push clients to hurry this process. The helper who chides a client, "If you really wanted to, you would make the necessary adjustments" is insensitive to the complexities of problem identification and altering established behavior.

3. **Clients who want to change may not know how or may feel threatened by the thought of changing.** Some persons with disabilities become obsessed with the fear that they will be publicly embarrassed or lose what little security they have if they behave differently. They know how to behave as cripples but are unsure what will happen to them if they stop playing the role of helpless, dependent persons. Some families structure their lives around taking care of members with disabilities. There is no denying the vulnerability inherent in trying new behavior. When persons with disabilities expose themselves this way, they may indeed lose something.

4. **It is imperative that helpers focus on problems they can help clients think through.** Helpers should do the job they are paid to do: focus on the problems their job description implies or delineates. It is helpful to focus on immediate crisis situations or the single most important issue at the moment but not to become a participant in a client's flight. Experienced helpers know when and where to refer clients when they are unable to deal with them.

POINTS FOR DISCUSSION AND SUGGESTED ACTIVITIES

1. Contact at least three rehabilitation professionals and discuss some of the techniques they use to assist persons with disabilities.

2. In your discussion with the rehabilitation professionals, ask them to describe some of the limitation they have experienced in attempting to assist persons with disabilities.

REFERENCES

Boyd, M. (1971). *Human Like Me, Jesus.* New York: Simon & Schuster.

Buber, M. (1957). *Pointing the Way.* New York: Harper & Row.

Carkhuff, R.R. (1969). *Helping and Human Relations.* Vol. 1. New York: Holt, Rinehart, & Winston.

Carney, J., and Cobia, D.C. (1994). Relationships of characteristics of counselors-intraining to their attitudes toward persons with disabilities. *Rehabilitation Counseling Bulletin, 38,* 72–76.

Hall, E.T. (1959). *The Silent Language.* New York: Doubleday.

Harding, M.E. (1965). *The "I" and the "Not I."* Princeton, NJ: Princeton University Press.

Huitt, K., & Elston, R.R. (1991). Attitudes toward persons with disabilities expressed by professional counselors. *Journal of Applied Rehabilitation Counseling, 22,* 42–43.

Ippolitti, C., Peppey, B., & Depoy, E. (1994). Promoting self determination for persons with developmental disabilities. *Disability & Society, 9,* 453–460.

Kiekegaard, S. (1962). *The works of love.* New York: Harper & Row.

Marini, I. (1992). The use of humor in counseling as a social skill for clients who are disabled. *Journal of Applied Rehabilitation Counseling, 23,* 30–36.

Maslow, A.H. (1962). *Motivation and Personality.* New York: Harper & Row.

Maslow, A.H. (1970). *The Further Reaches of Human Nature.* New York: Viking Press.

Menninger, K. (1942). *Love Against Hate.* New York: Harcourt, Brace & Word.

Perlman, H.H. (1957). *Social casework: A Problem-Solving Process.* Chicago: University of Chicago Press.

Tournier, P. (1957). *The Meaning of Persons.* New York: Harper & Row.

SUGGESTED READINGS

Bryan, W.V. (2006). *In Search of Freedom.* Springfield, IL: Charles C Thomas.

Bryan, W.V. (2007). *Multicultural Aspects of Disabilities.* Springfield, IL: Charles C Thomas.

Bryan, W.V. (2009). *The Professional Helper.* Springfield, IL: Charles C Thomas.

Bryan, W.V. (2010). *Sociopolitical Aspects of Disabilities.* Springfield, IL: Charles C Thomas.

Doty, P., Kasper, J., and Litvak, S. (1996). Consumer-directed models of personal care: Lessons from Medicaid. *The Milbank Quarterly, 74:* 377–409.

Hahn, H. (1984). Reconceptualizing disabilities, a political science perspective. *Rehabilitation Literature, 48:* 362–365.

Seelman, K. (1993). Assistive technology policy: A road to independence for individuals with disabilities. *Journal of Social Issues, 49:* 115–136.

Chapter 10

COPING STYLES

Outline

- Introduction
- The Quest for Acceptance
- Stress
- Maladjustment
- Summary
- Note to Helpers
- Points for Discussion and Suggested Activities

Objectives

- To identify some of the psychosocial ways individuals cope with life situations
- To identify how these coping mechanisms impact the rehabilitation process

INTRODUCTION

People with disabilities have as many social selves as there are distinct groups of people whose opinion they value. It is extremely painful for them to be rejected by individuals about whom they care. This is a normal reaction. Continued rejection may cause an individual to stop seeking recognition or to change reference groups. Cynical persons are created out of a series of rejections and put-downs. This condition suggests a centrality in which persons with disabilities who receive recognition conform to the peer norms or standards of persons without disabilities. These conformists also are likely to be individuals with disabilities who have high status within their communities. They are not treated the same as the masses of people with disabilities. Thus, differentiation of social status usually results in differentiation of conformity to group norms. Most people with physical disabilities are able to fit into majority group social and economic settings. Unfortunately, too few are allowed to do so; instead, they tend to be relegated to low social status and low-paying jobs.

Rather than focusing on individual needs, most people treat individuals with disabilities as an aggregate. As a whole, parents of children with disabilities are not much different. Instead of encouraging their children to assume responsibility for their own learning and personal growth, many parents cause them to be docile and dependent. Educators contribute to this process, too. Instead of helping these students to optimize their intellectual abilities, most teachers tend to focus on low-level cognitive activities. Employers also do their share of stunting individual skill development. Instead of being equal opportunity employers, most supervisors assign people with disabilities to dead-end, low-paying jobs. The final result is people with disabilities who fit the negative stereotypes discussed in earlier chapters.

THE QUEST FOR ACCEPTANCE

Within aggregates of persons with disabilities, however, are individuals who have various needs (Fowler & Wadsworth, 1991). Some of them have a *dependency need*, which is characterized by dependence on persons in positions of authority for succor. Others have a status need as exemplified by seeking recognition from nondisabled persons. The *dominance* need manifests itself in expressions of intellectual superiority. Still others clearly exhibit a combination of these needs. In order to succeed in the larger community, they usually learn to be overtly cooperative, covertly competitive, and publicly inconspicuous. In most instances, success means being accepted as peers by people who do not have disabilities.

Acceptance by significant others builds a positive self-concept; rejection builds a negative one. Succinctly, *self-concept* refers to the composite of attitudes, beliefs, and values that persons hold pertaining to themselves and the interrelating environmental forces. The self-concept determines an individual's reaction to other people and is shaped by their reaction to him or her. People who feel abused, neglected, or rejected tend to abuse, neglect, or reject other people, including their parents and relatives. Power seems to be a strong antecedent or predictor of the direction of self-concept changes. Individuals high in group or organizational power tend to have positive self-concepts; those who feel powerless have low self-concepts.

Individuals with disabilities who have a high need for achievement generally set goals of moderate difficulty so that they will succeed. For example, instead of setting a goal of getting a job commensurate with his or her college education, a person who has epilepsy sets his or her sights on getting a job as a clerk. The major emphasis is placed on the highest level of failure. This method of competing with their age-mates for employment is common among persons with disabilities. The fear of failure looms large in their minds. Internal dialogue that reflects the self-conception of a person with a disability includes these questions: "What type of person am I?" "How do I compare with the other persons?" "What do my friends think of me?" Answers to these questions affect the continuity of his or her mental functioning. Positive or negative responses tell the person: "This is what I am." "This is how I compare with others." "This is what my friends think of me."

Personality theorist Richard Lazarus (1961) noted that adjustment to life situations is always taking place because social, psychological, and biological needs are constantly changing. In addition, the environment is constantly changing, and this requires additional adaptive behavior. Change and the subsequent need to adjust to those changes are an integral and natural part of living. Coulter and Marrow (1978) refer to the manner in which people respond to change as coping. Whitman (1980) states that coping styles are pathological only if an individual uses excessive psychic energy to cope and distorts reality in the process.

Some of the responses of individuals with disabilities are appropriate; others are not. Furthermore, a response that is appropriate at one time may be totally inappropriate at another time, even under similar circumstances. If every day were the same as the preceding day, very few adjustments would be required. Survival within one's environment would not be a major concern because once a successful adaptation had been made, survival would be ensured. However, even though one may wish it, life is not that simple. Each day brings new anxieties and renewed stress situations for all people.

STRESS

Stress and anxiety are feelings all humans experience. Stress refers to any assault or demand placed on a person or a system. Stress is often thought of negatively; however, stress per se is not harmful. Rather, it is the *reaction* to stress that determines whether it is harmful. Consequently, reactions can produce either good or bad results. Simply stated, stress produces change in emotional state, and each person learns to tolerate, reduce, or eliminate the resultant uncomfortable feelings. If the person fails to respond adequately to stressful situations, his or her behavior may be considered psychologically unsafe. On the other hand, successful adaptation to stress or management of the stressful situation leads to personal growth.

Each person with a disability reacts to stressful situations differently. In fact, what is stressful for one person may not be stressful for another. Lazarus explained what happens when an individual's reactions or adjustment efforts are not successful: "The processes of adjustment are, therefore, important to us not only because under normal circumstances of living they determine our actions but also because when they fail under conditions of unusual demands, our welfare is in danger. When this happens we talk about the existence of a state of stress, an extreme instance of disturbed equilibrium" (p. 303).

All people strive to maintain a balance in their lives, and the struggle for equilibrium occurs at both the conscious and the subconscious levels. As an example of the conscious level, many people attempt to keep a proper balance between their social activities and work activities. Simultaneously, their subconscious tries to maintain a balance in emotions. Thus, people may become very elated over an event or find something extremely amusing, but their subconscious will not allow them to remain in an extreme state of euphoria. If they do, the behavior is labeled *abnormal.* Likewise, when they become depressed or unhappy, generally they do not remain in this state for extended periods either. If they do, the behavior is considered psychotic (Elliott, Witty, Herrick & Hoffman 1991). When people do not return to a state of equilibrium, they experience severe emotional or psychological problems. Sechrest and Wallace (1967) pointed out that most people try to minimize immediate discomfort.

The home is the primary source of security and emotional support or, conversely, stress for most persons with disabilities. A close-knit family is an effective insulation against stress. However, no family can effectively thwart the stress that an individual carries around in his or her subconscious, nor can the individual. Unless one is aware of the origins of a stressful situation, resolution is unlikely.

Stress is psychologically and physically draining on an individual's energies. Some stressful situations are accompanied by considerable physical pain. Kaplan (1965) documented the fact that sociopsychological disorders are not less real or less painful than physical injuries are. In fact, psychological stress is more painful to most persons with physical disabilities than their physical impairments are. Under conditions of extreme psychological stress, some of them experience adrenal production of desoxycorticosterone, which greatly reduces excitability of the nervous system. The result of desoxycorticosterone production is depression, apathy, and feelings of fatigue and weakness. The gastrointestinal system also responds to stress. For example, a socially or psychologically frightening situation may cause vomiting, nausea, or diarrhea.

During periods of anger, acid production doubles, and heartburn and ulcers are common. The bowel and the stomach are good indicators of how stressful a psychological situation is. Outwardly calm individuals often are burning and churning inside. Other important areas are the cardiovascular and respiratory systems. During conditions of extreme stress, the heart functions in an exaggerated manner, and the diaphragm is flattened and shortened, causing cramps in the chest and the inability to take a deep breath. Constant tension in the circulatory system can cause headaches as well as arteriosclerosis. The most serious effect of tension on the cardiovascular system is the formation of blood clots in the heart or brain. It is well known among medical practitioners that excessive stress can lead to asthma, rhinitis, and other allergic symptoms. The mucous membranes of the nose, mouth, throat, and upper respiratory system are extremely sensitive to psychological stress.

Numerous writers, including DeLoach and Greer (1981), observed that individuals with disabilities are more vulnerable to anxiety than are persons without them. The potential stress is greatly enhanced for individuals with disabilities because the environment has many barriers or restrictions that also create stressful situations. Depending on the severity of his or her disability, an individual may encounter stress associated with getting an education, participating in social events, securing access to buildings, dating and marriage, and obtaining gainful employment. These overt restrictions, added to numerous covert ones, create frustration and more stress for people with disabilities. Sawrey and Telford (1975) summarized these causes of stress in the following manner:

> The person with a disability is more likely to engage in fewer and simpler activities and functions in a more limited area. The restriction is dictated partly by the nature of the disability, but also partly is the result of social attitudes and cultural expectations. When any person has many things done for him, when he does not have to use his own initiative and when his social relations are limited and stereotyped, he has less opportunity and motivation for free and adventuresome idealism and activity. People who could learn to feed themselves are often spoon fed, both literally and figuratively, for many unnecessary years. Socially engendered fearfulness and low levels of self-expectancy promote excessive dependency on others. (p. 70)

Just as persons with disabilities are more vulnerable to stressful situations than are persons without disabilities, a person with a disability is more likely to react inappropriately. The reason for this is that social conditioning and the more limited responses available to the individual with a disability compound stressful situations. The unfortunate truth is that many of the appropriate ways of responding to stressful situations are not available to people with disabilities or, at best, are difficult for them to act out. Consider the case of a man who is capable of working (an important factor in establishing positive self-esteem) but is unable to do so because no employer will hire him.

This problem is partially created by societal attitudes that make it not only easy but also acceptable for employers to view a disability as one of the worst things that can happen to an individual. Most workers with disabilities can do much to improve their job skills but very little to alter the negative attitudes of some employers. Too often an employer's solution to the employment problem is to "help" persons with disabilities by providing charity and otherwise protecting them. When a society expects little productivity from people, however, it usually gets little in return. Moreover, those who refuse to be cared for as charity cases experience an inordinate amount of stress.

Methods of Coping

Although persons with disabilities as a group experience stressful situations more often and more intensively than persons without disabilities, the same methods of coping are used by both groups. *Coping mechanisms* are emotions and behaviors that allow an individual to adjust to problems. The survival of all people depends on their being able to regulate personal feelings, beliefs, and actions so that their anxiety remains at a manageable level.

There are three categories of coping or defense mechanisms: deception, substitution, and avoidance. Mechanisms of *deception* alter or hide an individual's perception of a threat so that he or she does not sense it. These mechanisms include repression, projection, and displacement. Mechanisms of *substitution* replace stressful goals with those that are safe and relatively tension free. Examples of these mechanisms include compensation and reaction formation. Mechanisms of *avoidance*–those that enable people to remove themselves psychologically from threatening situations–include fantasy and regression.

Freud (1938) defined *defense mechanisms* as unconscious, self-deceptive defenses against anxiety. However, Sawrey and Telford stated that it is the motivation behind an act rather than the act itself that is unconscious, for individuals using defense mechanisms may be aware of what they are doing but unaware of the motivation. As noted earlier, individuals with the same disability may not utilize the same defenses because what is stress for one person may not be for another. Also, there is a wide variety of factors that can influence an individual's coping styles, for example, age at the time of the disability, sex, severity of the disability, and visibility of the disability.

A male who has had polio that leaves him with a limp and one leg smaller than the other, for example, will experience less stress dealing with his disability than a female with the same disability and limitations. The reason is that the male can always wear pants in public to hide the leg, whereas a female is likely to encounter situations in which it is more socially acceptable for her to wear a dress (e.g. church and formal dinners). Also, the appearance of a female's legs probably will be a factor in her overall physical attractiveness, and a limp will draw attention to her leg and thus devalue her appearance.

With respect to age at the time of the disability, a person born with a disability handles stress quite differently than an adult recently disabled does. The person born with a disability or acquiring one early in life has not developed a strong nondisability identity that will have to be rethought and reshaped. Conversely, a recently disabled adult has a self-concept much more based on body image and, therefore, a more difficult adjustment.

The rest of this chapter consists of a discussion of defense mechanisms commonly used by persons with (and without) disabilities. The order of their listing should not be interpreted as the order in which they are employed, nor should the reader assume that one defense is more likely to be used than another or than others not mentioned. The major purpose of the discussion is to illuminate several coping styles.

Depression

Depression is a common defense reaction to loss of a body function; however, not all persons experiencing a physical loss immediately become depressed. When depression does occur, individuals generally become despondent over things they can no longer do or those they think they cannot do. Wright (1960) refers to depression as mourning a loss of a function or a limb no longer available. Depression often coincides with discovery that limitations are associated with the disability. An individual may become depressed because he or she feels that there is little chance of being independent and that his or her dreams for the future have been shattered, if not destroyed. This form of depressed thinking occurs because the individual continues to cling to the past and has not adapted to the new situation. Individuals who immediately become depressed experience their first serious bout with depression long before they enter the physical rehabilitation stage. Early or late, depression usually is part of the realization that returning to "normal" is going to be impossible or a long and difficult process. It is at this time that the person with disabilities comes face to face with reality.

IMPLICATIONS FOR THE REHABILITATION PROCESS. To say that depression is a state of mind that recurs is to state the obvious. However, this statement deserves attention because clients with disabilities have additional stressful situations during rehabilitation about which they seem to be able to do nothing except become depressed. While people with disabilities are in a state of depression, any progress made in the rehabilitation process will at best be limited. However, there are several things that need to be discussed with them during this period: (1) what is psychologically hurting them, (2) how they feel about themselves, (3) what their goals are, what they think they can do, and (4) what lies ahead for them in rehabilitation.

These discussions will probably have to be repeated several times. If an individual is in a state of deep depression, he or she may not hear, or at least not give much attention to, what is being said. Therefore, reinforcement is very important. Even though it may appear that the person is not responding adequately, it is wise to continue communication efforts. Questions oriented to the present and future may gradually shift the individual out of the past. In human relations jargon, this is the process of focusing on the here and now (present) rather than the there and then (past). Leaving the past may not relieve the depression, but it will change it to a different and more manageable form.

Denial

There are two major forms of denial: rationalization and reaction formation. *Rationalization* is the process by which people justify their behavior by replacing the true reasons for it with reasons that are more ego satisfying. The person who rationalizes usually is not trying to distort the truth and is quite unaware of doing so. Rationalization serves to justify what a person thinks, does, and believes. There are several forms of rationalizations; the two that are most relevant to this discussion are "sour grapes" and "sweet lemon."

Devaluing something, for example saying that an unattainable goal is not worthy of interest, is called sour grapes. A person who explains not being hired for a job he or she wanted by saying, "I was glad I didn't get the job after I heard that the company is racist" is demonstrating sour grapes. Sweet lemon rationalization is the opposite, finding something worthwhile in a situation that is undesirable: "Since I have been deaf and learned to read lips, I pay more attention to people. I observe their body language, and so, since being disabled, I understand people better."

Reaction formation is a special type of substitution. This occurs when the original activity is heavily laden with social sanctions and guilt feelings. The person who fears being permanently impaired but jokes about his or her disability and the rehabilitated person who denounces the helpless cripples of the world are exhibiting reaction formation.

IMPLICATIONS FOR THE REHABILITATION PROCESS. After overcoming the shock of discovering that they have a disability, many individuals with permanent disabilities then move to an equally dangerous mind game: denying that they are likely to be physically impaired for the rest of their lives. When people refuse to accept the reality of their disabilities, they often exhibit unproductive behavior such as trying a number of unproven remedies and miracle cures. They become easy marks for unscrupulous con artists who prey on distraught people in order to make money. People in this frame of mind are difficult to assist in the rehabilitation process. They do not want to take on the roles of persons with disabilities restoring themselves to a productive life but instead believe that with one more nontraditional and non–medically proven treatment they will find the cure that will make them "whole" again.

If not carried to an extreme, denial can be beneficial in the rehabilitation process. Sawrey and Telford (1975) observed that, if it is not excessive, denial can help a person with a disability to regain his or her psychological equilibrium: "Following the initial period of denial there normally occurs the emergence of a more realistic attitude toward disability. This more realistic and accepting attitude requires an integration of the previous nondisabled self and roles with the individual's changed status. One personality trait that has been shown to be related to this transition is tolerance of ambiguity" (p. 325). Professional and paraprofessional helpers must be alert for denials such as rationalization. Clients may rationalize their lack of initiative by saying that the rehabilitation professionals and paraprofessionals are the experts and know what is best. Through rationalization, they may try to get others to make decisions for them.

Repression

Repression is an unconscious process wherein painful, distasteful, or guilt-producing memories are removed from awareness. An example of repression is the difficulty that might be experienced by a man who balks at discussing sexual intercourse with his therapist because as a child he was severely beaten by his father for exploring a female playmate's sex organs.

IMPLICATIONS FOR THE REHABILITATION PROCESS. Individuals who repress unpleasant thoughts should be encouraged to discuss them. Failure to do so will not only stall or prevent emotional development with regard to their disabilities but also negatively affect other aspects of their lives in which disabilities have minimal or no impact. As Whitman (1980) pointed out, "Repression can create a snowball effect, as time passes and new things occur which might be associated with anxiety provoking thoughts, these new events and thoughts also must be repressed" (p. 152). The old adage that one cannot solve what one does not know is true. A problem is a puzzle, and repressed thoughts are missing pieces of the rehabilitation puzzle. However, the authors give one final caution: Only well-trained persons should encourage individuals to open up painful, repressed thoughts.

Projection

The process of shifting the responsibility for an act or thought from oneself to another person is called *projection*. This enables an individual to avoid dealing with his or her failures or aggression. For example, a woman who loses her hearing does not admit that she dislikes people who have disabilities but instead cites their hatred and jealousy of her. (It is especially difficult for individuals who were previously able-bodied to accept having a disability.)

IMPLICATIONS FOR THE REHABILITATION PROCESS. Persons with a disability are a product of their environment. Individuals who were not born with a disability but acquired one probably share many of the negative perceptions of people with disabilities that are commonly held by the nondisabled. Now that they have a disability and "one of them," they may project their previous (nondisabled) feelings about disabilities to those around them. Regardless of the fact that their disabilities may not create severe limitations, the knowledge that they no longer are, in their opinion, physically whole causes many persons to ascribe negative attitudes to individuals trying to help them.

Helpers must be aware that people may project an impulse that is threatening onto someone else and attribute it to the external world rather than to themselves. Much of a helper's time and energy may be devoted to getting people with disabilities to own their feelings, getting them to send "I" messages instead of "you," "those people," "them," and "the system" messages. Only by accepting responsibility for their feelings can they gain control of their rehabilitation.

Displacement

Displacement is the process by which an individual releases energy associated with a specific individual or thing onto a secondary target. Displacement is occurring when a woman who is upset with her whining husband who has a disability scolds her children instead of confronting him. The reason is quite simple: The children are less threatening than her husband is and are less able to retaliate. In this situation, it is likely that both the wife and the children will be upset with the husband/father. The process of scapegoating is common in homes where persons with disabilities are protected from ill feelings.

IMPLICATIONS FOR THE REHABILITATION PROCESS. Anger, frustration, fear, and hostility are a few of the emotions felt by persons with disabilities and their loved ones as they attempt to deal with their problems. In many cases, people do not know whom to blame for their disabilities; thus, the release of negative emotions usually is directed at the people around them—spouse, parents, siblings, friends, and medical and rehabilitation staff. This scattergun approach of dispensing hostile feelings is indiscriminate. In some instances, persons with disabilities will displace their anger on themselves, or, stated another way, the anger becomes internalized, and this leads to depression. In the early stages of adjustment to a disability, the individual with a disability frequently vacillates between depression and displacing anger onto others.

An effective method of working with individuals exhibiting this behavior is to confront them about their actions, making them aware of what the displacement is doing to the people around them and to themselves. A disability does not give an individual license to be insensitive to others or cruel to them. Sometimes people aimlessly lash out at others because of their own pain, not from malicious intent. However, not even pain absolves them of incivility. Furthermore, assessing blame is seldom helpful. Sometimes, in addition to rehabilitation of the body, there also must be rehabilitation of interpersonal relations.

Sublimation

By channeling energy from prohibited goals or desires to socially acceptable ones, people move one step closer to normalcy. Examples of this process are exercising instead of fighting with a spouse, painting instead of breaking dishes, and lifting weights instead of having sexual intercourse with a friend's girlfriend.

IMPLICATIONS FOR THE REHABILITATION PROCESS. Anger and aggression channeled into constructive activities are integral aspects of all rehabilitation programs. A danger, however, is that the displaced activities could replace interaction with people. No amount of exercising, painting, or lifting weights, for example, is an adequate substitute for resolving conflicts between people. There is a tendency to avoid encounters if they have embodied socially unacceptable thoughts. Yet, this is the stuff out of which rehabilitation takes shape. People making is seldom without risks.

Aggression

Aggression can be defined as the first attack or act of hostility, an offensive action. Hostility can be directed inward or outward. Battered and abused children and spouses are but one example of inappropriate, outward-directed aggression.

IMPLICATIONS FOR THE REHABILITATION PROCESS. To make sense of aggression as a coping style, *hostile aggression* and *aggressive behavior* must be distinguished. Hostile aggression serves no useful purpose in the rehabilitation process, and in reality it is a disruptive force that can undo progress that has been made. On the other hand, aggressive behavior can be either productive or unproductive. Aggressively pursuing a rehabilitation program is quite different from hostile aggression.

Aggression is the opposite of passivity, and just as there are times when passive behavior is appropriate, so there are times when being aggressive is the correct behavior. Certainly, there are times when aggressive behavior means asserting oneself. In the case of some people with disabilities, assertive behavior often is not only a desired response but also actively encouraged by rehabilitation personnel.

Dependency

A brief definition of *dependency* is relying on someone or something for help in carrying out activities of daily living. This is the "poor little helpless me" attitude and corresponding behavior. Dependency is a natural state. Whether or not they admit it, all people depend on other people to some degree. As the saying goes, "no person is an island," which simply means that no one is capable of meeting 100 percent of his or her needs without help. In fact, even with help, all needs are not met. People need assistance in a variety of areas; therefore, throughout their lives they continually move in and out of stages of dependency.

There is a tendency for most people to think of being dependent in negative terms: Dependent people are sometimes considered lazy, lacking initiative, and possessing very little character. However, what is really being referred to when negative connotations are attributed to dependency is the group of people that Sechrest and Wallace (1967) refer to as "those who have abandoned attempts to solve their problems and have entrusted the solution of the problems to others" (p. 321). Frequently, persons with disabilities bait this trap by presenting themselves to rehabilitation personnel with a disclaimer of their ability to do anything about their problems, and they catch lots of rehabilitation personnel with this posture.

IMPLICATIONS FOR THE REHABILITATION PROCESS. Rehabilitation personnel and others trying to assist individuals with disabilities must not allow physical disabilities to cloud their vision and distort the helping process. In short, they should not allow persons with disabilities to become overly dependent on them. A balance must be kept between assisting and controlling. One must not lose sight of the ultimate goal in working with persons who have a disability: helping them to help themselves.

Sympathetic emotions are aroused in most people when they see someone whom they believe to be less fortunate than themselves. No matter how noble these feelings are, a person with a disability does not need sympathy. *Sympathy* implies feeling sorry for someone. People with disabilities are capable of producing enough sorrow for themselves; they should be spared additional doses. What they need, and it is in short supply, are empathetic feelings. Empathy implies an appreciation of another person's feelings or life situation. Without empathy, rehabilitation becomes an abortion in the helping process: Weak and budding relationships die prematurely.

Self-Abasement

Self-abasement is a passive coping mechanism of which the major characteristic is humbling and denigrating oneself. This is a frequently used survival technique, and it is a viable mechanism for several reasons. (1) Persons with disabilities need assistance from others, and one of this society's unspoken norms is that in order to receive help people should humble themselves. (2) As discussed in earlier chapters, many people believe that a disability is the result of sin; therefore, self-abasement is retribution. (3) In some cases, individuals with disabilities believe that they are inferior to other people.

IMPLICATIONS FOR THE REHABILITATION PROCESS. It is important that individuals helping people with disabilities not engage in actions that further devalue them. The old adage "beauty is in the eye of the beholder" is certainly appropriate. *Disability* is not a synonym for *ugliness* or *ineptness*. Much of the helper's energies initially may have to be spent accentuating the positive attributes of the person being helped before focusing on behavior that needs change. In the end, rehabilitation will succeed or fail based on the ability of a person with a disability to accept himself or herself as a human being of equal worth and dignity.

Regression

Regression is the mechanism of relieving anxiety or stress by reverting to thoughts, feelings, and behavior that worked well during an earlier period of life. When under mild stress, some adults engage in childlike playing. In extreme stress, they regress to an infantile stage and become unable to wash or feed themselves or control their excretion.

IMPLICATIONS FOR THE REHABILITATION PROCESS. Regression is an attempt to deny reality by distorting it. Helpers may be perceived as parents or lovers or friends who met the person's needs several years ago. Although it may be ego gratifying to be considered able to replace an individual's significant others, this does little to cement present relationships. By not accepting helpers for themselves, the person also fails to accept his or her disabilities for what they are. Regression is analogous to taking a detour when going on a mission; it may be interesting and even fun, but it delays the mission.

Compensation

Compensation is the process of enhancing one's self-esteem by excelling in one area to cover up weakness or failure in another. Some people with physical disabilities, for example, become academic achievers in order to compensate for their physical impairments.

IMPLICATIONS FOR THE REHABILITATION PROCESS. Whether the motivation producing the compensatory act is a feeling of inferiority or a desire to succeed, it is an unconscious decision and must be brought to consciousness. It is helpful for clients to take inventory of themselves in order to know their strengths and weaknesses as well as their coping styles and life goals. Like other defense mechanisms, compensation can be helpful and wholesome when the adjustment is personally and socially beneficial. The first step is, of course, self-knowledge.

Fantasy

The ability to substitute imaginary activities for real ones allows some people with physical disabilities to hang on to fragile lifelines, but DeLoach and Greer (1981) took exception to the statement that there is nothing wrong with fantasy. Like the other defenses, there is something very wrong when fantasy is continuous.

IMPLICATIONS FOR THE REHABILITATION PROCESS. All people spend a portion of their lives in fantasy places. The fictitious world of the imagination is certainly a haven for persons with disabilities, but this form of flight does nothing to relieve the stresses and barriers in the real world. Fantasy is the "what if" and "I wish" portion of a person's existence. However, one should not abandon the real world for fantasy. Helpers must place this mechanism of coping in proper perspective. Although no defense mechanism can in itself solve problems, fantasy may allow an individual to cope until better solutions are found.

Passing

Passing is the process of denying one's difference and attempting to conceal it. This process is most popularly associated with ethnic minorities who have physical appearances approximating whites and who live as whites to avoid discriminatory treatment. Technically, passing is not a defense mechanism since it is a conscious behavior. For the person with a physical disability, passing consists of using cosmetic devices and isolation and not disclosing the disability. Passing extracts a high price. Sawrey and Telford (1975) wrote, "Concealment indicates shame and involves strain. Despite external vigilance and constant work, the person with a disability often cannot get away from his disability. The price of passing is high and the effort is often futile. When a person must constantly be vigilant in order to deny his disability it becomes the central focus of his life. He may resort to partial social isolation in order to help conceal his defect and thus fend off possible discussion" (pp. 71–72).

IMPLICATIONS FOR THE REHABILITATION PROCESS. Rather than deny their limitations, people with disabilities should accept them, not as badges of courage but as reality. Those who pass as nondisabled persons are living a lie that tends to multiply and spread to all areas of their lives. Until they have accepted their disabilities, people with disabilities will not be able to build freely on the resources available within and outside themselves. The freeing dimension of acknowledging that "I have a disability" is the beginning of rehabilitation.

MALADJUSTMENT

When defense mechanisms cease to relieve stress, people may turn to behavior that is called *maladjustment* or *maladaption*. A few words of caution are in order at this time. There is a thin line between normal behavior and psychotic and neurotic behaviors. Except for extreme psychoses, what is normal and what is not normal are difficult to ascertain. Most normal people have periods of maladjustive behavior; most maladjusted people have periods of rational behavior. According to Milt (1960), borderline personality types exhibit the following behavior:

1. *Belligerence*–walking around continuously with a chip on the shoulder, ready to argue or quarrel at the slightest excuse, or even without an excuse.
2. *Excessive moodiness*–spells of blues or feeling down in the dumps, feeling a great deal of time that nothing is worthwhile or really matters.
3. *Exaggerated worry*–continuous anxiety about nothing at all or entirely out of proportion to the cause.
4. *Suspiciousness and mistrust*–a persistent feeling that the world is full of dishonest, conniving people, that everyone is "trying to take advantage of me."
5. *Selfishness and greediness*–lack of consideration of the needs of others, a "what's in it for me" attitude about almost everything.
6. *Helplessness and dependency*–a tendency to let others carry the burden, difficulty in making decisions.
7. *Poor emotional control*–exaggerated emotional outbursts out of proportion to their cause and/or at inappropriate times.
8. *Daydreaming and fantasy*–spending a good part of the time imagining how things could be rather than dealing with them the way they are.
9. *Hypochondria*–worrying a great deal about minor physical ailments, experiencing imaginary symptoms of illness.

Transference

Transference occurs when a client projects onto the counselor or helper feelings he or she holds for someone else. Generally the feelings occur as a result of interaction with significant others.

Implication for the Rehabilitation Process

The feelings that clients or patients transfer onto the helper may be either positive or negative. In most cases, the client is unaware that he or she is transferring these feelings. The helper may remind the client of someone who is significant or has been significant in his or her life. This familiarity often is not based on physical appearance; rather, it may be grounded in such things as mannerisms, attitudes, and position of authority. Once helpers recognize or suspect that transference is occurring, they should explore with the clients its origin in order to help them understand what it means and how it may also be occurring with others. Above all, helpers must not take the transference personally. In the case of transference of negative feelings, helpers must guard against becoming defensive. Again, exploring it will help both the client and the helper.

At this point, a good question is how does one know when transference is occurring? In most cases the beginning of transference is difficult to detect; however, a general rule in recognizing transference is when the clients'/patients' reactions to the helper are not in proportion to the issues being discussed. In other words, if the clients'/patients' reactions to the helper are exaggerated in relation to what should be reasonable reactions, the helper should explore the issues of transference with the client/patient.

Countertransference

Countertransference occurs when the helper transfers onto the client/patient feelings she or he holds for someone else.

Implication for the Rehabilitation Process

In most professional helping relationships, the helper is in the "power position." Therefore, it is incumbent upon professional helpers to recognize when they are projecting feelings to the client, who generally will not have any idea what is happening. If countertransference occurs and the helper recognizes it and attempts to eliminate it but it continues to occur, he or she should consult with a colleague who has a background in dealing with such psychological and emotional issues. The repeated occurrence of countertransference probably is a signal that the helper has some psychological or emotional issues with which she needs help.

SUMMARY

People with disabilities who are continuously characterized by all or some of the previously conditions are desperate, lonely, and cynical. Indeed, they are alienated from themselves and their significant others. The anomic aspects of their alienation are fourfold. They believe that (1) community leaders are indifferent to their needs, (2) their living conditions are getting progressively worse, (3) life is meaningless, and (4) their immediate circle of relationships is not supportive or comfortable. The life theme of alienated people includes a preference for fatalism and an orientation to the past. Feeling helpless in an unpredictable world controlled by people who are not disabled, they resort to a "live for today" philosophy that leaves little room for projecting long-range rehabilitation goals. Fortunately, a growing number of agencies are providing psychological services for people with disabilities and their families (Elliott et al., 1991). Equally fortunate is the fact that most people with physical disabilities are well-adjusted individuals.

NOTE TO HELPERS

Persons with disabilities are simultaneously persons with identities apart from their disabilities. They can best cope with their disabilities when their helpers cope with them. The following observations may help helpers to do this:

1. Helpers cannot solve clients' problems, but they may be able to help them solve their own problems.
2. Every client's problems have more than one possible solution.
3. The easiest, least-creative response to disabilities is to pretend they do not exist.
4. Every client behaves according to unwritten ethnic group customs and traditions.
5. The family is the most important group in rehabilitation.
6. Client knowledge of scientific aspects of his or her disability may help or hinder adjustment.
7. Humor can help helpers and people with disabilities over rough spots; people must be able to laugh at themselves and with other people.
8. Previous experience with people with disabilities is a valuable asset if it is used as a general guide. However, if viewed as offering the correct view of every person with a disability, experience (as well as the information in this book) will be a liability.
9. All helpers make mistakes when working with people with disabilities. They should learn from their mistakes and try not to repeat them.

POINTS FOR DISCUSSION AND SUGGESTED ACTIVITIES

1. How do you handle stress?
2. Make a list of agencies in your community that help people with disabilities who have psychological problems. Visit one of the agencies and interview a counselor in order to find out what he or she recommends for others who have stressful life situations.

REFERENCES

Coulter, W.A., and Marrow, H.W (1978). *Adaptive Behavior.* New York: Grune & Stratton.

DeLoach, C., and Greer, B.G. (1981). *Adjustment of Severe Physical Disability.* New York: McGraw-Hill.

Elliott, T.R., Witty, T.E., Herrick, S.M., and Hoffman, J.T. (1991). Negotiating reality after physical loss: Hope, depression and disability. *Journal of Personality & Social Psychology, 61,* 608–613.

Fowler, C.A., and Wadsworth, J.S. (1991). Individualism and equality: Critical values in North American culture and the impact on disability. *Journal of Applied Rehabilitation Counseling, 22,* 19–23.

Freud, S. (1938). *Basic Writings of Sigmund Freud.* New York: Modern Library.

Kaplan, L. (1965). *Foundations of Human Behavior.* New York: Harper & Row.

Lazarus, R.S. (1961). *Adjustment and personality.* New York: McGraw-Hill.

Milt, H. (1960). *How to Deal with Mental Problems.* New York: National Association for Mental Health.

Sawrey, J.M., & Telford, C.W. (1975). *Psychology of Adjustment.* Boston: Allyn & Bacon.

Sechrest, L., & Wallace, J. Jr. (1967). *Psychology and Human Problems.* Columbus, OH: Charles E. Merrill.

Whitman, R.D. (1980). A*djustment: The Development and Organization of Human Behavior.* New York: Oxford University Press.

Wright, B.A. (1960). *Physical Disability: A Psychological Approach.* New York: Harper & Row.

SUGGESTED READINGS

Elliott, A. (1994). *Psychoanalytic Theory: An Introduction,* Oxford: Blackwell.

Freud, S. (1949). *An Outline of Psychoanalysis.* New York: Norton.

Schultz, D., and Schultz, S.E. (1998). *Theories of Personality.* (6th ed.). Pacific Grove, CA: Brooks/Cole.

Searless, H.F. (1979). *Countertransference and Related Subjects: Selected Papers.* New York: International University Press.

Chapter 11

HELPING PROFESSIONALS

Outline

- Introduction
- The Helping Relationship
- Becoming an Effective Helper
- Summary
- Points for Discussion and Suggested Activities

Objectives

- To emphasize steps in building an effective helping relationship
- To identify important areas of understanding a professional helper must master to be an effective helper

INTRODUCTION

In a previous chapter we discussed the need for empowerment of persons with disabilities, and we have made clear the fact that no person, one with a disability or not, is capable of meeting all of his or her needs. Therefore, seeking and receiving help is not a sign of weakness, nor should it, in most cases, be considered as identifying a dependent personality. Most people take care of as many of their needs as they are capable and seek assistance for those needs they are unable to meet satisfactorily. This belief was the underlying concept that the founders of the disability rights movement used in developing ILC. Accepting help did not make them or mark them as dependent; rather, it identified them as realistic and innovative individuals. Another principle that persons with disabilities should understand from the independent living movement is that whenever reasonable and possible, even though they are receiving assistance, they should maintain as much control of their lives as possible. What is being suggested is that as often as possible persons with disabilities should make decisions that affect their lives rather than defer the decision making to others. This is a very important concept that helping professionals should remember when rendering assistance to persons with disabilities. Equally important as helping professionals remembering this concept they should encourage persons with disabilities to control their lives and destiny as much as possible.

THE HELPING RELATIONSHIP

Establishing Trust and Rapport

As previously stated, all persons need assistance at various points in their lives. Some need considerable and frequent help; others need periodic assistance. This statement is true for both persons with disabilities and those considered nondisabled. The most important factor in being a helper is not necessarily the frequency of assistance given, but rather the quality of the assistance. First we will discuss the process of helping from the helper's standpoint, and following that discussion we will discuss receiving help from the standpoint of persons with disabilities.

With regard to the helping relationship, to be successful, the relationship requires individuals, often strangers to each other, to develop a dialogue based on understanding and mutual respect. Respect does not always require all parties to agree with each other; rather, all parties should respect each other's point of view. To accomplish this most important task, trust must be established among those involved in the helping process. With the following comments Brammer and MacDonald (2003) emphasized the importance of trust in the helping relationship.

> A crucial relationship dimension is that of trust-distrust. Helpees are willing generally to accept help from people they trust. For trust to develop, helpees must have confidence in their helpers and must be able to believe what they say. Certain specific helper behaviors, such as clear motives for helping, create trust. The motives of the helper must be apparent and attractive to the helpee, and they must not be a cover for helper efforts to control, manipulate, or punish. (p. 51)

Egan (1994) points out that an effective way of developing trust with a client is through attending. Egan interprets attending as actively being with clients. He further explains the concept of attending as well as identifies what active attending does for the helping relationship with the following comments.

> Helping and other deep interpersonal transactions demand a certain intensity of presence. Attending, or the way you orient yourself physically and psychologically to clients, contributes to the presence. Effective attending does two things: it tells clients that you are with them, and it puts you in a position to listen carefully to their concerns. Attentive presence can invite or encourage them to trust you, open up, and explore the significant dimensions of their problem situations. Half hearted presence can promote distrust and lead to clients' reluctance to reveal themselves to you. (p.91)

Okun (2002) expands upon Egan's discussion of developing trust with concrete ways of establishing trust.

> To establish trust and support, it is necessary that the helper provide a meeting place where client confidentiality can be ensured. If you do have a private office, try to arrange the furniture so that you can sit facing the helpee without any barriers between you. For example, you can sit on one side of your desk close to the helpee, rather than across from him or her. Some people prefer to work away from their desks and arrange chairs facing each other in another part of the room. (p. 93)

Given the numerous concerns the client may have, it is incumbent upon the helper to establish a comfort level within which the helpee is able to interact. This comfort level is often called establishing rapport. Many positive results occur as a result of developing trust such as increased cooperation from the client, positive verbal and/or nonverbal interaction, and respect from the client to mention only three.

Confidentiality

One of the most important parts of establishing an effective working relationship with your clients is maintaining confidentiality. Maintaining confidentiality is a major way of maintaining the trust of your clients. The first point to be made with regard to confidentiality is to know your limitations with regard to keeping client information confidential. Depending on the type of helper, as well as local, state, and federal laws, some information, such as child abuse, and some types of threat must be disclosed to certain officials, such as courts of law and law enforcement officers. Additionally, all helping professions must be aware of whether they have privileged communication and if so the limitation of the privileged communication. As a helper you must be knowledgeable of limits with regard to confidentiality and you must explain those limitations to your clients.

Identifying and Clarification of Issues

Clients seek the assistance of helpers for a variety of reasons, some of which may appear to be clear, whereas others may appear to be convoluted. In working with persons who have a disability there may be additional elements involved in issue identification and clarification. For persons who have cognitive disabilities and/or mental disabilities as well as children with learning disabilities and some adults with severe physical disabilities, parents and other family members may have significant involvement with the person with the disability seeking help. Stated in other terms, the helper may need to consult with family members of the person with the disability in an effort to identify the central problem(s) to be addressed. Certainly, in situations in which the client is capable of assisting with discussion of what assistance is needed and how that assistance should be applied, he or she should have the most input with regard to the relationship with the helper.

As a helper one should not minimize the thoughts and beliefs of the person with a disability. Although you as the helper may have what you consider to be an accurate view of the situations being encountered by the person with a disability, you must always keep in mind that you are viewing the client's situation as an outsider. To be more specific, you do not live in the client's body and mind. How you perceive life events is based on your observations and personal viewpoints. Regardless of how convinced you are that your perceptions are on target and that the client's perceptions are distorted, this does not take into consideration that the client's viewpoints have been and are being filtered through his experiences and/or perception of how the experiences are affecting his life.

The client's mind may be flooded with many issues, all of which have some degree of concern to him. Your role as his helper is not to make value judgments with regard to the right or wrong of his perceptions, rather to help him understand how his perceptions are affecting him. Without this understanding it will be difficult for the client to develop lasting solutions to his issues. With the clarification of his feelings and perceptions, appropriate lasting solutions can be put into place. Likewise, clarification of issues will help in establishing goals sufficient to helping solve or at least effectively deal with the problems being encountered by the client.

Establishment of Goals

The establishment of goals should be a joint effort between the client and the helper. It is certain that in many situations the helper is inviting failure if she dictates the goals to the client because the goals become the helper's goals, not the client's goals. Some clients may attempt to abdicate their responsibility in deciding which goals are the most important to be addressed in the helping relationship. When this happens, the helper will be wise to assist the client with regard to appropriate decision-making procedures. Assisting the client in developing confidence in her decision-making abilities will benefit the helpee in making future life decisions. In situations in which the client with a disability is not intellectually or mentally capable of making the decisions, the helper should obtain the assistance of family, friends, and/or caregivers who will be affected by the decisions to be made.

Goals should serve as directional signs for both the client and the helper. Well-established goals can be the cement that bonds the helping process together. Both short- and long-term goals should be established. The short-term goals should be formulated so their accomplishment will serve as motivation and lead to the attainment of the long-term goals. In this manner, meeting short-term goals will have served as motivation that drives the helpee toward the conquest of the long-term goals. Bryan (2009, pp. 34–35) discussed four rules with regard to establishing short- and long-term goals:

1. **Goals should be stated in clear and specific terms.** To identify a goal such as "The individual will be better able to deal with personal problems" is too general and does not mean much. Being specific with regard to which problem(s) or the kind of problems the helpee will be better able to handle is much more meaningful and adds direction to the helping process. An example of a specific goal for a person with a learning disability could be, within two weeks, identify a tutor to assist with specific reading skills.

2. **Goals should be stated in measurable terms.** Granted, it is much easier to establish measurable goals when dealing with a quantifiable product than it is when assisting with interpersonal relationships. However, goals that relate to interpersonal relationships that are carefully conceived can be measured. Goals such as spending specific amounts of time with a particular family member or the family in general can be measured. Again these goals have to be specific, such as identifying a specific amount of time and/or particular activities.

3. **Goals should be realistic.** One should take into consideration the helpee's resources when establishing goals. It is senseless to assist the helpee formulate goals the helpee will not be able to attain for lack of adequate resources (i.e. time, money, and educational background, to mention only three needed resources).

4. **Helpees must have input in the establishment of goals.** As previously stated, the establishment of goals is primarily for the benefit of the helpee. Helpees should be discouraged from turning over their responsibilities for providing solutions to their problems to the helpers. This is a major reason why helpers should encourage helpees to take ownership of their issues as well as the possible solutions to those issues.

Egan (1994, pp. 262–265) added to the list of things to do when assisting clients establish goals:

1. **Help clients set goals that can be sustained.** Egan points out that clients need to commit themselves to goals with staying power. He further points out that goals are more sustainable if they are flexible.

2. **Help clients choose goals consistent with their values.** Egan explains this point by stating that "although helping is a process of social influence, it remains ethical only if

it respects, within reason, the values of the client. Values are criteria we use to make decisions. Although helpers may challenge clients to reexamine their values, they should in no way encourage clients to perform actions that are not in keeping with their values.

3. **Help clients establish realistic time frames for the accomplishment of goals.** Egan expands this thought by stating that "goals that are to be accomplished 'sometime' probably won't be accomplished at all. Therefore, helping clients put some time frames in their goals can add value."

As much as possible the goals should be the goals of the client not of the helper. Once engaged in the helping process, helpees too frequently look to the helper to solve their problems. Some falsely believe the reason that they are participating in the helping process is to turn over the problem portion of their lives to the helper. Although it may be flattering to the helper to be considered that powerful, it is not productive. Establishment of realistic, understandable, specific, and achievable goals can best be accomplished with full participation of the client.

Identifying and Implementing Solutions

After assisting the client in selecting goals the helper believes will regulate the client's issues, the next step in the helping process is to engage the client in exploring possible solutions to the issues of most urgency. In most cases, there is going to be more than one possible resolution to issues confronting the client. A critical component of the part of the helping process is the helper working with the client to explore the various possibilities for relief and resolution of the confronting situation. This phase is considered the **exploration stage** of identifying possible solutions.

Once the exploration stage has produced results that the client and the helper believe has the potential of providing relief to the helpee, the next **stage of implementing** the results of the exploration occurs. A word of caution is warranted because during the process of implementing the solutions, it may be necessary to revisit the exploration stage if the desired results do not occur. Both the helper and the client should review the need to rethink the solutions once considered appropriate, because there may have been a number of variables that cause a potentially good solution to no longer be appropriate. Variables such as timing of implementation and unexpected impact on others are only two of several possibilities. Additionally, the failure of some goals to meet Egan's (1994) test of flexible and sustainable can also be a variable that makes once-attractive goals less desirable and attractive. Therefore, **testing the impact** of the solutions is necessary to make a determination of whether they are appropriate.

Bryan (2009) warns us that in the process of testing, two events may occur: one is what he calls the **eureka effect**, which occurs when the client begins to understand her or his situation better as well as understand what is causing the discomfort associated with the situation. He further explains that with this increased understanding of the situation often comes the feeling that "at last I know what is bothering me; therefore I can now handle the situation." Too often when clients have this eureka moment they are ready to discontinue the hunt for solutions because they believe that they know all that is needed to know to apply appropriate solutions to the problem. In some cases this may be an accurate assessment on the part of the client; however, in many cases the clients have just begun to "scratch the surface" of understanding the issues confronting them. Therefore, the helper should explore with the client the possibility of testing the solution to determine the degree to which the client understands.

The second event Bryan describes is the problem of the client's **resistance to change**. Bryan elaborates on this second point:

> From a psychological standpoint, we become accepting of routines even if those routines create some discomfort and are emotionally unhealthy. Requests for change often create additional discomfort and uncertainty, and when faced with living with the familiar or venturing into the unknown, too often we choose the familiar. Offered as an example is obesity that is caused by the lack of will power to curb overeating rather than obesity resulting from genetics. Although we know that overeating and eating certain foods causes us to gain weight and is not healthy for us, we too frequently choose to continue this unhealthy lifestyle rather than change our eating habits. It appears that sometimes the unwillingness to change is stronger than being rational and doing those things that are most productive for our well-being. (p. 36)

One of the responsibilities of the helper is to assist clients to feel comfortable with making decisions to change behavior and believe in their ability to live with those changes. When clients make decisions to change and experience the positive results of those changes, they will become confident in their ability to make appropriate life decisions; as a result of this self-confidence, the helper will have helped to empower the client.

Termination

In some situations of working with persons with disabilities there may not be a point where services are terminated. In other instances, certain services may be terminated but others are begun as an extension of the overall rehabilitation and maintenance services for the client. Some social work services are examples of not completely terminating services to a client but instead, transitioning from one type of service to another.

The operational procedure for either total termination of services or transitioning from one service to another is **planning and preparation**. Effective helpers will communicate each step of the rehabilitation process with the client. This communication should include a detail discussion of how various aspects of the rehabilitation process will be administered. Another key to effective communication is to frequently repeat information with regard to the various steps. The repetition of information is important because clients may not only forget what was said but also fear and anxiety may cause clients to hear but not absorb the information that has been given. Helpers must take into consideration that the prospect of certain medical procedures, including having to spend time in hospitals and rehabilitation facilities can be frightening, causing considerable anxiety. Therefore, if the client is in a state of anxiety, carefully explained information can easily be forgotten. Thus, as previously stated, information should be frequently repeated. Additionally, if providing information to family members and/or significant others is not a breach of confidentiality, this information should be provided to them. The best way to avoid breaches of confidentiality is to simply ask the client if you may provide the information to whomever needs it.

With regard to psychological counseling, there are certain steps to take in terminating counseling. The mechanics of termination should include phasing in termination. Each session should begin with an overview of progress that has been made in previous sessions of the relationship, and each session should end with both an evaluation of the session and a discussion of what is to occur at the next session. Events may change what actually occurs at the next session; however, it is better to have a plan for the next session than to wait for events to dictate what will happen.

Generally speaking, there are four steps to an effective termination of psychological counseling:

1. **Begin discussion of termination early** in the encounters, no later than the second session. It is a good idea to mention the fact that counseling is not a process that lasts forever and at some point the encounter will end. The discussion of when the counseling encounters will end may be predicated on the number of sessions a third-party payer will support. In other situations, the number of sessions may be determined by the counselor, social worker, or other psychological helper. Regardless of the determining source, the client should be informed early that there eventually will be an end to counseling services.

2. **Termination should be phased in.** An example of how this could occur follows: If the helping session has been occurring once a week, it could be changed to two-week intervals; if progress continues, the session could be changed to three-week intervals; and so on until the relationship reaches the point that the client and helper feel that the client can function without the counseling sessions. An advantage of changing the intervals of the counseling relationship relates to the fact that in some cases clients begin to depend on the counseling relationship and become reluctant to end the relationship. Changing the intervals can help break the dependency that may occur. Moreover, as the client devotes more time and effort to working on issues without the helper, the client gains self-confidence.

3. **Provide community resources.** As the counseling process is being transitioned toward termination, the counselor should provide the client with community resources to use in dealing with issues. This will also help eliminate the client becoming dependent on the counselor.

4. **Provide follow-up.** The counselor should provide follow-up; at certain intervals the counselor should contact the client to learn the progress or lack thereof. It is impossible for us to prescribe a certain time for follow-up; each situation has its own merits with regard to when to provide follow-up.

BECOMING AN EFFECTIVE HELPER

The survival of humankind to a large extent depends on humans helping each other in a variety of settings and ways. In some countries, including the United States, many people pride themselves on being independent. Some may think that their survival and destiny are determined by their own thinking and actions. However, a truth of life is that no matter how independent and self-sufficient we may think we are the reality is that all humans, to a major degree, dependent on each other for survival in this world.

Many humans recognize the importance of being helped and the nobleness of being a helper; thus they choose to dedicate significant portions of their lives to providing assistance to their fellow human beings. Although most humans in various ways render assistance to others, there are some people who choose to devote significant portions of their lives helping others. In this text, we will call them helping professionals, regardless of whether the job for which they are rendering assistance is called professional, paraprofessional, or nonprofessional.

The authors of this text firmly believe that dedicating one's life to assisting others is one of the noblest professions in which one could be engaged. We further believe that it takes a special sensitivity to give of oneself in this noble profession of helping. Likewise, to be effective as a professional helper there are some important professional characteristics one must possess and/or develop to be successful in this profession. We will briefly discuss the following personal characteristics: **trustworthy, effective communicator/listener, caring and compassionate, and empathic**. Certainly, there are a number of other characteristics that could be added to this list for discussion; however, if the helper possesses these characteristics, it is our belief, he or she also possesses many of the other notable characteristics we have omitted. Following this discussion we will present the following professional understandings a professional helper must have to be effective in assisting his/her clients: **understanding self, understanding human behavior, understanding resources, understanding family dynamics, understanding cultural differences and understanding disabilities, and persons with disabilities**.

Trustworthy.

For a professional helper, being trustworthy is vital because, in many if not most cases, clients that come to a professional helper or are referred to the helper are at a vulnerable state in their lives. Quite often some situations in their lives are beyond their control or have been deemed by someone to be beyond their control, thus significant and personal information, some of which maybe psychologically painful, is exposed or will be exposed. The professional helper must be ethical and not take advantage of the client's state of vulnerability. As will be discussed in "Understanding one's self" the helper must not use clients and the information that they share, or is provided by a third party, for his or her personal and/or psychological advantage or gratification.

A successful outcome of a helping relationship is increased significantly if the client has trust in more than the helper's skills in assisting in the resolution of issues. The chances of being successful are also increased if the client can trust the helper to not take advantages of his or her weakened situation. The helper must remember that, within the encounter between the helper and the client, the helper is in the power position and the client recognizes this fact. Therefore, it is incumbent on the helper to make the client feel assured that the helper has the client's best interest and welfare as the primary concern in the helping relationship.

Effective Communicator.

Communication is a key ingredient that will help determine whether the helping relationship is a success or failure. Virtually all aspects of the helping relationship depend on communication between the helper and the client. Although the previous statement is obvious, the real fact is that we tend to overlook the various ways we communicate. As much as 80 percent of our communication is nonverbal. Therefore, much of our interaction in a helping relationship involves such actions as body posture and facial expression, or lack thereof, to mention only two.

It is essential that the helper master the art of effective communicating nonverbally as well as verbally. Equally important, the helper must become proficient with regard to understanding the client's verbal and nonverbal communication.

With regard to effective communication, it is one thing to recognize various forms of communication; however, understanding and being comfortable with various expressions of communication is another. For example, understanding and being comfortable with clients' silence is also important. Some helpers begin to feel discomfort when a client becomes silent. Some helpers tend to feel that every moment within the helping relationship should be filled with conversation, and unfortunately when there is silence they interject words to fill the perceived void. Experienced helpers who are comfortable with silence and recognize the possible benefit of this silence will allow a reasonable period of time to pass and, if the silence continues, may remind the client that he or she has ceased talking and inquire what the client thinks his or her silence means. In most cases, silence has meaning; therefore, rushing in with his, the helper's, conversation may relieve the client of having to explain what is or is not causing the silence. Bryan (2009) contends that silence is another form of communication.

For a helping professional, another critical form of communication is listening. As previously stated, some beginning and/or inexperienced helpers feel that every moment in the helping relationship has to be filled with conversation, primarily the helper's conversation. Considerable information and direction for possible solutions can be obtained by listening to the client. It is our opinion that most persons, unless there is a disability that impairs cognitive ability, have solutions to their problems; therefore, the more the client talks and the helper listens, the greater the likelihood of solutions being found.

To some nonprofessional helpers the assumption may be that listening is an easy technique to master; however, effective listening can be as difficult as mastering the art of understanding nonverbal communication. In a helping relationship when a client is talking, often the helper is engaged in a number of activities such as attempting to observe body language, listening to detect underlying meaning of the conversation, taking notes mentally or physically, thinking of the next appropriate response, as well as attempting to demonstrate to the client a serious degree of being fully present while she or he is discussing immediate concerns, and lastly thinking about the next question or line of inquiry to present to the client. While all of these things are occurring in the helper's mind at the same time the client is speaking, important bits of information may be missed by the helper.

Given the many things that occur in a helping setting that may distract the helper from the task of being an effective listener, one may ask the obvious question of "how does one become an effective listener." Bryan (2009, pp. 9–11) has offered the following suggestions with regard to being an effective listener:

1. **Ask questions.** Listening does not always mean silence. By asking for clarification with regard to things the helpee is saying, one will get a clearer understanding of what one is hearing. Considerable information can be lost by assuming understanding of what is being said. Seeking clarification aids the helper with regard to underlying meanings of the messages being verbally expressed. Also, asking questions demonstrates to the helpee that the helper is interested and attentive to what is being said; thus the flow of information may increase.

2. **Observe body language.** Notice the level of comfort the client exhibits as he or she speaks. Being uncomfortable in a helping setting is a natural reaction for the helpee; however, careful observation of the level of discomfort as the helpee speaks can provide clues with regard to significant or sensitive information. To be more specific, by recognizing when the helpee's discomfort level goes beyond the normal or baseline discomfort, an astute helper can identify when the conversation of the helpee ventures into sensitive territory.

3. **Listen for logic in the helpee's conversation.** It is normal for clients to become nervous and forget facts as well as get confused in discussing some issues. However, being confused and illogical are often two different acts. When clients begin to leave out relevant facts and the information being presented does not tie together or, stated another way, does not make sense, it is often an indication that the client is more than confused. Quite often this means that the client, for a variety of possible reasons, is trying to avoid discussing significant issues. Carefully listening to the client's conversation will aid in making this observation.

4. **Listen to the client's tone of voice.** Change in the tone of voice often means that the client has significant emotional attachment to what is being discussed. This should be a signal to the helper that additional attention should be given to the topic. Because this indicates an increase in the emotional level, the helper should be careful with regard to exploring the issues. This does not mean not to explore the issues; rather, it means to carefully process information or the lack thereof.

5. **Listen to determine whether the helpee takes any responsibility for her or his actions.** As human beings, we are not responsible for others' behavior. However, we are responsible for our own behavior; thus the helper should listen to determine whether the helpee takes responsibility or blames other for the situation. It may be true that others have significant responsibility for some or all of the issues being discussed; however, blaming others, generally speaking, does not solve problems. Taking responsibility for one's own actions goes a long way toward resolutions to significant life issues. Taking responsibility for one's behavior, as previously stated, is important; however, the helper also has to be aware of some clients' tendencies to become martyrs and take responsibility for others' behavior. Just as avoiding responsibility for one's behavior meets some psychological need, the helper must realize that assuming responsibility for others' actions also meets a psychological need. Therefore, in the case of the martyr, it is important to understand why the client is assuming undeserved responsibility and help him or her understand what he or she is doing and why.

6. **Listen to the client's responses to your questions.** How the client responds to questions can provide considerable information with regard to how willing the client is to put forth efforts to solve the issues. If a helper consistently hears the helpee refer to others as the ones to deal with the issues, it should be a flag alerting the helper to the fact that she or he must work with the client to accept her share of the responsibilities in solving the problems.

Caring and Compassionate.

Some may think that being caring and compassionate is an obvious quality that all helpers possess. Unfortunately, this is not always the case. Sometimes, hopefully not frequently, one will hear a helper state that the client's need for help is the result of his or her wrong doing. If one has been in the helping business for a reasonable period of time she or he has heard "he is getting what he deserves," referring to the belief that the client has done something wrong and is being punished for his actions.

Professional helpers must posses the quality Rogers was referring to when he said an essential quality of a helper must be unconditional positive regard. What Rogers meant by unconditional positive regard is that a helper must accept people as they are and not wait until they become what the helper thinks they should be before the helper accepts the client. In some cases, this is a difficult undertaking but a necessary one to be an effective helper. One should have the professional philosophy that unless clients have some intellectual and/or cognitive disorder they have the ability to understand their issues and make appropriate changes.

A word of caution for all helpers: One has to be careful in being a compassionate caring individual and not allow that caring to digress into sympathy.

Sympathy and caring are two totally separate emotions and have two significantly different impacts on clients.

Empathic.

Most if not all academic training programs that concentrate on helping clients adjust to or deal with personal issues emphasize being empathic in working with clients rather than having a sympathetic tone to the helping approach. This certainly is good and constructive advice. However, too frequently when working with persons who have experienced tragedy or other events that cause their lives to deviate from what society considers as normal, the best trained and educated helpers slip into a sympathetic mood rather than empathetic approach to working with the clients. This certainly is too often the case in working with some persons with disabilities, especially those persons with very visual disabilities. Stated in other terms, the more a person's disability appear to distinguish him or her from what we consider normal appearance and/or normal behavior—such as walking, talking, seeing and hearing—the greater the likelihood that sympathetic feelings will occur in the helper and paternalistic applications of helping occur. It has been stated many times and bears repeating many more times that persons with disabilities want and need understanding, not sympathy. A major problem with displaying sympathetic feelings toward persons with disabilities is that sympathy, albeit in many cases unintentional, places the persons receiving it in an inferior position. Sympathy too often causes persons who are the recipient of the sympathy to feel inferior and be treated as less than those who are considered as not having a disability.

To be an effective professional helper assisting persons with disabilities, the helper must have the intellectual view that no one is perfect and that everyone has some limitations; therefore, persons with disabilities are persons with limitations and in some cases their limitations maybe more noticeable than for other persons. One of the best ways to treat all persons that one is assisting is to have a good understanding of oneself.

Understanding Self

To be an effective helper, one must have a high level of self-awareness and self-confidence, as well as a good understanding of one's strengths, weaknesses, prejudices, and the things about which one feels strongly, either pro or con. Self-awareness assists the helper in understanding his or her idiosyncratic views and actions. This understanding makes taking responsibility for beliefs and actions much easier, hopefully not allowing the helper to deny and/or overlook her or his limitations. Confidence in one's abilities helps the helper to project a sense of leadership as well as display feelings of comfort in assisting the client. Self-confidence aids the helper in establishing strong boundaries within the helping relationship. Boundaries are necessary for developing and maintaining the professional distance required for an ethical and effective helping relationship skills. This way the helper will not slip into the habit of trying to always please the client, especially when sensitive discussion occurs and there is a need for direct and forthright opinions to be expressed.

An additional component of self-confidence is to love oneself. Professional helpers must care deeply about themselves—their abilities as both an ordinary human being and someone who has chosen to be a helper as his profession. To be effective at helping and caring for others and their problems, they must care passionately about themselves and have a good perspective with regard to their life situations. Professional helpers must be content with who they are before they can make someone else content. This fact is important because, without personal contentment, focusing on someone else's life issues becomes difficult. Professional helpers must learn to separate their personal lives from their professional lives. When this appears to not be possible, helpers must move away from the helping relationship and refer the client to someone else.

Understanding Human Behavior

To be successful in most life ventures, it is imperative that one has a well-thought-out plan of action. Similarly, to be an effective helper, one must have a basic helping plan of action supported by a theory or concept of what motivates human behavior. Recognizing inappropriate behavior is not sufficient to ensure a successful helping relationship. As a professional helper one must have a concept of what motivates inappropriate behavior as well as an understanding of what causes humans to react in the variety of ways we react.

The professional helpers must study human behavior through observations and readings to be effective and hopefully over a period of time will develop their own beliefs with regard to human behavior. Through application, helpers can refine their theory so that it is their approach to helping, not a copy of a prominent theorist and/or mentor. Once their theory is sufficiently developed, they will hopefully be able to develop effective goals and techniques that are extensions of the theory.

Understanding Resources

Knowledge of appropriate resources is one of the most important things a professional helper can possess, especially social workers, case managers, and rehabilitation counselors, to mention only three. Most clients come to a helper with specific needs and expectations. Many of those needs relate to community and other resources. Knowledge of resources and being able to connect the client with the appropriate agency or persons to supply those resources can be one of the most helpful things helpers can do for their clients. Rarely do helpers have knowledge of the variety of resources available in a large community; however, it is imperative that helpers develop a file of resources and keep the file updated. Additionally, as much as possible, helpers should keep in touch with resources so they are on a first-name basis with the potential helpers.

Understanding Family Dynamics

Most, if not all, issues for which a client needs professional assistance do not occur in a vacuum. They occur as a result of interactions with—and generally speaking will have an impact on—other people. In many cases, those who are affected are family members. Therefore, it is important that professional helpers have an understanding of family dynamics.

Understanding Cultural Differences

The professional helper must realize that for most situations there are a variety of ways to perceive those situations; therefore, there are an equal number of solutions to the situation. Thus the helper's view of the situation and subsequent ideas of how to solve the problem may not be the result the client is seeking. There may be numerous acceptable solutions to a situation, and the solution or solutions acceptable to the client may be affected by her cultural views. It is imperative that the professional helper become sensitive to cultural differences. It is impossible to know all things with regard to all cultural issues, but it is possible to be sensitive enough to allow for different ideas and patterns of thoughts other than your own. The following insightful comments by Drennan (2007) provide an excellent summary of the importance of being sensitive to cultural differences:

> An effective helper must be tolerant, knowledgeable, and equipped to assist individuals outside their own ethnic group. Each client should be regarded as an individual with a distinct history, social, and familial environment that may or may not be related to the client's reason for requesting help. Therefore, a helper must not assume a universal broad spectrum approach, but rather must adapt her helping methods to reflect the specific needs of each autonomous individual. It is essential that a helper listen and be attentive to a client's nonverbal behavior to identify problems; a dilemma that would normally be of no consequence in one culture might be considered a crisis in another.

Understanding Disabilities and Persons with Disabilities

One of the most effective ways of explaining how to interact with persons with disabilities is to take the reverse approach and explain what not to do when helping persons with disabilities.

Do not use a paternalistic attitude in assisting persons with disabilities. One of the things that has hindered the progress of effectively integrating persons with disabilities into society is the well-meaning but overprotective attitudes and actions of persons without disabilities. Many persons without disabilities, because of their lack of knowledge of the potentials, desires, and abilities of persons with disabilities, tend to either avoid contact with persons with disabilities or overcompensate and inhibit their emotional growth by trying to protect them from failing.

Do not be afraid to ask about the person's disability and how it has affected his or her life. Part of the lack of personal contact between persons with disabilities and those whom are considered as not having a disability is the fact that many persons without a disability are reluctant to get to know persons with disabilities on a more than superficial level. Part of getting to know persons with disabilities is becoming aware of their disability and some things about their life situations as a result of having a disability.

Do not express sympathy to the person for having a disability. Although it is acceptable to express sympathy to a person on the death of a family member or close friend, generally speaking, it is unacceptable to show expressions of sympathy because a person has a disability. Persons with disabilities do not need sympathy; they need understanding and assistance to overcome some of the stumbling blocks of negative attitudes and paternalistic attitudes toward their life situations.

Expressions of sympathy may make some persons with disabilities feel good temporarily, but sympathy does nothing to improve the person's self-esteem. In fact, sympathy, in the long term, lowers one's self-esteem because it has a negative impact on one's self-concept.

Do not treat the person with a disability as being a special person for having

the disability. The opposite of expressing sympathy is to praise the person for moving forward with life despite the fact that he or she has a disability. Everyone, with or without disabilities, faces obstacles and difficult times in their lives. Most people overcome their obstacles with or without professional help. Treating persons with disabilities as special tends to set them apart from other people who have overcome or learned to live with obstacles. The most important thing a professional helper can do with regard to persons with disabilities is to treat them as human beings, no better or worse than any other human.

Do not stare. If you want to know something about the person and his or her disability, ask. Curiosity is a normal trait. Therefore, it is not inappropriate to want to know the whys and hows of the situation. However, what is inappropriate is staring at people as if they are freaks of nature. Equally insulting is to move away from the people as if they had a contagious disease. Most persons with disabilities are willing to discuss their disability.

When communicating, talk directly to the person with the disability, not to the person or persons accompanying her or him. A mistake that some helping professionals make when verbally assisting persons with disabilities, particularly persons who have a hearing impairment or some mental limitation (thus they have an interpreter or someone to speak for them accompanying them) is to talk directly to the accompanying person. Even if the person with the disability cannot hear what is being said or cannot completely understand what is being said, it is appropriate and best to address comments to the client rather than to the interpreter. By doing this, you are acknowledging the person with the disability as a human being. It is inappropriate to talk directly to the accompanying person or persons, as if the client is not in the room.

Do not be afraid to say the word disability or handicap to a person with a disability. Some professional helpers avoid saying the word disability or handicap as if these words represent death or nonexistence. These are words that describe a condition of life. If the person with a disability is not in denial of his or her life condition, the uttering of these words should not place the client in a state of shock.

There is some debate with regard to whether to say disability or handicap to describe the person's condition. Some prefer the phase person with a disability, others prefer the phase person who has a handicap, and others have no preference. The thing on which most people agree is to emphasize the person rather than the disability, thus the term **person comes first**. To be more specific, say person with a disability, rather than a disabled person, or say person with a handicap rather than a handicapped person.

SUMMARY

Everyone needs assistance dealing with the myriad things we encounter at various points in our lives. Persons with disabilities are no exception. In fact, some tend to believe that persons with disabilities are in constant need of assistance, which is not true for the majority of persons with disabilities. However, when persons with disabilities do need assistance with physical, mental, and emotional issues, to mention only three, it is imperative that they receive assistance from knowledgeable, empathetic, and well-trained professional helpers. Professional helpers must walk a fine line between being helpful and being helpful to the point at which the client becomes dependent. The professional helper in the process of helping persons with disabilities must provide assistance associated with promoting independence. Promoting independence does not mean that the person with a disability must learn to take care of all his or her needs. However, the professional helper must encourage and allow the person to take care of those needs for which she has the capability to do so.

Part of the responsibility of rehabilitation professional helpers is to help boost the self-esteem of their clients/patients. Professional helpers often are looked on by the clients/patients as knowing what is best with regard to their rehabilitation. Therefore, it is the moral and professional responsibility of the helpers to not take advantage of that trust and boost their egos by doing everything for the patients, rather than help boost the patient's ego by helping them attain their maximum potential.

POINTS FOR DISCUSSION AND SUGGESTED ACTIVITIES

1. Identify the steps discussed in this chapter with regard to the establishment of goals.
2. Identify the stages of termination discussed in this chapter.
3. List at least five things you can do to become an effective helper.
4. Explain what understanding yourself means to you?
5. Explain how you think understanding human behavior will help you be an effective helper.
6. Explain how you think understanding resources will help you be an effective helper.
7. Explain how you think understanding cultural differences will help you be an effective helper.

REFERENCES

Brammer, L.M. and MacDonald, G. (2003). *The Helping Relationship: Process and Skills* (8th ed.). Boston: Allyn and Bacon.

Bryan, W.V. (2009). *The Professional Helper: The Fundamentals of Being a Professional Helper.* Springfield, IL: Charles C Thomas.

Drennan, A. (2007). *Understanding Culture.* Unpublished paper, University of Oklahoma.

Egan, G. (1994). *The Skilled Helper* (5th ed.). Pacific Grove, CA: Brooks/Cole.

Okun, B. F. (2002). *Effective Helping* (6th ed.). Pacific Grove, CA: Brooks/Cole.

SUGGESTED READINGS

Corey, G., Corey, C., and Callanan, P. (1998). *Issues and Ethics in the Helping Professions.* (4th ed.). Pacific Grove, CA: Brooks/Cole.

Fong, M.L., and Cox, B.G. (1983). Trust as an underlying dynamic in the counseling process: How clients test trust. *The Personnel and Guidance Journal,* 163–166.

Ratliff, N. (1988). Stress and burnout in the helping professions. *Social Casework: The Journal of Contemporary Social Work, 69:* 147–154.

Chapter 12

CULTURAL SENSITIVITY

Outline

- Introduction
- Culture, Race and Ethnicity
- Become Aware of the Whole Person
- Become Culturally Competent
- Disability Culture
- Disability Cultural Sensitivity
- Deaf Culture
- Summary
- Points for Discussion and Suggested Activities

Objectives

- To define what culture is
- To emphasize the importance of being culturally competent
- To emphasize that there is a disability culture
- To emphasize the importance of being sensitive to the cultures of disability
- To explain deaf culture

INTRODUCTION

Effective rehabilitation efforts for persons with disabilities require not only comprehensive and well-conceived rehabilitation plans, but also an understanding of human behavior. That is, optimum rehabilitation is based on understanding and devising treatment plans for each client. This is obvious of course, but effective helping is predicated on knowledge of human behaviors and cultural differences. As an example, with regard to racial, ethnic, and gender minorities people are consistently lumped together and categorized into "ethnic and racial" groups. Next, certain characteristics are attributed to these groups and their cultures—African American culture; Hispanic, Latino/Latina cultures; Asian culture; and American Indian culture. Moreover, interaction with them is based upon these assigned characteristics and cultural attributes, and everyone in the respective group is treated essentially the same. Categorizing individuals may never stop because it is such an easy way to define people. Despite this reality, professional rehabilitation helpers must remember that there are more differences within groups than among them. To be more specific, persons from different racial or ethnic groups reared in similar environments will have many similar attitudes, beliefs, and behaviors.

In this chapter the authors will briefly provide some definitions of culture and discuss culture from a racial and ethnic prospective. We will follow that discussion with a discussion of disability culture and provide some information with regard to effectively working with persons with disabilities as cultural groups.

CULTURE, RACE AND ETHNICITY

Defining and Dissecting Culture

A cursory review of some of the numerous definitions of culture reveals that there is no unified concept of what constitutes culture. In fact, a definition of culture will depend on the professional orientation of the describer. As an example, anthropologists, generally speaking, define culture in the context of being part of the environment humans have made, including artifacts, myths, and the special ways of perceiving the environment. Other social scientist such as Lee (1989) and Axelson (1993) add to anthropological definitions by indicating that culture is the collective reality of a group of people and it is from this collective reality that attitudes, behaviors, and values are formed and become reinforced among a group of people. Triandis (1972) stated that culture is learned through socialization rather than through an active teaching process. These and other definitions of culture led Bryan (1999) to the following definition: "Culture is commonly held characteristics such as attitudes, beliefs, values, customs and patterns of behavior possessed by a group of people, which has been learned and reinforced through a socialization process" (p. 39). From this definition several points become clear: (1) culture is learned behavior, attitudes, beliefs, and values; (2) it is learned as a result of group interaction; and (3) it is learned via socialization rather than through a formal teaching process. Because we are not born with a culture, environmental factors play the major role in our cultural development. Therefore, culture is not based on an individual's race or ethnic background; it is a product of our environment. A major reason some people appear to act and think alike is because they have been influenced by similar environmental stimuli, rather than because there is some inherent racial or ethnic cultural predisposition to do so. Bryan (2007) provides further information with regard to the composition of culture.

Humans Create Culture

As previously mentioned, culture is not inherited but is developed through a socialization process. Therefore, the premise that by classifying persons into ethnic, racial, and religious groups (to mention only three groups) and declaring that they have the same culture, thus we can explain their existence is false. There are several facts about culture that makes this belief untrue: (1) culture is influenced by proximity, (2) culture is not restricted by race or ethnicity, and (3) culture is mobile.

Regardless of ethnicity or racial background, the local social and environmental atmosphere will have an influence on a person's cultural development. Offered as an example is the fact that native New Yorkers who are black have similar mannerisms, such as speech patterns, as well as beliefs and attitudes, as native New Yorkers who are white. Blacks in the southwestern part of the United States have similar speech patterns and attitudes as white counterparts in the southwest, and these cultural differences often are strikingly different than those of blacks in the northeast part of the United States. When people move, they take with them many aspects of their current culture; however over time, being influenced by the new cultural environment, they will gradually adopt the new prevailing culture.

Each Group Develops its Own Culture

Each individual is part of many cultures and if she or he intends to be accepted by those cultures, she or he incorporates many of that group's cultural values. If the group's values are contrary to the person's values, hopefully she or he removes herself or himself from the group and associates with a group that has values, beliefs, and attitudes that are congruent with her or his cultural beliefs. Unfortunately, this does not always happen, in too many instances, to be accepted by the majority some people compromise their standards.

Everyone Has Some Degree of Ethnocentrism

Ethnocentrism is the belief that one's culture is superior to all other cultures. At first glance, to some, this statement may seem absurd; however, as we give closer and deeper thought to what is being said the truth of this statement is revealed. As Americans, most of us, out of pride in our country and belief in our system of laws and government, think that the cultures of America are superior to other cultures. Harmful ethnocentrism occurs when a group is told it is better than other groups and this message is constantly reinforced through various forms of propaganda. For example, if the group with which one associates one's cultural identity is constantly referred to as being gifted athletically and academically then over a period of time, one begins to believe the message. Pride in one's group is not bad; however, when we act upon our feelings of superiority, then our actions go beyond pride and become prejudice.

No One Knows All Things About All Cultures

In an age when most helping professionals are sincerely concerned about not being offensive to any person or group of people, much concern exists with regard to how much professionals should know about cultures other than their own. Unless a helping professional has a very limited practice, it is impossible to know about every aspect of a person's culture. Honesty is the key word in discussing cultural awareness. Being honest with oneself that one does not know and will not know all aspects of a client's culture and being honest by explaining that one does not know but is willing and interested in learning is not only important but also essential (Bryan, pp. 5–7)

BECOME AWARE OF THE WHOLE PERSON

Each environment causes people to adopt both formal and informal rules to which its members are required to adhere in order to survive. To a large extent, these environmental rules frame belief systems. As an example, if people are reared in an environment that leads them to believe in divine healing this will significantly influence their beliefs with regard to medical and rehabilitation interventions. Therefore, rehabilitation professionals must not exclusively focus on a client's race or ethnic background to understand his or her cultures. They must understand the client as a whole person who is influenced by many factors, some of which may have very little to do with race or ethnic background per se.

The issues of race, ethnicity, and culture are very difficult to address when trying to determine how helping professions should use these variables in the helping process. In attempting to determine the appropriate ways to utilize these variables in the helping process, sometimes conflicting messages are sent. On the one hand, they say that a helping professional must take into consideration a patient's or client's racial and ethnic background. By saying this, they make a strong case for treatment based on racial identity and cultural background. Bryan (1999) set forth the argument that when working with minority clients or patients, practitioners must consider the racial or ethnic backgrounds of the helpees and also their disabilities. The professional helper must not consider the person's disability to the exclusion of his or her race, or vice versa. This approach may lead one to believe that race is a major factor in the rehabilitation process. On the other hand, there is a point of view that race is an arbitrary concept. Many social scientists and biologists argue that race is an arbitrary designator (Harrison, Tanner, Pibeam & Baker, 1988; Lieberman & Jackson, 1995; Montague, 1997). Loveland (2001) explained why some scientists do not use the term race.

> Typically, racial categorization is done on the basis of appearance or stereotype, and the physical trait that is given most importance is skin color. This is so arbitrary and the variation within so-called races is so extensive that many scientists no longer use the term race. The association of specific physical traits with ethnic and racial groups is arbitrary (for example, what if height or eye color was used to define races rather than skin color?) and is not based on science, and should not be used to stereotype people in any cultural setting. Both race and ethnicity are cultural categories. If people in a particular subculture tend to speak and behave in a distinct and consistent way, it is because they learned the behavior, not because it is innate or genetically based. (p. 19)

Earlier we stated that culture does not evolve from race or ethnicity but is a product of environment. Loveland (2001) makes what we consider to be the correct observation about race and ethnicity and cultural categories. Even though most scientists believe that the only race of any significance is the human race, we persist in categorizing each other into racial and ethnic groups. It is unlikely that this behavior will be discontinued. Therefore, helping professionals will be on relatively safe ground if they consider race and ethnicity as variables that help make cultures somewhat different but not the major or sole factor in cultural development.

The essence of the authors' thoughts regarding race, ethnicity, and culture is not meant to be double-talk or psychobabble; rather, it is our attempt to give careful and considerate thought to a difficult and complicated issue. Perhaps, Bryan (1999) provides a good summary of how helping professionals should consider race and ethnicity in the helping relationship:

> As helping professionals increase their efforts to work more effectively with minority clients and patients, an understanding of factors, which have played significant roles in shaping a person and/or group's culture, is essential. An awareness of factors, which have had an impact upon a person's culture, will bring to the forefront of the helping professional mind that there is no single culture for any minority group. In other words, there is not African American culture, Native American culture, Hispanic/Latino American culture, or Asian Pacific American culture. However, there are African American cultures, etc. If the helping professional learns little about minorities other than this point he will have made significant progress in his quest to become a more effective helper of people, because being aware of individuals' within group difference will help eliminate from his mind stereotypes and prejudices. (p. 90)

To accomplish what Bryan (1999) recommends, the helper practitioner must become culturally competent. Leavitt (2001) offers some suggestions with regard to the helping professional's becoming culturally competent. The culturally competent practitioner must:

1. Have the capacity for cultural self-assessment. Practitioners must recognize the immense influence of culture and be able to assess the effect it has on their own and other people's life views and actions.
2. Value diversity, with an awareness, acceptance, and even celebration of differences in life view, health systems, communication styles and other life sustaining elements.
3. Be conscious of the dynamics of difference. With cultural interaction comes the possibility of misjudging the other's intentions and actions. One must be vigilant to minimize misperceptions, misinterpretations and misjudgment.
4. Institutionalize cultural knowledge. Cultural knowledge must be accessed and incorporated into the delivery of services. It is impossible, and not necessary, to learn all there is to know about all cultural sub-groups, but clinicians must be aware of the ethnographic information related to the community and relevant beliefs and behaviors of their clients and theirs clients' families.
5. Adapt to diversity. A system is adapted to create a better fit between the needs of the people requiring services and those facilitating the process, which can meet the needs. (p. 20)

Certainly becoming culturally knowledgeable and competent are as important as becoming knowledgeable and competent in rehabilitation theories, techniques, and human behaviors. In fact, a thorough understanding of cultures will be invaluable in understanding theories, techniques, and human behavior.

Davila (1995) stated that in the past, persons with disabilities were viewed one-dimensionally; that is, they were seen only in terms of their disability. The result has been a disregard of their other needs. To avoid this mistake, Davila cautions practitioners to recognize persons with disabilities from all backgrounds, to ensure that all their human rights concerns are placed on the national agenda, and to provide persons with disabilities with the skills and knowledge they need to succeed in life.

DISABILITY CULTURE

There are differing opinions with regard to whether there is a disability culture. If one views culture from an anthropological standpoint, one might conclude that there is no disability culture. This assumption may be rooted in the theory that persons with disabilities are part of every ethnic and racial and each gender group; therefore, their cultural identity is related to the previously mentioned groups. In part, this is a true assumption. However, the assumption does not take into consideration some of the social discrimination, isolation, and disregard that many persons with disabilities experience, often on a daily basis that nondisabled persons do not experience. Therefore, most persons with disabilities receive similar treatment and must overcome similar obstacles to their pursuit of independence and self-determination. Barnes and Mercer (2007) hypothesize that "disability presumes a sense of common identity and interest that unite disable people and separate them from their non-disabled counterparts."

In the following comments, Bryan (1999) summarizes his point of view with regard to whether there is a disability culture.

> While it is true that persons with disabilities as a group do not have a mother language that distinguishes them from other groups and thousands of years into the future archeologists will not unearth artifacts that relate to a society of disable persons; however, persons with disabilities have experienced not only within America, but throughout the world, treatment and attitudes that have cause them to be treated differently than the so-called "non-disabled." Both society-at-large and persons with disabilities have been socialized to think of persons with disabilities as being different from others. People with disabilities have a long and unique history as a group of people. The reality is that a person with a disability has more in common with his "non-disabled" neighbors than he does with another person with a disability; he nevertheless is perceived to have a common bond with other persons with disabilities and as a result have been classified and characterized as being part of a different and unique group of people. (p. 42)

To base one's opinion of persons with disabilities as not having a disability culture because they are part of other cultural groups would be similar to disregarding women as being in a cultural group of their own because they are part of each ethnic and racial group. Dismissing women as a cultural group would also disregard the fact that women through out the world have been and continue to be discriminated against based on their gender. Therefore it is the conclusion of these authors that there is a disability culture. In the remainder of this chapter we will discuss in general terms disability culture and will also discuss a disability subculture–the deaf culture.

DISABILITY CULTURAL SENSITIVITY

When discussing interacting with persons of different ethnic, racial, and/or gender backgrounds we generally refer to the approach as cultural sensitivity. When discussing appropriate ways of interacting with persons with disabilities the term often used is disability etiquette; however, we are calling the approaches disability cultural sensitivity.

The first and perhaps most important approach when working with and/or encountering persons with a disability is to **treat them as human beings**. Stated in other terms, do not treat them as a different type human. Do not avoid interacting with them because of their disability. Do not patronize them with false comments of how brave and courageous they are. One should realize that everyone, disabled or nondisabled, has some limitations. Many persons with disabilities have visible limitations; because they are interacting in society does not make them any braver or more courageous than any other person.

An equally important point to make with regard to disability cultural sensitivity is to **be aware of terminology used** to identify persons with disabilities. One may be inclined to think that in the twenty-first century we have as a society banished from our vocabulary derogatory words such as idiots, freaks, morons, retards, gimps, cripples, lame brains, and numerous other useless and insensitive words used to describe persons with disabilities. The fact is that some, if not all, of these words remain in the vocabulary of some uninformed and inadequately sensitive persons. These persons may not use the terms when speaking to a person with a visible disability but may do so during what the person may consider as safe conversations, such as with family members and friends. Similar to most racial or ethnic bigots who will not use epithets when talking with a racial or ethnic person, likewise the uninformed and insensitive nondisabled person will not utter the derogatory disability words to a person with a disability. However, the fact that these words remain part of the person's vocabulary indicates not only insensitivity but also a lack of respect for the human rights of persons with disabilities.

A very important point to remember with regard to communicating with and about persons with disabilities is to follow the rule that disability advocates have promoted for a number of years and that is to **emphasize the person before the disability**. As we have done in this text, we refer to **persons with a disability** rather than disabled persons. The point being made is that the person is more important than his or her condition. Some may think that this is a minor difference; from a human rights standpoint, however, this is a major difference. We should always consider the person as being more important than his or her condition. Very few people, if any, would prefer to be known for their limitations rather than their humanity.

Do not stare when meeting a person with a visible disability. This point is somewhat tricky in that it is human nature to be curious when experiencing something that one does not experience on a daily or regular basis. It is natural to want to satisfy one's curiosity. On the other side of this situation, one should not act as though the person does not exist by trying so hard to not appear curious that you avoid looking at the person. The answer to this complex dilemma leads to the next point.

Do not be afraid to ask a person with a disability questions with regard to his or her disability. Most persons with disabilities are not ashamed of their disability and are willing to talk about the same. In fact most persons with disabilities prefer that if you have questions you ask them. Discussing the disability allows the person with the disability and you to get that part of the interaction completed so that all concerned can move onto other discussions. Thus the normal human interactions can proceed without fear of either party offending the other party. Most persons with disabilities are sensitive to nondisabled persons' body language and can easily identify when the nondisabled person is uncomfortable and/or curious; therefore, as previously stated, it is best to address curiosity early so that other human relations can effectively proceed.

When encountering persons with a disability and you, as a nondisabled person think the person needs help in accomplishing a task, **do not be aggressive and begin to help without asking if the person needs assistance**. If the person says that he or she would like to have assistance, you should ask how you can assist. As an example, do not assume because a person appears to be blind or has a visual disability that he or she needs assistance crossing a busy street. The answer is to ask and if the person says yes ask how can you assist him or her. Do not grab the person by the arm and rush him or her across the street. If the person says no, do not feel insulted. In most cases, the person probably is very experienced at being independent, the refusal of assistance is based on not needing assistance.

Do not be afraid to interact with a person with a disability because you are afraid that you will make a mistake in the conversation and "say the wrong thing." If you make a mistake it is not going to be the ending of the world. Most persons with disabilities are not so sensitive and fragile that a few misplaced words or inquiries are going to emotionally destroy them. If you make a mistake, apologize by pointing out that you did not intend to be offensive. Most persons with disabilities are aware that every conversation is not going to be prefect, and when imperfection in the conversation occurs they will correct you if they feel correction is important to the conversation or they may overlook the mistake. When one considers the many conversations or interactions one has with nondisabled persons one realizes that not all of those conversations are flawless and in most cases the mistakes made do not end the conversation or the friendship.

A mistake too frequently made when communicating with persons with a disability who have someone accompanying them either as a friend or as an interpreter is to speak directly to the person accompanying the person with the disability rather than speaking directly to the person with the disability. If the conversation is with or about the person with the disability, it is rude to avoid speaking to the person with the disability. Even if the person with the disability has a hearing disability comments should be directed to him or her. Think about how you would feel if someone were talking about you but directing the conversation to a third party. Unfortunately, too often, this is done when the person with the disability has a mental and/or emotional disability. Also, this mode of communication is frequently used when speaking to an elderly person. When this type of communication occurs it has a tendency to make the person with the disability feel irrelevant—a nonbeing.

When communicating with a person who has a hearing disability, do not yell. Let the person take the lead by indicating to you how she or he would like to receive communication, for example, lip reading, sign language, or written notes. Obviously, if you do not know sign language, you must communicate that to the person. This can be done by simply writing a note to the person. If the person indicates that she or he reads lips, you should directly face the person and maintain eye contact and make sure that nothing is obstructing the view of your lips. If the person has partial hearing, maintain a constant vocal level of your voice as much as possible. Also be aware of any background noises and try to eliminate such distractions.

When communicating with a person who has a visual disability, especially if the person is legally blind, remember that there are various levels of blindness. Legally blind is 20 over 200, which means the person has some vision. Therefore it is important to be aware of the level of vision the person has. The best way to determine the level of vision is to ask. Most persons with visual disabilities will not be offended. In fact, most will be glad you asked so that appropriate interaction can occur. If the person is without vision or her or his vision is to the point she or he cannot identify human faces and other objects, when speaking with this person, first identify yourself, do not begin talking without identifying who you are. To avoid having the person talking to empty space, when you move inform the person that you have moved and where you are. When the conversation has ended, excuse yourself.

When interacting with persons with disabilities who have mobility and other type of helping devices, be respectful of the devices. Do not pet the dog belonging to a person with a visual disability or any other service animal. The service animal is not a pet; it is there to assist the person with the disability. Likewise, do not touch or ask to examine the person's mobility device, such as a wheelchair, cane or mobility aid. Although these may be items of curiosity to you, they are personal items for the person with a disability, thus you should treat the items with respect, as you treat the person with the disability with respect.

A final point we wish to make is to not be afraid to ask questions of persons with disabilities. As previously stated, most persons with disabilities are not so emotionally fragile that any questions you ask will destroy their hold on reality. If you are asking reasonable questions that cause a person with a disability to become emotionally upset, generally speaking, it was not the question that caused the problem; other problems exist that have nothing to do with the question you asked. The reality is that most persons with disabilities prefer that you ask any questions you may have with regard to their disability. By asking your questions and receiving an answer, you and the person can progress to other areas of conversation. Words of advice with regard to asking questions; unless you are in a therapeutic setting or asking questions to complete a project, do not devote your entire conversation to questions about the person's disability. Remember the person is more than the disability.

There are many more tips with regard to being disability culturally sensitive. Every state has an agency or agencies as well as private organizations that publish information with regard to disability etiquette. The reader is directed to those resources for additional information. Next we will discuss what some consider a disability subculture.

DEAF CULTURE

As previously discussed, defining what constitutes culture is a difficult undertaking. Understanding why some choose some aspect of culture as opposed to another is equally challenging. Persons who are deaf or have severe hearing impairments are examples of cultural choices that represent difficult decisions that have to be made. To be more specific, over significant periods of time there have been major improvements in technology designed to assist persons who have difficulties hearing. Miniaturization of electronic hearing aids as well as miniaturization and improvement in the lasting power of batteries used in hearing aids have revolutionized hearing aid devices and made them more comfortable and practical to use. Additionally, the development of the cochlear implant device that bypasses damaged portions of the ear and sends electrical impulses directly to the auditory nerve has provided improved hearing for thousands of persons.

The cultural choice to which we previously alluded is that some persons with severe hearing impairment make the choice, for themselves or for their children, to either use a hearing device such as those previously mentioned or not to use such a device. For those persons who choose or have chosen for them not to use any technological hearing device, their mode of communication is, generally speaking, through sign language. In America, it is called American Sign Language (ASL). From the vantage point of some deaf persons, this means that they have a language of their own. Additionally, this allows them to socialize together and share many of the same things that nondeaf persons as well as deaf persons who use technological devices enjoy. Cartwright (2010) helps us understand components that compose the deaf culture.

> The hearing culture have a shared communication mode, oral speech; they have shared traditions of music appreciation; they share the sense of hearing and all it entails. Nonhearing individuals of the deaf community also share a culture. They do not consider themselves to be impaired; they consider themselves different in that they do not have the sense of hearing. They have a mode of communication, sign language. In the United States the official language of the deaf community is American Sign Language (ASL). They have shared experiences; sometimes those

include life at a school for the deaf. The deaf community value system favors the well being of the group over individual justification. The deaf also pass their traditions on to the next generation, but in an untraditional manner. Over 90 percent of deaf children are born to hearing parents. If hearing parents allow their deaf children to become part of the deaf community then those traditions are passed on to the children. When deaf children are born to deaf parents their membership in the community is automatic. More importantly, deaf individuals acknowledge themselves as having a culture and being members of that culture.

Moore and Levitan (2003) provide the following explanation of deaf culture: "Deaf culture is social, communal, and creative force of, by, and for deaf people base on ASL. It encompasses communication, social protocol, art, entertainment, recreation (e.g., sports, travel and deaf clubs), and (to a point) worship" (p. 325) Lane, Hoffmeister, and Bohan (1996) further explain deaf culture: "For unlike other cultures, deaf culture is not associated with a single place, a native land; rather, it is a culture based on relationships among people for whom a number of places and associations may provide a common ground" (p. 5).

In further explaining deaf culture, Lane and associates inform us that there are deaf clubs, and they are tiny reservations of deaf culture where deaf people govern, socialize and communicate fluently in ASL" (p. 127). Within the world of the deaf club the deaf and their families are free to share their community aspiration away from the hearing culture.

Cartwright (2010) provides some examples of nondeaf culture social norms and corresponding deaf culture social norms. Social norms dictate that it is impolite to stare; for persons who receive most of their cues visually, staring in deaf culture is paying attention. Social norms dictate it is impolite to point; the deaf point. A hearing person would signal with a look or a nod, but deaf people point as part of signifying the object or person. Social norms dictate that if people are having a conversation in an area through which another person needs to pass, that person should stop and ask permission to interrupt and pass through; deaf culture dictates that the person should just pass through so as not to interrupt the conversation. If the person stops to ask permission to pass through, he or she is being rude. Social norms dictate that unless one is intimately familiar with another person there is a distance of personal space that should not be invaded. Deaf culture dictates that it is sociably acceptable to tap a person on the shoulder to get his or her attention no matter how familiar one is to the other; this is for communication reasons. Social norms allow, but rarely encourage, a person to interrupt another during communication. Deaf culture greatly discourages this behavior, if one wish to say something he or she waits until the speaker has signaled he or she has finished speaking. Social norms for the hearing dictate that personal questions are not asked of people one just met. Deaf culture is very direct; therefore, members ask questions to which they want answers.

SUMMARY

To be successful with regard to giving all of its citizens opportunities to participate in the daily activities of its society, the society must be open to and accepting of cultural differences. Part of accepting cultural differences is to recognize that each person has many cultures that contribute to his or her personality. When we stereotype people and use those stereotypes to place them into certain groups based on erroneous concepts and beliefs, not only do we perpetuate an injustice upon the individual but also as a society we stifle potential valuable contributions the person could make to society.

Persons with disabilities are part of every ethnic and racial and gender group; thus, their cultural identity is often associated with the previously mentioned group or groups. The reality is that disability culture does exist, and this culture is an important part of the composition of persons with disabilities. To be more specific, the discrimination, neglect, and paternalistic treatments that many persons with disabilities experience have an impact on the psychological and emotional well-being of those who experience the treatment. Therefore, as a society, it is very important that everyone recognize the impact some of the previously mentioned cultural traits have on the daily lives of persons with disabilities. It is incumbent on each of us to be aware of how we interact with persons with disabilities, so that we do not help create poor self-esteem for them.

POINTS FOR DISCUSSION AND SUGGESTED ACTIVITIES

1. What is your definition of culture?
2. Do you believe that there is a disability culture? Explain your belief.
3. What are your opinions of deaf culture?
4. What can you do to become more sensitive to the needs of persons with disabilities?

REFERENCES

Axelson, J.A. (1993). *Counseling and Development in a Multicultural Society* (2nd ed.). Pacific Grove, CA. Brooks/Cole.

Barnes, C. and Mercer, G. (2007) Disability culture: Assimilation or inclusion? In G.L. Albrecht, K.D. Seelman, and M. Bury (Eds.), *Handbook of Disability Studies*. Thousand Oaks, CA: Sage.

Bryan, W.V. (2007). *Multicultural Aspects of Disabilities* (2nd ed.). Springfield, IL: Charles C Thomas.

Bryan, W.V. (1999). *Multicultural Aspects of Disabilities*. Springfield, IL: Charles C Thomas.

Cartwright, L. (2010). *Being Deaf in the Hearing World*. Unpublished paper. University of Oklahoma.

Davila, R.R. (1995). *Leadership for a New Era: Disability and Diversity: New Leadership for a New Era*. President's Committee on Employment of People with Disabilities.

Harrison, G., Tanner, J., Pibeam, D., and Baker, P. (1998). *Human Biology* (3rd ed.). Oxford: Oxford University Press.

Lane, H., Hoffmeister, R., and Bohan, B. (1966). *A Journey Into the Deaf-World*. San Diego, CA: Dawn Sign Press.

Leavitt, R. (Ed.). (2001). *Introduction to Cross Cultural Rehabilitation: An International Perspective*. London: W. B. Saunders.

Lee, C.C. (1989). Multicultural counseling: New direction for counseling professionals. *Virginia Counselors Journal, 17*: 3–8.

Lieberman, L., and Jackson, F. (1995). Race and three models of human origin. *American Anthropologist, 97*: 231–242

Loveland, C. (2001). The concept of culture. In R. L. Leavitt (Ed.), *Cross-Cultural Rehabilitation: An International Perspective*. London: W. B. Saunders.

Montague, A. (1997). *Man's Most Dangerous Myth: The Fallacy of Race*. Walnut Creek, CA. AltaMira.

Moore, M.S., and Levitan, L. (2003). *For Hearing People Only* (3rd ed.). New York: Deaf Life Press.

Triandis, H.C. (1972). *The Analysis of Subjective Culture*. New York: John Wiley.

SUGGESTED READING

Allport, G. (1958). *The Nature of Predjudice.* New York: Doubleday/Anchor Books.

Betancourt, H., and Lopez, S.R. (1993). The study of culture, ethnicity and race in American psychology. *American Psychologist, June,* 629–636.

Gellman, W. (1959). Roots of prejudice against the handicapped. *Journal of Rehabilitation, 40:* 4–6.

Pape, D.A., Walker, G.R., and Quinn, F.H. (1983). Ethnicity and disability: Two minority statuses. *Journal of Applied Rehabilitation Counseling, 14,*(4): 18–23.

Roeher, G.A. (1966). Significance of public attitudes on the rehabilitation of the disabled. *Rehabilitation Literature, 22*: 66–72.

Walker, S., Orange, C., and Rackley, R. (1993). A formidable challenge: The preparation of minority personnel. *Journal of Vocational Rehabilitation, 2,* (1): 46–53.

Part 4

PSYCHOSOCIAL ISSUES

Chapter 13

HUMAN RIGHTS FOR ALL

Outline

- Introduction
- Protecting the Human Rights of Persons with Disabilities
- Mental Health Human Rights Pioneers
- New Considerations of Human Rights for Some Persons with Mental and Emotional Disabilities
- Employment–A Human Right for Persons with Severe Disabilities
- Helping–Part of the Solution
- Summary
- Points for Discussion and Suggested Activities

Objectives

- To emphasize that the human rights of some persons with disabilities have improved in the United States and some other developed countries.
- To emphasize that the human rights of some persons with severe disabilities have not improved much as persons with less severe disabilities.
- To emphasize how innovations in employment has improved the human rights of some persons with disabilities.
- To emphasize how professional helpers can help persons with disabilities obtain and maintain their human rights.

INTRODUCTION

In 1948, the United Nations Declaration of Human Rights affirmed the "equal and inalienable rights of all members of the human family." Specifically concerning people with disabilities, this principle of human rights is applicable to medical, psychological, sociological, and economic well-being. A relevant question is what is meant by inalienable rights of humans? The authors of this book believe a succinct answer is that it means the opportunity to develop to one's maximum potential. Most goal-oriented individuals seek to obtain the knowledge and skills to reach what the noted psychotherapist Alfred Adler called the ideal self. In the not too distance past, some nondisabled persons, and to a lesser degree some of the current generation of nondisabled people, developed attitudinal barriers that became restrictions and stumbling blocks for persons with disabilities' achieving their full complements of human rights.

Bickenbach (2001) provides us with additional information with regard to the United Nations' position on human rights for persons with disabilities:

> The evolution of recognizing human rights for persons with disabilities by the United Nations exemplifies a different development of disabil-

ity rights. After World War II, the United Nations sought to promote the rights of persons with disabilities by assisting governments in improving social welfare programs, particularly rehabilitation and training. Then, in direct response to initiatives from within the community of persons with disabilities in the 1960s, the United Nations initiatives embraced the notion of human rights for persons with disabilities, their full participation in all areas of society through an equalization of opportunities. In 1971, the General Assembly adopted the Declaration on the Rights of Mental Retarded Persons as the first international statement of disability human rights. This was followed in 1975 by the more inclusive rights document, the Declaration on the Rights of Disabled Persons. This proclaims the equal civil and political rights of persons with disabilities around the world and sets the standard for equal treatment and access to services to further social integration. (p. 573)

Although some paternalistic attitudes continue to exist, for a variety of reasons, which have been discussed in this book, attitudes toward persons with disabilities are changing and becoming more realistic with regard to the desires and capabilities of most persons with disabilities. Because of the improved attitudes of the nondisabled toward persons with disabilities, as well as persons with disabilities having pride in themselves and legislative actions guaranteeing and protecting the rights of persons with disabilities, many persons with disabilities are enjoying greater freedoms and improved living conditions in the United States and a number of other human rights–oriented countries. Despite the progress that has been made with regard to improved human relationships between the nondisabled and persons with disabilities and the nation's increased dedication to equality of human rights for all of its citizens, there can be no question that within the United States there still are areas that need improvement. Throughout this book we have discussed the need for better access for persons with disabilities to gainful employment. The fact that currently, at a minimum, one third of persons with disabilities are unemployed and approximately two thirds are underemployed speaks poorly for a nation with the resources of the United States. One method that has been used effectively to enhance the chances of protecting and highlighting human rights is the passage and enactment of legislation that mandates fair and equal treatment of disenfranchised populations. Within the United States, antidiscrimination legislation to ensure women's rights, civil rights for ethnic and racial minorities, and disability legislation are only three examples of human rights legislation that have been successful in providing increased opportunities and to a great extent transformed many people's attitudes with regard to the rights of persons targeted by the legislation.

Bickenbach (2001) takes a two-pronged approach in explaining antidiscrimination legislation and how such legislation affects persons with disabilities.

First, antidiscrimination legislation takes pains to identify the difference between discriminatory and non discriminatory unequal treatment. The key to this distinction resides in a formula that has gained acceptance wherever antidiscrimination law applicable to disability is in effect. If an individual with a disability is treated differently for reasons that relate to the disability, that is discrimination if it can be argued that there is no reasonable way of accommodating the difference that the disability creates so as to allow equal participation.

Second, by its nature, antidiscrimination legislation is primary reactive and complaint driven. That is, the legislation seeks to protect human rights by giving people a legal tool to use when they feel that their rights to equal participation and equal respect are being infringed. Antidiscrimination is individualistic legislation since the onus is on the individual to take the initiative to use the power it provides. It is assumed that, if they are given the legal mechanism for doing so, people will identify discrimination and take the necessary steps to redress it. (p. 569)

As previously stated, improvements have been made and continue to be made with regard to equalization of human rights for persons with disabilities within the United States. Considerable credit for the changes can be given to grassroots movements of persons with disabilities and their advocates that have led to the United States Congress passing legislation that is designed to make society's goods and services available and accessible to persons with disabilities. Three pieces of legislation we refer to as the three legislative pillars that support the human rights of all persons with disabilities in the United States: 1973 Rehabilitation Act, the Americans with Disabilities Act and its 2008 Amendments, and the Individuals Disability Education Act. The centerpiece of the 1973 Rehabilitation Act as it relates to human rights for persons with disabilities is Section 504, which states "no otherwise qualified handicapped individual shall, solely by reason of his handicap be discriminated against in any program or activity receiving federal financial assistance." Similarly, the ADA and its amendments prohibit discrimination against persons with disability in the following five areas listed in the act: employment, access to public services, access to public accommodations, access to telecommunication relay services, and access to a variety of other services such as access to public recreational facilities. The IDEA ensures children with disabilities have access to appropriate education in the least restrictive environment. As a result of America's leadership in these areas of human rights Bickenbach (2001) points out that similar pieces of legislation have been enacted in several countries including Australia (Disability Discrimination Act, 1992), United Kingdom (Disability Discrimination Act, 1995), New Zealand (Human Rights Act, 1993), India (Disabled Persons Act), Israel (Disabled Persons Act 1998), and Canada (Human Rights Act) (p. 569).

Arguably, persons with physical disabilities, to be more specific persons with nonsevere disabilities, have been the biggest beneficiaries of the changing attitudes toward persons with disabilities. The less severe and less visible a person's disability, the better his or her chances of being accepted by the nondisabled, and a result of this acceptance is decreased discrimination based on the disability. Currently, and unfortunately, a group of people with disabilities that continues to experience significant discrimination and, to some extent, denial of their human rights are persons with mental and emotional disabilities. In previous years, and to some extent today, persons with mental and emotional disabilities who were unable to remain with their families were placed in institutions. Today there is a movement within some states of the United States to deinstitutionalize persons with mental and emotional disabilities and place them in various types of facilities within communities. At this point in the discussion of care of persons with mental and emotional disabilities it is appropriate to discuss the history of institutional care as well as the deinstitutionalization movement. Also we will discuss possible implications of deinstitutionalization.

Prior to the development of state-operated mental institutions, persons with mental and/or emotional disabilities received arguably the worst treatment by society of any persons with disabilities. In some instances, they were thought, by some segments of society, to be mentally and emotionally like animals and were treated accordingly. Some uninformed persons believed that persons with mental and emotional disabilities had no feelings or that intellectually they were incapable of experiencing mental and physical pain, joy, and other human emotions; therefore, society was justified in inflicting pain and placing these persons in inhumane and disgusting living conditions.

As one reviews information with regard to those who have championed the rights of persons with mental and emotional disabilities two names emerge: Dorothea Dix and Clifford Beers. Dix began her crusade for more humane treatment of persons with mental and emotional illness in the mid-1800s. As previously stated, the living conditions prior to and during the 1800s for most persons with mental illness including intellectual disabilities were deplorable. During most of the 1800s Americans who were considered to be mentally ill were placed in prisons, jails, and almshouses, where they were subjected to beatings, chained to walls and/or the floor, and left in cold damp rooms with little if any clothing. At best, that condition could be described as custodial care because little if any effort was put forth to cure or treat them professionally and humanely. Pelka (1997) provides a vivid description of the living conditions that Dix observed:

> Americans with mental illness or mental retardation were incarcerated in prisons, jails and poorhouses. Others were turned over to private individuals who would provide food and accommodations for a fee. In almost all cases the treatment ranged from callous neglect to outright physical sexual torture. The treatment was made worse by the common myths of the time that mental illness and mental retardation were God's punishment for sin and that people who were mentally disabled were impervious to pain, cold and hunger. (p. 107)

Dix began her advocacy efforts by reviewing the living conditions of many of the jails, almshouses, and prisons in the state of Massachusetts. She presented the results of her efforts to the political leaders of the state of Massachusetts. According to Pelka (1997), Dix pressed the power structure of Massachusetts to discontinue the jailing of persons with mental illness and to develop instead a system of mental institutions.

Dix expanded her efforts by encouraging other states to abandon the practice of incarcerating persons considered to have a mental disability and replace this practice with placing them in mental institutions. Pelka (1997) informs us that in 1854 Dix convinced some U. S. institutions to care for persons with mental disabilities as well as people who were deaf, mute, or blind. The bill, however, was vetoed by President Franklin Pierce because he believed the care of persons with disabilities was the responsibility of the states, not the federal government. Despite this defeat, Dix's efforts remain as remarkable accomplishments, especially as one considers two facts: one, the negative attitudes and beliefs society held about mentally ill persons, and two, the fact that Dix was a woman. One must remember that in the 1800s women did not have many rights especially in the area of politics—women did not gain voting rights until 1920.

As we review the recent efforts to deinstitutionalize persons with mental disabilities and the reasons for those efforts, Dix's crusade and accomplishments may begin to pale in some persons' eyes. However, as we contemplate Dix's contributions, we should take into consideration that the establishment of institutions, at that time, represented forward steps. Although, as we now know, in some instances, the treatment that patients received in a mental institution was not much different than what they received when being placed in jail. In contrast, medical and psychological treatment did occur for some patients. Finally, we must always remember that Dix's primary goal was humane treatment for persons with mental disabilities (Bryan, 2001).

Clifford Beers, similar to Dorothea Dix, advocated for humane treatment of persons with mental disabilities. Whereas Dix's primary efforts were to improve the living conditions, Beers' primary efforts were to provide competent professional psychological treatment of mental patients.

Beers was born in New Haven, Connecticut, and was educated at Yale University. He began to display signs of having a mental disability in his early twenties. He eventually attempted suicide and was placed in a mental institution. While a resident of the mental institution, Beers observed the deplorable treatment of the patients, many of whom were treated similarly to what Dix observed some sixty years earlier. Beers observed physical and sexual abuse as well as neglect, and he began to maintain a record of what was occurring at his institution. The information that he maintained became the foundation of his book, *A Mind That Found Itself* (1908).

After being released from the mental institution, Beers used his book and the information he had obtained from his stay in the institution, to advocate for professional psychological treatment of mental patients. He and some of his family members established the Connecticut Committee for Mental Hygiene. Clifford Beers' tireless efforts resulted in the establishment of Mental Hygiene Committees in many American states, as well as some foreign countries.

Pelka's (1997) research emphasizes the influence of Clifford Beers' efforts.

> After 1918, the national Committee for Mental Hygiene, together with American Legion, pushed the federal government into providing psychiatric care for World War I veterans suffering from "shell shock"—now know as post-traumatic stress disorder. In the 1920s, the committee began a campaign for the founding of children's community mental health (or "child guidance") clinics. By 1937, there were 631 such clinics across the country. The most significant legislative achievement of the committee was the passage of the National Mental Health Act of 1946, which dramatically increased the availability of federal funding for mental health programs. (p. 40).

Perhaps the lasting tribute to the accomplishments of Clifford Beers was the merging of several mental health organizations in 1950, including the one Beers helped establish, the National Committee for Mental Hygiene to form the National Association for Mental Health (Bryan, 2001)

Without doubt the efforts of Dorothea Dix and Clifford Beers improved the lives and living conditions of thousands of persons with mental and emotional disabilities. As the short biography of the accomplishments of Dix and Beers reveals they were able to get mental institutions built. Additionally, they helped improve living conditions for persons with mental and emotional disabilities. This without question was an improvement in the human rights of persons with mental and emotional disabilities. Unfortunately, in the decades that have passed since the two mental health pioneer advocates put forth their exemplary works, the living conditions at many mental institutions have deteriorated. Some have referred to mental institutions of the twentieth century as "warehousing of patients." Overcrowding, lack of mental and emotional stimulation, lack of physical activities, and improper and sometimes abusive punishment describe the living conditions of some mental and emotional patients being warehoused. Because of the previously mentioned condition in which many mentally and emotionally disabled persons were living during the twentieth century, family members of persons with mental and emotional disabilities and their advocates as well as some inhabitants of these mental institutions began to push for relocation of patients from mental institutions to facilities within communities, where they could be part of a community and engage in appropriate employment as well as community activities. Because of this push, several states have closed all or most of their mental institutions, preferring to have the former patients living in community-based group homes. Griffin (2010) succinctly summarizes the evolution of institutional mental and emotional care in the United States:

> The evolution that has occurred in the area of care and treatment for persons with developmental disabilities in modern history is remarkable. Within the span of a few hundred years society has moved from perceiving these persons as mad or possessed by demons to the general recognition that all individuals have the fundamental rights of self-determination and human dignity. Advances in the available residential options for those with developmental disabilities are similarly impressive. Once hidden away in attics or bedrooms and later relegated to huge impersonal institutions, many individuals with developmental disabilities now live in ordinary residential neighborhoods across America. (p. 3)

For a large portion of the mentally and emotionally disabled population placement in community-based group homes has represented increased freedom and increased opportunities to return to the mainstream of American life. Unfortunately, for others the transition from institutions to community-based housing has not meet their needs. James Griffin (2010) explains why some persons with mental and emotional disabilities have not been as blessed by the movement to community-based housing: "Amid this transition and advancement there is another, less visible, population of individuals, often with more severe mental and physical limitations, whose care and quality of life has been negatively affected by the push for universal community care." He continues by explaining "in community based group homes, it is frequently impossible to meet the often extensive medical needs required by this group of patients" (pp. 3–4). In addition to an inability to meet medical needs, too often these patients as well as other patients who have mental and emotional disabilities are difficult to place in any kind of employment, not to mention gainful employment. As previously mentioned in this book, within the United States, at almost any time period, at least 30 percent of persons with disabilities are unemployed. Many of the persons with mental and emotional disabilities are classified as severely disabled and within that classification the unemployment increases to more than 60 percent.

Employment is a basic and important human right in the United States, as well as many other industrialized countries. For persons who want to be employed but for reasons beyond their control cannot secure employment, considerable self-esteem is lost. Likewise, to be employed in a job that is not emotionally rewarding and does not provide enough financial benefits to meet many basic needs is demoralizing.

There are many reasons for some of the severely mentally, emotionally, and physically disabled persons being either unemployed or underemployed; some are the negative attitudes of some employers, as well as lack of confidence on the part of the unemployed persons with disabilities. Fortunately, there are at least two types of programs that specialize in providing employment opportunities for persons with disabilities who have difficulties in securing employment: sheltered workshops and supported employment. These two programs are important from the standpoint of assisting persons with disabilities obtain and maintain their human rights.

Sheltered workshops have been around for many years, providing employment, training, and other rehabilitation services to persons with disabilities. As the name implies, sheltered workshops were initially established to provide protected employment for some persons with disabilities. Due to the severity and/or nature of the disability, some individuals with disabilities were unable to secure gainful employment in private industry; therefore, these workshops were established. In 1837, the first sheltered workshop for persons with disabilities was established. The Perkins Institute of Boston trained people who were blind so they could work in the community. Toward the end of the nineteenth century, a group of women from Cleveland, Ohio, known as the Sunbeam Circle, made and sold handiwork and used the profits to help Cleveland's children with disabilities.

Other well-known private organizations that had or later developed sheltered workshops began during this period. The Salvation Army began in 1878 in England and expanded to the United States in 1880. In 1902, the Goodwill Industries was organized in the United States by Edgar J. Helms, a Methodist minister. The early history of sheltered workshops indicates it was primarily individual religious or social groups that instituted major efforts to get persons with disabilities employment.

Today, there are many types of sheltered workshops, most organized locally and funded from a variety of sources, including community contributions, contracts, grants, church missionary support and, federal and state support. Many of these workshops are exempt from paying minimum wages because, in some instances, the productivity level of the persons employed is considered to be below industry standards. Some sheltered workshops use "piecemeal" method as one way of employing persons with severe disabilities. Piecemeal refers to paying the individuals for the number (pieces) of items assembled or completed. Others may use a form of supported employment to fulfill work contracts they have obtained. Most sheltered workshops make available a variety of jobs to their clients/employees. In addition to employment, many sheltered workshops provide training, in some cases to help the individuals perform their workshop jobs better. In other instances, the training is designed to help the individuals prepare for work outside the sheltered environment.

In past years, some sheltered workshops employed persons with disabilities in menial tasks, training them in areas with few chances of securing employment in the private sector (Bryan, 1996). Today, some sheltered workshops have taken a progressive approach to employment opportunities by structuring their training to the local market needs. In addition, some sheltered workshops aggressively seek and successfully compete with the private sector for employment contracts. The successful completion of these contracts is proving to private and public industry that persons with disabilities can perform job tasks as efficiently as their nondisabled counterparts. This success has also improved the economic status of the sheltered workshop employees because their performance warrants it, and they have received at least minimum wage. In some instances, they are paid according to industry standards. In addition to providing meaningful employment, the progressive workshops have begun to provide employment training, commonly called work adjustment training. This is designed to teach good work habits such as punctuality, cooperation, interpersonal relations skills, communication, and effective listening skills to mention a few. The ultimate objective is to prepare the individual for employment outside the sheltered workshop environment. The success of these individuals is very important to helping change attitudes about the employability of persons with disabilities, especially those with disabilities that are considered severe.

In the past, and to a lesser extent today, some sheltered workshops have been criticized for low pay, inadequate training, and work that does not lead to employment outside the sheltered environment. Although in some instances this criticism is warranted, however for some workshops this is unfair criticism. Many of these sheltered workshops operate on a very limited budget and work with individuals who have limited skills and/or limited abilities to utilized skills they may have possessed prior to their disability. Furthermore, we must keep in mind that for some individuals this is the only employment they will be able to obtain. An important point that is too often overlooked when evaluating the usefulness of sheltered workshops is the fact that they are helping some persons with disabilities retain and, in some instances, regain their dignity and feeling of self-worth.

Supported employment is defined as work performed on a full- or part-time basis averaging twenty hours per week and for which an individual is compensated in accordance with the Fair Labor Standards Act. According to the Developmental Disabilities Act of 1984, supported employment is

> for persons with developmental disabilities for whom competitive employment at or above the minimum wage is unlikely and who because of their disabilities, need intensive ongoing support to perform in a work setting; conducted in a variety of settings, particularly worksites in which persons without disabilities are employed; and supported by any activity need to sustain paid work by persons with disabilities, including supervision, training and transportation.

Supported employment represents a service strategy that enables people with significant disabilities a chance to obtain and maintain meaningful community employment. By definition, supported employment has three essential features: (1) opportunity for paid productive work, (2) ongoing support and training to ensure continued employment, and (3) employment in socially integrated environments (Sinnott-Oswald, Gliner & Spencer, 1991).

Sheltered employment and supported employment are two examples of creative and compassionate efforts to assist persons with severe disabilities obtain and maintain their human rights. Without these and other types of employment for persons with severe disabilities, a significant number of people would have difficulty meeting some of their self-esteem needs.

HELPING–PART OF THE SOLUTION

There are many types of helpers who have and continue to assist persons with disabilities. Some are professionally trained; others are concerned friends, family, neighbors, and advocates, all of whom have varying backgrounds. The following are some suggestions for anyone who desires to be of assistance to persons with disabilities. Successfully helping clients with disabilities does not require gimmicks or tricks. Furthermore, effective helpers use different techniques. There is not just one right approach, and there are many wrong approaches. Indifference or condescension, for example, is an ineffective way to help; concern and respect have proved to be better. Many persons with disabilities have been both disappointed and psychologically deprived by professional, paraprofessional, and other types of helpers. When this happens, persons with a disability quickly learn to consider a helper guilty of disliking them until he or she proves otherwise. However, once most clients accept a helper, it is almost impossible for the helper to do anything wrong in their eyes.

Generally speaking, low achievement by persons with disabilities is encouraged by the low expectations held by the helpers. In many instances, this attitude is fostered by the conscious or unconscious belief in the notion of the physiological and intellectual inferiority of all people with disabilities. Such an attitude can be completely destructive to the education and rehabilitation processes. One thing of which helpers should not become guilty is what the authors call a no win situation for persons with disabilities. If individuals with disabilities do poorly in a task, some helpers may erroneously perceive the cause of the performance as internal to the clients and thus attribute negative characteristics to them. However, if the clients do well the helper may take credit for having helped persons with disabilities overcome formidable odds and succeed.

It is behavior, not physical difference that is the crucial quality of rehabilitation. As previously noted, helpers should treat all clients fairly. Hostile clients frequently are provoked to aggressive acts by hostile helpers. The initial error committed by helpers is usually to assume that persons with disabilities and those without them are biologically and psychologically different. Each client wants to be treated with respect. Through their behavior, helpers demonstrate the extent of their recognition that each client has worth and dignity. In spite of how difficult it may be to assist some persons with disabilities, helpers must view these persons as individuals who deserve the same opportunity to succeed as those who are believed to be easier to reach. Besides, there is a way to help every client effectively, and each helper must find that way.

Clients with disabilities who have been treated with respect and dignity are likely to reciprocate with similar behavior. Most people learn best by example. Children who hate have been conditioned by adults who hate them, whereas those who love have been the recipients of love. With regard to education, the authors wish to point how important it is that educators consciously seek to minimize unfair treatment and maximize fair treatment. Showing favoritism to some students and constantly punishing and/or ignoring others is enough to suggest to class members that the teacher is attracted to some students more than to others. When students see a teacher reject students with disabilities, they may imagine that in order to be liked by the teacher they must also reject those students. There is nothing creative or imaginative about most forms of rejection. They are merely old-fashioned ways of hatred.

If they wish to be successful working with their clients, helpers must convey the fact that they are concerned with and interested in each of them. Clearly, this should have nothing to do with physiological attributes. It is a matter of equity and professionalism. Helpers who maintain an attitude of fairness to all clients and whose behavior demonstrates it will find their clients with disabilities most receptive to them as helpers and, perhaps, friends. All clients want desperately to be assisted by helpers who care about them.

In many instances, helpers will discover that they must first build confidence in their clients. Believing that clients with disabilities are capable of learning and succeeding is not sufficient. The clients also must believe the same. There are many ways helpers can assist in raising clients' levels of aspiration. It would be cruel to raise them above the point of their realization, but, then who except persons who really know the clients' condition should make such a crucial determination? Commenting on levels of aspiration of school children, Wattenberg (1959) provided the following:

The ideal situation for normal children is for their level of aspiration to be just high enough so that they have to put forth effort to reach it, and yet for them to achieve success. In school, at least in the beginning for any subject, children tend to accept the teachers' expectations and standards as their level of aspiration. Therefore, we can influence this level quite effectively. Now, when the level favors success with effort, a number of fine things happen.

The situation itself is satisfying. The child will want to return to the type of task. So to speak, now he is motivated, shows interest, and puts out effort. Moreover, unless he is emotionally disturbed, he will begin to raise his sights. He will set himself after each success a somewhat higher level of aspiration. If the task at hand is clearly beyond his ability, he fails. What does failure do? Not only does it rob the task of interest, but it can have a depressant effect on his future level of aspiration. His ambitions for himself will curve sharply downward. He sets himself a level considerably below his true ability. (p. 231)

Thus, levels of aspiration are similar to an automobile's governor: on the one hand, protecting the individuals with disabilities against demoralizing failures but, on the other hand, allowing them to experience safe, moral-building success. Also like a governor, when the mechanism of levels of aspiration is thrown out of balance, it fails to perform its protective function. Under this condition, aspirations may be maintained consistently above or below achievement.

SUMMARY

With regard to understanding the true meaning of human rights for all, we refer to the African proverb "it takes a village to raise a child" and paraphrase by stating "it takes everyone to protect the human rights of everyone else." When a group of individuals lose or are denied their human rights, everyone is in danger of losing some of their human rights. Each atrocity that lessens the rights of any group in some way diminishes the rights of all human beings. Laws can be eloquently written to identify and correct mistreatment and denial of person's human rights, but they have little effect if many chose to ignore and/or circumvent the mandates of the laws. This is why it is important that everyone becomes sensitive and responsive to the needs of persons who may not be as privileged as we are.

As previously stated in this chapter, several countries have followed the lead of the United States in passing and enacting laws designed to increase and protect the human and civil rights of persons with disabilities. Because of laws such as the ADA and its amendments, persons with disabilities within the United States enjoy a more open and accepting society. Although significant progress has been made with regard to breaking negative attitudinal barriers, there remains much more work to be done before life's playing field becomes level for all persons with disabilities and we can proclaim that "human rights for all" has been achieved.

POINTS FOR DISCUSSION AND SUGGESTED ACTIVITIES

1. Research the difference between human rights and civil rights.
2. Research some human rights advocates in your state and/or community.
3. Research the employment rate of persons with disabilities in your state.

REFERENCES

Bickenbach, J.E. (2001). Disability human rights law and policy. In K. Albrecht, D, Seelman, and M. Bury (Eds.). Thousand Oaks, Sage.

Bryan, W.V. (2001). *Sociopolitical Aspects of Disabilities.* Springfield, IL. Charles C Thomas.

Bryan, W.V. (1996). *In Search of Freedom.* Springfield, IL: Charles C Thomas

Griffin, J. (2010). *Community Based Care and the Developmentally Disabled.* Unpublished paper. University of Oklahoma.

Pelka, F. (1997). *The Disability Rights Movement.* Santa Barbara. ABC-CLIO.

Sinnott-Oswald, M.S., Gliner, J.A., and Spencer, K.C. (1991). Supported and sheltered employment: Quality of life issues among workers with disabilities. *Education and Training in Mental Retardation, Dec,* 280–284.

Wattenberg, W.W. (1959). Levels of aspiration. *Michigan Education Journal, 37,* 231–240.

SUGGESTED READINGS

Arendt, H. (1958). *The Human Condition.* Chicago: University of Chicago Press.

Charlton, J. (1998). *Nothing about us without us: Disability, oppression and empowerment.* Berkeley: University of California Press.

Doyle, B. (1996). *Disability Discrimination: The New Law.* London: Jordans.

Driedger, D. (1989). *The Last Civil Rights Movement.* London: Hurst.

Chapter 14

DISABILITY ISSUES FOR THE TWENTY-FIRST CENTURY

Outline

- Introduction
- When Is a Disability a Disability?–An Update
- Fate of Persons With Severe Disabilities
- Inclusion
- End of Life Decisions
- Personal Assistive Services
- Are Accommodations Preferential Treatment?
- How Much Should Be Spent on Rehabilitation?–An Update
- Prenatal Testing and Genetics
- A Suggested Activity

Objectives

- To identify some important disability issues to be discussed in the twenty-first century
- To identify some important disability issues that will require some answers during the twenty-first century

INTRODUCTION

As we have pointed out throughout this text, there have been significant improvements in the human relationship interaction between persons without disabilities and persons with disabilities. Nondisabled persons have begun to better understand some of the needs of persons with disabilities. Additionally, nondisabled persons have begun to recognize that it is their negative and paternalistic attitudes, not the person with disabilities' physical and/or limited mental abilities, that have been one of the biggest handicaps limiting the progress of many persons with disabilities. Likewise many persons with disabilities have learned that one of the most productive ways of making the United States aware of their strengths and what they have to contribute to the productivity and growth of society is to vocalize their feelings and desires. Also, persons with disabilities have become more aggressive with regard to insisting that their demands be heard and their needs met.

In the third edition of this book, we pointed out that as persons with disabilities become more visible in society and vocal with regard to their rights, American society will begin to raise questions about the extent to which those rights should be granted. This certainly has been the case over the past half decade, and in our opinion this is good. If we as persons with disabilities want to be treated as equals with nondisabled persons, we have to be willing to accept the fact that if the playing field becomes a level playing field (to the extent that is possible) we have to be willing to compete with our nondisabled brothers and sisters without special rules for our participation. We are not attempting to say that society has reached the point that there no longer exist disadvantages for persons with disabilities in areas such as employment, education, and economics to mention only three societal areas of important human relationships. Anyone knowledgeable about the interaction of persons with disabilities and nondisabled persons knows that we have not reached nirvana in this relationship. What we are saying is that for those of us who have disabilities, as we continue to demand equal and fair treatment and once we receive the same, we have to be prepared through our actions and attitudes to show that is all we expect and want.

In this chapter, we will update some of the issues raised in the third edition; additionally, we will raise some new issues and reemphasize some issues that were discussed in the previous edition. The issues which will be discussed are an update of when a disability is a disability, what is going to happen to persons with severe disabilities, whether accommodations are preferential treatment, an update of how much should be spent on rehabilitation, service animals, the ultimate decision, prenatal testing and genetics, and inclusion.

WHEN IS A DISABILITY A DISABILITY?–AN UPDATE

Before we provide an update to this question, we shall review what was identified as the issue in the third edition. In that edition, we wrote that, the ADA defines a disability in the following ways:

1. a person with a physical or mental impairment that substantially limits one or more major life activities such as walking, seeing, hearing, speaking, breathing, learning, working or caring for oneself;
2. a person who has a record of such a physical or mental impairment
3. a person who is regarded as having such an impairment.

Bryan (2002) posed the following relevant questions with regard to the subject of when is a disability a disability:

1. If a person is considered to have a disability if she has a physical or mental impairment that substantially limits one or more major life activities, then is she rehabilitated when there is no longer a limitation to a major life activity?
2. Is the person rehabilitated when he is gainfully employed, thus able to provide for his basic needs?
3. Is a person to be considered rehabilitated when through the use of assistive devices or personal assistance she is able to carry through with her major life activities? (p. 224)

As noted by (Disability Right Education and Defense Fund, 2002), DREDF members of the U.S. Supreme Court have ruled on some of these questions, and their opinions have narrowed the definition of a disability. This assessment is based on at least three cases: *Sutton v. United Airlines, Inc.* (1999), *Murphy v. United Parcel Services, Inc.* (1999), and *Albertson's Inc. v. Kirkingburg* (1999). The central issue of the Sutton case was whether two sisters who had very poor uncorrected vision were disabled once their vision had been corrected to 20/20 with corrective lenses. The Court ruled that when the corrective lenses restored their vision to normal, they did not have a substantial limitation of a major life activity. The Court had essentially the same ruling in *Murphy v. United Parcel Services, Inc.*, when it ruled that Murphy no longer had a substantial limitation once his high blood pressure was controllable with medication. In the third case, *Albertson's Inc. v. Kirkingburg, the Supreme Court took the position that if* a person could subconsciously make physical adjustment to control his or her limitation, this must be considered in deciding whether the person has a disability as defined by the ADA.

These decisions raise serious questions about when a disability is in fact legally a disability. Are persons with disabilities and their advocates presenting inconsistent arguments? Are they saying on the one hand that persons with disabilities should be protected from discrimination by laws because the so-called playing field is not level? If so, why do they also say, on the other hand, that persons with disabilities should continue to be in a legally protected class once the playing field is level.

UPDATE. Many persons with disabilities, their advocates, and the U.S. Congress believed that the previously mentioned rulings, as well as other rulings, by the U.S. Supreme Court were narrowing Congress' intent for the ADA. Therefore, in 2008 the U.S. Congress passed the Americans with Disabilities Act Amendments, and they became law January 1, 2009. The Congress answered through the previously mentioned amendments Bryan's questions one and three Bryan (2002). If a person is considered to have a disability because she has a physical or mental impairment that substantially limits one or more major life activities, then is she rehabilitated when there is no longer a limitation to a major life activity? Is a person to be considered rehabilitated when through the use of assistive devices or personal assistance he is able to carry through with his major life activities? 2008 amendments address the two questions Bryan (2002) raised and the overall question of when is a disability a disability. (1) Mitigating measures are no longer to be used to disqualify a person for reasonable accommodations. The ADA has five titles: Title I, Employment; Title II, Public Service; Title III, Public Accommodations; Title IV; Telecommunica- tion Relay Services; and Title V, Miscellaneous Provisions. As previously stated, the U.S. Supreme Court in *Sutton v. United Airlines Inc.* ruled if medication or other measures control or significantly lessen the impact of the disability or cause the person to be able to function to the extent that a major life activity is not substantially limited, the person does not qualify for a reasonable accommodation. The 2008 ADA Amendments proclaim that with the exception of regular eyeglasses and contact lens, mitigating and corrective measures are not to be considered in determining whether services are to be provided. Thus with the previously mention exception, when a person has been hired and it is determined that she has a disability, the disability is to be considered when determining whether a reasonable accommodation is to be provided–not whether her disability is mitigated by medication, assistive devices, and/or other rehabilitation aids. (2) The ADA indicates that a person is considered to have a disability if he or she has a physical or mental impairment that substantially limits one or more major life activities. The 2008 Amendments lessen the proof needed to prove "substantially limited"; therefore, as previously stated, the amendments address the overall question of "when is a disability a disability?"

FATE OF PERSONS WITH SEVERE DISABILITIES

We have mentioned several times that attitudes toward and beliefs about the abilities of persons with disabilities, as well as their place within American society, is changing to a more positive view of this large and important population. The improved positioning within the United States population has meant increased opportunities for persons within areas such as employment, education, and economics. Although the transformation from being viewed as charitable dependent persons to persons who are capable of charting much of their own destiny is far from being complete, the opportunities for completing the transformation and the willingness to complete the transformation is evident. The evidence can be seen in the fact that thousands of persons with disabilities are living independent lives, sometimes with minimal assistance from nondisabled persons and at other times with considerable assistance from their nondisabled family, friends, and advocates.

More persons with developmental disabilities and severe disabilities who heretofore have had an extremely difficult and sometimes impossible time securing employment are now being employed by sheltered workshops and well-devised employment opportunities such as supported employment. These and other forward thinking employment opportunities are allowing some persons with disabilities to become independent. Likewise, advanced teaching techniques and increased involvement of parents and other family members of students with what is termed learning disabilities have been a catalyst for many students with learning and/or developmental disabilities to obtain many of the skills necessary to succeed within American society.

Also as previously mentioned, a number of states have either closed or are in the process of closing their mental institutions and transitioning the patients into community living arrangements. This can be a positive step for some persons with mental, behavioral, and/or developmental disabilities but can also present some major problems for other patients who may not be emotionally and/or physically prepared for this type of arrangement.

All of the previously mentioned advancements in the human relationships between nondisabled persons and persons with disabilities are very good and as previously stated mark an improvement and important societal change with regard to attitudes toward and opportunities for persons with disabilities. These changes are the background for an important issue for the twenty-first century. The issue concerns what will happen to persons with severe disabilities who, because of the severity of their disabilities, cannot significantly benefit from the previously mentioned advancements as well as from others that undoubtedly will occur in the future. To be more specific, what will happen to persons who are incapable of functioning outside an institutional setting? What type of living arrangements will be provided to those persons who cannot live or function outside of an institutional setting when all or most of the institutions are closed and the emphasis is on community living? This is not meant to imply that institutional living is preferable to community living, but the question is being raised as to whether we are giving adequate consideration to those who cannot benefit from noninstitutional living. Another part of the overall question of what we are going to do for persons with severe disabilities is what efforts will be put forth to educate those students who do not benefit from "regular" or special education? What efforts will be put forth to provide employment for persons who may have difficulties adjusting to sheltered employment and supported employment?

These, in our opinion, are questions we will face during the twenty-first century as we attempt to provide opportunities for all of our citizens. Persons with disabilities, regardless of the severity of their disabilities, deserve opportunities to feel pride in themselves. We can develop devices to probe deep space; we can also develop devices to communicate with persons throughout the world. Certainly if we apply resources and dedication we can find ways to overcome most severe disabilities to the point that those persons can function at levels where they feel pride in being human.

INCLUSION

Closely related to the question of the fate of persons with disabilities is how we will ensure inclusion of persons with disabilities. By inclusion we are referring to all persons with disabilities, not just persons with severe disabilities.

Perhaps the biggest issue facing rehabilitation helping professionals and perhaps all Americans with regard to interaction with persons with disabilities is how to ensure inclusion of all persons with disabilities in the everyday functions of American society. This is a task that is so monumental that it requires the effort and dedication of all concerned Americans. Not only will more attitudes have to change, but also additional actions will have to reflect the dedication and desire to have persons with disabilities receive the same opportunities as persons without disabilities: to be educated to their maximum potential, to be trained and employed at maximum potential, and to live wholesome and productive lives. To be truly included in American society, physical, attitudinal, and behavioral barriers must be removed. Removal of barriers opens opportunities to be educated; to be employed; to be involved in community, state, and national activities; to enjoy social events; and to enjoy recreational activities.

END OF LIFE DECISIONS

The subject of death, especially our own or that of our significant others, is generally difficult to address. Although we realize the certainty of death, in many cases, the topic is placed in the "to be dealt with later" category. Unfortunately, in some instances, later is too late, as is the case for people who have a degenerative or terminal illness. From a healthcare standpoint, the kind of care these individuals may need to keep them as comfortable as possible while their quality of life decreases requires careful planning. In some cases, the question becomes whether the patient should have the right to have his or her life terminated when there is no medical hope of improvement and the quality of his or her life is greatly diminished.

Opponents of someone's taking her or his own life, assisted suicide, or mercy killing currently point to the fact that these acts are illegal; others frame their objections in moral terms. Those who favor such acts make their arguments on the basis of freedom of choice, insisting that all persons should have the right to decide not to live when the quality of their life has been reduced to a level they believe is not worth continuing. Certainly these are powerful arguments on both sides of the issue. If the act of ending one's life is made legal, additional questions must be answered. Where should the line be drawn? What is sufficient justification for such an act? Who would be responsible for carrying out the act? How will the act be accomplished? What are your thoughts on this issue?

PERSONAL ASSISTIVE SERVICES

As we learn more about human and animal behavior, it is evident that humans and animals can benefit each other. For a number of years it has been recognized that some animals, such as dogs, can be of tremendous benefit to persons with disabilities, particularly those with visual disabilities. Dogs can also be of assistance and comfort to seriously ill individuals and persons who have cognitive disabilities. As our scientific studies revealed additional information about humans and animals assisting each other, we have found that other animals, such as monkeys and small ponies, can be of tremendous assistance to some persons with disabilities. With the increased understanding of human and animal helping relationships undoubtedly we will discover that other animals can be of assistance to some persons with disabilities. With this knowledge, some social issues will be raised: (1) What type of access should be given to service animals? (2) What are the types of disabilities persons may have that would qualify them to use service animals? (3) What license and/or training must a person have to have and maintain a service animal? (4) What are the responsibilities of the owners of these service animals? These and other questions will no doubt be issues to be addressed in the twenty-first century.

ARE ACCOMMODATIONS PREFERENTIAL TREATMENT?

The question of preferential treatment may surface when a person with an "invisible" disability, such as a hearing condition, diabetes, or a learning disability, to mention only three, is provided "reasonable accommodations." In most instances, individuals with hidden disabilities are not being given preferential treatment, at least not without good reasons. The fact that coworkers may believe that favoritism is taking place could be handled by explaining to them the circumstances; however, employers or supervisors may be muted by laws of confidentiality. Neither the persons with disabilities nor their supervisors should be compelled to disclose personal information.

The education profession, particularly higher education, is an area where there may be concern with regard to preferential treatment of persons who are identified as having a learning disability. For example, a student identified as having a learning disability may request, as a reasonable accommodation, extra time for taking tests, a relative stress-free testing environment, or assistance with note taking. There is a very fine line separating a learning disability such as difficulty in comprehending material being taught from not having an aptitude for mastering the subject matter. The point being made is that it is not uncommon for student to experience difficulties in comprehending subject materials in challenging academic fields such as allied health, medicine, and engineering, to mention only three. Therefore, the question is whether giving some students extra assistance constitutes giving them an unfair advantage. What do you think?

With regard to employment-related accommodations, Bryan (2002) offers the following comments providing a good overview of what some employers must sort out when their employees request accommodations:

> Despite the fact it has been shown that most job related accommodations cost less than $500, there continues to be concern about providing accommodations. If providing an accommodation creates an undue burden the

employer does not have to comply with the employee's request. An issue of concern is what constitutes an undue burden. Employers may be required to document why and/or how the requested accommodations create a hardship on the business or company. One can easily see the point of contention if the employer is required to provide the requested accommodation when the employer strongly believes the request is unreasonable. Some employers feel that the "red tape" they have to encounter is not worth the effort, therefore, they provide the accommodation despite their beliefs the request constitutes a burden. This attitude can cause employers to avoid hiring persons with a disability. (p. 225)

What do you think?

HOW MUCH SHOULD BE SPENT ON REHABILITATION?– AN UPDATE

Some of the issues raised in the third edition of this text with regard to this subject will be answered by the 2010 The Patient Protection and Affordable Care Act that the U.S. Congress passed and President Barak Obama signed into law. As of this writing, all of the details with regard to who pays for what and how much, as well as the various types of services to be provided, specifically regarding rehabilitation efforts will be made clear as regulations are written and the new law is fully implemented. However, a point we wish to make is that we predicted that some issues that are addressed in the law would be issues that would have to be addressed in the twenty-first century. Some of the issues raised in the third edition are (1) is health care a right or privilege? In our opinion The Patient Protection and Affordable Care Act makes health care a right for all. Another issue was (2) How extensive should health care be? To our knowledge the Health Care law to a major extent addresses this issue. (3) Who should be responsible for paying for health care? The previously mentioned law addresses this issue. As previously stated, in the previous edition of this text we predicted that these issues would have to be addressed during the twenty-first century, and they have been addres-sed.

Although portions of our third edition predictions have been addressed, there remains an issue we raised that, to a major extent, is an ethical issue that has not been addressed. Most ethical issues take considerable time to address because they often involve societal attitude changes. The following discussion represents the issue.

With regard to persons with disabilities and rehabilitation, how much health care should be provided? One thing that makes this question difficult to answer is the fact that arguably it should be addressed on a case by case basis. Some health care professionals argue that the extent of service to be provided should be based on disease or medical procedure priorities. In other words, third-party payers such as insurance companies will pay for a predetermined number of treatments and/or days spent in a health care facility based on the type of disease or medical procedures required. Some critics of this approach say that the insurers do not take into consideration an individual's optimum health care needs. Perhaps the new health care law will address this issue.

Additional concerns with regard to the extent of services to be provided relate to whether those services should be based on the prognosis of recovery, including how likely is the patient's recovery with the approved treatment. This should be of considerable concern for persons with disabilities, their families, advocates, and in fact, everyone. This kind of decision making devalues the lives of persons with severe disabilities. To be more specific, how much value to society is a person with a disability? What are your thoughts?

PRENATAL TESTING AND GENETICS

Advances in prenatal screening have made it possible for early detection of some possible birth defects, as well as providing a variety of other information, such as gender identification. Garver and Garver (1991) state that traditionally one of the goals of prenatal screening was to provide the parents with information about genetic diseases and the risk of having an afflicted child, or their chances of having a "normal" child. Hatchett (1991) poses this question: Could prenatal screening lead to genetic perfection? Other questions can also be raised; namely, in an attempt to have genetic perfection, would fetuses be aborted because they are not the parents' desired gender? Would abortion be allowed if there is a determination that the unborn child may have a predisposition toward obesity, visual problems, or perhaps be short of stature? Will parents go as far as terminating a pregnancy because of the "wrong" eye color? One might think these things are absurd: however, Lamb (1994) reported that 11 percent of New England couples polled indicated they would abort a fetus predisposed to obesity. Bryan (2002) summarizes some of the issues and questions that should be addressed with regard to the subject of prenatal screening and genetics:

> For the sake of discussion, let's assume scientific advances make possible ninety to ninety-five percent accuracy of prenatal information (one doubts if we will ever reach 100 percent). With this high level of assurance, there will continue to be some significant questions such as, what will happen to the five or ten percent that are missed? Will we have built such an idea of perfection that persons born with a disability will be treated as "freaks of nature?" What kind of life will they have, and what limitations will they experience, not so much from their physical and/or mental condition, rather from societal attitudes? Eventually, we will have ninety-five percent accuracy on whether there will be a disability; this will probably not answer the question of, if the person has a disability, what level of involvement of the disability? Nor does it provide an answer to the questions of how well the person will be able to adjust to the disability or how productive will the person be? One must keep in mind that there are various levels of developmental disabilities, and that persons missing limbs or who have visual problems have over the years accomplished many things. Who is capable of determining the individual's worth to himself or herself, the family, and society? There can be no question that attempting to prevent and eliminate problems as well as possible suffering is a noble undertaking. However, in doing so, we must be careful about the message we are sending about disabilities. Are we devaluing persons who have a disability? Despite our best scientific, medical, and any other efforts there is a very high probability that for the foreseeable future the best science can offer in prenatal screening, there will be at least five to ten percent genetic problems that will go undetected. Should we reach the unlikely possibility of 100 percent accuracy of prenatal screening, we will continue to have persons with disabilities because of accidents and diseases after birth. Thus in our efforts to reach perfection have we not established a bias or at least our bias against persons with disabilities? Given this bias, then how will these persons be treated in society? (pp. 228–229)

Privacy fears could be real issues with regard to employment. In this case, the fears revolve around the possibility of employers' requiring genetic testing and using the results as part of their employment decisions.

A related issue, which is not an exclusive disability issue, relates to everyone who may be subject to genetic testing. That is, who owns your genes? The answer to the question may seem to be that each individual owns his or her genes. Despite the apparent obviousness of the situation, there is currently some question as to whether medical research companies can use an individual's genes without his or her consent. To be more specific, let us assume that through genetic testing it is determined that Mary has a rare gene that provides immunity to a certain disease. Does the company that found the gene have the right to use it without Mary's consent" None of the previously mentioned issues have easy answers; there are legal, moral, and in some cases religious implications. Over time, as technology continues to make advances, there will be other issues that will have to be addressed. What are your thoughts?

A SUGGESTED ACTIVITY

List at least three disability issues not discussed in this chapter that you think will be discussed during the twenty-first century.

REFERENCES

Bryan, W.V. (2002). *Sociopolitical Aspects of Disabilities.* Springfield, IL: Charles C Thomas.

Disability Rights Education and Defense Fund. (2002). Disability Rights Education and Defense Fund, CA.

Garver, K., and Garver, B. (1991). Historical perspective of eugenics: Past, present and the future. *American Journal of Human Genetics, 49*: 1109–118

Hatchett, R. (1991). Brave new world: perspectives on the American experience of eugenics. *The Pharos, Fall,* 13–18.

Lamb, L. (1994). Selecting for perfection. *UTNE Reader, 66,* 26–28

Appendix A

FAMOUS DECEASED PERSONS WITH DISABILITIES: A BRIEF SAMPLE

Clinton P. Anderson (1895-1975) served as Secretary of Agriculture and later as a United States Senator from New Mexico. He had diabetes.

Susan B. Anthony (1820–1906) was a leading advocate for women's rights and is the first woman honored on a United States coin. She had arthritis.

Aristotle (384–322 B.C.) was one of the world's greatest philosophers and teachers. He stuttered.

Thomas R. Armitage (1795–1842), a physician, introduced braille into England and also spearheaded legislation that mandated compulsory education for the blind between the ages of five and sixteen years. He was partially sighted.

Bernard M. Baruch (1870–1965) was a successful businessman, elder statesman, and presidential adviser. He was hearing impaired.

Thomas A. Becket (1117–1170) was a member of the clergy who became Archbishop of Canterbury and, after his death, a saint. He stuttered.

Joachim du Bellay (1522–1560) was a talented poet. He was hearing impaired.

Louis Braille (1800–1852) invented the braille system by which blind people can read and write through a planned series of raised dots. He was visually impaired.

Elizabeth Barrett Browning (1806–1861) was a world-renowned poetess. She had a spinal injury.

Ralph Bunche (1904–1971), a physician, served as undersecretary-general of the United Nations and in 1950 won the Nobel peace prize. He had diabetes.

Julius Caesar (100–44 B.C.) was one of the world's greatest military leaders and a Roman emperor. He had epilepsy.

George Washington Carver (1864–1943) was an outstanding scientist and educator. He is best known for developing hundreds of uses for the peanut. He stuttered.

Irene Chavarria (1941–1974) was an instructor at East Los Angeles College. She had a physical disability.

Fanny Crosby (1820–1915) was a much-acclaimed teacher of the blind at the New York Institute for the Blind. She was visually impaired.

William Oh Douglas (1898–1980) was a successful lawyer who became an associate justice of the U.S. Supreme Court. He had poliomyelitis as a child.

Thomas A. Edison (1847–1930) was a famous inventor whose inventions included the incandescent electric lamp and the receiver and transmitter for the automatic telegraph. He was hearing impaired.

St. John Ervine (1883–1971) was a well-known writer of novels, plays, biographies, and reviews. He had one leg.

Leonard Euler (1707–1783) was one of the founders of the science of pure mathematics. He was visually impaired.

Henry Fawcett (1833–1884) was an economist and statesman who became postmaster general of Britain. He was visually impaired.

Gustave Flaubert (1821–1880) was a famous French novelist. He had epilepsy.

Galileo Galilei (1564–1642) was a famous astronomer and physicist who wrote The Laws of Motion. He was visually impaired.

Charles Gounod (1818–1893) was a celebrated composer whose music includes "Ave Maria" and "Faust." He was visually impaired.

Francisco Goya (1746–1828) was a royal painter to the King of Spain. He was hearing impaired.

Edwin Grasse (1884–1954) was a composer, violinist, and organist. He was visually impaired.

Hannibal (247–183 B.C.) led his army with its elephants across the Alps in an unsuccessful attempt to defeat the Romans. He had a visual impairment in one eye.

Francois Huber (1750–1831) gained fame as a naturalist who became an authority on the honeybee. He was visually impaired.

Elizabeth Inchbald (1753–1821) was an actress and writer in England. She stuttered.

Isaac II (1155–1204) ruled the Eastern Roman Empire. He was visually impaired.

James Joyce (1881–1941) gained world recognition as a novelist. He was visually impaired.

Philip Kearney (1814–1862) was a much-decorated Civil War general. He had one arm.

Rudyard Kipling (1865–1936) was a successful writer who received a Nobel Prize for literature in 1907. He was visually impaired.

Caspar Krumbhorn (1542–1621) was a director of the Academy of St. Peter's in Rome. He was visually impaired.

Fritz Lang (1890–1976) was a director of motion pictures. He was visually impaired in one eye.

Canada Lee (1907–1951) was one of the most successful black actors in the United States in the early twentieth century. He was visually impaired in one eye.

Maxim Litvinoff (1876–1951) was Russian Ambassador to the United States in 1941. He had diabetes.

Henry Luce (1898–1976) founded and published *Fortune, Time*, and other magazines. He stuttered.

Anne Sullivan Macy (1887–1936) was a teacher and life companion of Helen Keller. She was visually impaired in one eye.

Edward Marshall (1856–1937) founded the *Harvard Lampoon* and *Life Magazine*. He was hearing impaired.

Herbert Marshall (1890–1966) was a star of radio, theatre, movies, and television. He had one leg.

Harriet Martineau (1802–1876) was an English economist and novelist. She was hearing impaired.

John Metcalf (1717–1810), a road builder, was one of the first persons to use crushed stone in roads. He was visually impaired.

Horatio Nelson (1758–1805) was a distinguished English admiral. He was visually impaired in one eye and had one arm amputated.

Louis Pasteur (1822–1895) verified the germ theory of disease and developed the process of pasteurization. He was a paralytic.

- **Wiley Post** (1900–1935) was a pioneer in aviation. He was visually impaired in one eye.
- **William Prescott** (1796–1859) was a famous historian who wrote classic volumes of Spanish-American history. He was visually impaired in one eye and partially sighted in the other.
- **Joseph Pulitzer** (1847–1911) endowed Columbia University's School of Journalism, which in turn established the Pulitzer prizes. He was visually impaired.
- **Joshua Reynolds** (1732–1792) was a famous portrait painter. He was hearing impaired.
- **Anne Eleanor Roosevelt** (1884–1962) is considered by many writers to have been America's greatest first lady. She was hearing impaired.
- **Franklin Delano Roosevelt** (1882–1945) was the thirty-second president of the United States and the only president elected to four terms. He had poliomyelitis.
- **Edward Scripps** (1854–1926) organized a chain of newspapers throughout the United States and endowed the Scripps Institute of Oceanography in San Diego. He was visually impaired.
- **Maurice de la Sizeranne** (1857–1924) taught blind students and was a founder of a library and a museum that featured the cultural contributions of visually impaired persons. He was visually impaired.
- **Thomas Sydenham** (1624–1689) was the founder of modern clinical medicine. He had gout.
- **Norman Thomas** (1884–1968) was an American Socialist leader and candidate for president of the United States six times. He was vision impaired.
- **Edgar Wallace** (1875–1932) was a prolific novelist who wrote *Ben Hur*. He was hearing impaired.

Final Note

This list of abbreviated achievements is not meant to be exhaustive. Rather, it is presented to show various ways individual efforts can overshadow physical disabilities. The authors encourage readers to try to familiarize themselves with the total achievements of the persons on this list and others who are not included. There are thousands of success stories: Fill in some of the missing ones.

Appendix B

RESOURCES FOR PEOPLE WITH DISABILITIES

Alcoholism

National Council on Alcoholism and Drug Dependence, Inc.
244 East 58th Street
4th Floor
New York, NY 10022
Email: national@ncadd.org

Amputation

National Amputation Foundation
40 Church Street
Malverne, NY 11565
Phone: 516-887-3600
Email: amps76@aol.com

Arthritis

Arthritis Foundation
PO Box 7669
Atlanta, GA 30357-0669
Phone: 800-283-7800

Assistive Technology

Alliance for Technology
1304 Southpoint Boulevard
Suite 240
Petaluma, CA 94954

National Center for Accessible Media
Carl and Ruth Shapiro Family National Center for Accessible Media
One Guest Street
Boston, MA 02135
Phone: 617-300-3400
TTY: 617-300-2489
Email: access@wgbn.org

National Dissemination Center for Children with Disabilities (NICHCY)
1825 Connecticut Avenue NW
Suite 700
Washington, DC 2009
Phone: 800-695-0285
Email: nichcy@aed.org

Attention Deficit Disorder

ADDA
PO Box 7557
Willmington, DE 19803-9997
Email: info@add.org

Children and Adults with Attention Deficit Hyperactivity Disorder (CHADD)
CHADD National Office
8181 Professional Place
Suite 150
Landover, MD 20785
Phone: 301-306-7070

Autism

Autism Society of America
4340 East-West Highway
Suite 350
Bethesda, MD 20814
Phone: 800-3AUTISM

US Autism and Asperger Association (USAAH)
888-9AUTISM

Bipolar

Depression and Bipolar Support Alliance (DBSA)
730 N. Franklin Street
Suite 501
Chicago, IL 60654-7225
Phone: 800-826-3632

Blindness or Visual Impairment

Blinded Veterans Association (DVA)
Phone: 800-669-7079
Email: bva@bva.org

Guiding Eyes for the Blind
611 Granite Springs Road
Yorktown Heights, NY 10598
Phone: 800-942-0149

Leader Dogs for the Blind
1039 S. Rochester Road
Rochester Hills, MI 48307

Lions World Services for the Blind
2811 Fair Park Boulevard
Little Rock, Arkansas 72204
Phone: 501-664-7100
Phone: 800-248-0734
Email: training@lwsb.org

National Association for Parents of Children with Visual Impairments
PO Box 317
Watertown, MA 0247
Phone: 800-562-6265
Phone: 617-972-7441
Email: napvi@perkins.org

Cerebral Palsy

United Cerebral Palsy (UCP)
1660 L Street NW
Suite 700
Washington, DC 20036
Phone: 800- 872-5827
Phone: 202-776-0406

March of Dimes
1275k Mamaroneck Avenue
White Plains, NY 10605
Phone: 914-997-448

Easter Seals
233 South Wacker Drive
Suite 2400
Chicago, IL 60606

Deafness and Hearing Impairment

League for the Hard of Hearing
71 West 23rd Street
New York, NY 10010-4167
Phone: 917-305-7700
TTY: 917-305-7999

Telecommunication for the Deaf Inc.
8630 Fenton Street
Suite 604
Silver Spring, MD 20910
Phone: 301-589-3786
TTY: 301-589-3006

Diabetes

American Diabetes Association (ADA)
1701 North Beauregard Street
Alexandria, VA 22311
Phone: 800-342-2383
Email: askada@diabetes.org

American Dietetic Association (ADA)
120 South Riverside Plaza
Suite 200
Chicago, IL 60606-6995

National Diabetes Information
Clearinghouse (NDIC)
1 Information Way
Bethesda, MD 20892-3560
Phone: 800-860-8747
Email: ndic@info.niddk.nih.gov

National Diabetes Education Program (NDEP)
1 Diabetes Way
Bethesda, MD 20814-9692
Phone: 800-438-5383
Email: ndep@mail.nih.gov

Epilepsy

Epilepsy Foundation of America
8301 Professional Place
Landover, MD 20785
Phone: 800-332-1000

National Institute of Neurological Disorders and Stroke
NIH Neurological Institute
PO Box 5801
Bethesda, MD 20824
Phone: 800-352-9424

Fibromyalgia

National Fibromyalgia Association
2200 N. Glassell Street
Suite A
Orange CA 92865
Phone: 714-931-0150

Heart

American Heart Association
National Center
7272 Greenville Avenue
Dallas, TX 75321
Phone: 800-242-8721

National Heart, Lung and Blood Institute
Information Center
PO Box 30105
Bethesda, MD 20824-0105
Phone: 301-592-8573
TTY: 240-629-3255

Kidney

National Kidney Foundation
30 East 33rd Street
New York, NY 10016
Phone: 800-622-9010

National Kidney and Urologic Disease
Information Clearinghouse
3 Information Way
Bethesda, MD 20892-3580
Phone: 800-891-5390
TTY: 703-738-4929

Lung

American Lung Association
1301 Pennsylvania Aveue, NW
Washington, DC 20004
Phone: 202-785-3355

Mental Health

Mental Health America
2000 N. Beauregard Street
6th Floor
Alexandria, VA 22311
Phone: 703-684-7722
Phone: 800-969-6642

Multiple Sclerosis

National Multiple Sclerosis Society
New York Office
733 Third Avenue
3rd Floor
New York, NY 10017
Phone: 800-344-4867

Washington, DC Office
1100 New York Avenue NW
Suite 660
Washington, DC 20005
Phone: 800-344-4867

Multiple Sclerosis Foundation
6350 Andrews Avenue
Fort Lauderdale, FL 33309-2130
Phone: 800-225-6495

Muscular Dystrophy

Muscular Dystrophy Association–USA
National Headquarters
3300 E. Sunrise Drive
Tucson, AZ 85718
Phone: 800-572-1717

Occupational Therapy

American Occupational Therapy
Association
4720 Montgomery Lane
PO Box 31220
Bethesda, MD 20824-1220
Phone: 301-852-2682
TDD: 800-377-8555

Parkinson's Disease

American Parkinson's Disease Association
135 Parkinson Avenue
Staten Island, NY 10305
Phone: 718-981-8001
Phone: 800-223-2732

Physical Therapy

American Physical Therapy Association
1111 North Fairfax Street
Alexandria, VA 22314-1488
Phone: 800-999-2782
TDD: 703-683-6748

Rehabilitation

National Rehabilitation Counseling
Association
PO Box 4480
Manassas, VA. 20108
Phone: 703-361-2077

American Rehabilitation Counseling
Association
5999 Stevenson Avenue
Alexandria, VA 22304-3300
Phone: 800-347-6647
TTY: 703-823-6862

Respite Care Watch

National Respite Locator
800 Eastowne Drive
Suite 105
Chapel Hill, North Carolina 27514
Phone: 919-490-5577

Sickle Cell Disease

Center for Sickle Cell Disease
1840 7th Street NW
Washington DC 2001
Phone: 202-865-8292

Speech and Hearing

American Speech-Language Hearing
Association
2200 Research Boulevard
Rockville, MD 20850-3289
Phone: 301-296-5700

The Stuttering Foundation of America
3100 Walnut Grove Road
Suite 603
PO Box 11749
Memphis, TN 38111-0749
Phone: 901-452-3931

Spina Bifida

Spina Bifida Association
4590 MacArthur Boulevard NW
Suite 250
Washington, DC
Phone: 800-621-3141
Email: sbaa@sbaa.org

Tourette Syndrome
Tourette Syndrome Association Inc.
42-40 Bell Boulevard
Bayside, NY 11361
Phone: 718-224-2999

Veterans

Disabled American Veterans (DAV)
3725 Alexandria Pike
Cold Spring, KY 41076
Phone: 877-426-2838

Paralyzed Veterans of America
801 Eighteenth Street, NW
Washington, DC 2006-3517
Phone: 1-800-555-9140
Email: info@pva.org

Other Resources

National Clearinghouse of Rehabilitation
Training Material
6524 Old Main Hill
Utah State University
Logan, UT 84322-6524
Phone: 866-821-5355
Email: ncrtm@usu.edu

National Organization on Disability
888 Sixteenth Street NW
Suite 800
Washington, DC 2006
Phone: 202-293-5980
TTY: 202-293-5968

Appendix C

RECREATION ASSOCIATIONS

American Association of Adapted Sport
Programs
PO Box 5338
Pine Lake, GA 30072
Phone: 404-294-0070

America's Athletes with Disabilities
8630 Fenton Street, Suite 920
Silver Spring, MD 20910
Phone: 800-238-7632
Fax: 301-589-9052

American Camping Association
5000 State Road 67 North
Martinsville, IN 46151-7902
Phone: 765-342-8456
Fax: 765-342-2065

American Camping Association Project on
Science Technology and Disability
1333 H Street, NW
Washington, DC 20005
Phone: 800-653-1409

American Sled Hockey Association
21 Summerwood Court
Buffalo, NY 14223
Phone: 716-876-7390

American Water Ski Association Adaptive
Aquatics
PO Box 21
Jacksons Gap, AL 36861

Phone: 205-825-9091
Fax: 205-825-8332

American Wheelchair Table Tennis
Association
23 Parker Street
Port Chester, NY 10573
Phone: 914-937-3932

Association for Theatre and Disability
Access Theatre
527 Garden Street
Santa Barbara, CA 93101
Phone: 805-564-2063 Fax: 805-564-0051

Camp Holiday Trails
PO Box 5806
Charlottesville, VA 22905-0806
Phone: 804-977-3781

The Deaf Bowler
PO Box 171786
Arlington, TX 76003

Disability Net International Sports
http://www.disabilitynet.co.uk/info/
sport/index.html

Disabled Sports USA
451 Hungerford Drive, #100
Rockville, MD 20850
Phone: 301-217-9840

Easter Seal's Camping and Recreation List
Easter Seal's National Office
230 West Monroe Street, Suite 1800
Chicago, IL 60606
Phone: 800-221-6817
TTY 312-726-4258

International Wheelchair Aviators
Big Bear Airport
PO Box 2700
Big Bear City, CA 92314
Phone: 909-585-9663
Fax: 909-585-7156

International Wheelchair Road Racers Club
30 Myano Lane
Stamford, CT 06902
Phone: 203-967-2231
Fax: 203-327-7999

National Ability Center
PO Box 6827999
Park City, UT 84068
Phone: 435-649-3991
Fax: 435-658-3992

National Amputee Golf Association
1454 West Business Park Drive
Orem, UT 84508
Phone: 801-226-5587

National Association for Disabled Athletes
17 Lindley Avenue
Tenafly, NJ 07670-2816

National Deaf Bowling Association
9244 Ex Mansfield Avenue
Denver, CO 80237

National Wheelchair Shooting Federation
102 Park Avenue
Rockledge, PA 19046
Phone: 215-379-2359
Fax: 215-663-9662

National Theatre Workshop for the Handicapped
354 Broome Street, Loft 5-F
New York, NY 10013
Phone: 212-941-9511
Fax: 212-941-9486

Special Olympics International
1325 G Street, NW, Suite 500
Washington, DC 20005
Phone: 202-628-3630
Fax: 202-824-0200

National Deaf Education Network and Clearinghouse
Gallaudet University
800 Florida Ave, NE
Washington, DC 20002-3695
Phone: 202-651-5051
TTY: 202-651-5052

United States Association of Blind Athletes
33 North Institute Street
Colorado Springs, CO 80903
Phone: 719-630-0422
Fax: 719-630-0616

USA Deaf Sports Federation
3607 Washington, Boulevard, Suite 4
Ogden, UT 84403-1737
Fax: 801-393-2263

US Blind Golfers
3094 Shamrock Street N
Tallahassee, FL 32308
Phone: 904-893-4511

US Deaf Ski & Snowboard Association (USDSSA)
5053 Kenmore Drive
Concord, CA 94521
http://www.usdssa.org/

US Disabled Ski Team
PO Box 100

Park City, UT 84060
Phone: 435-649-9090
Fax: 435-649-3613

US Electric Wheelchair Hockey Association
7216 39th Avenue No
Minneapolis, MN 55427
Phone: 763-535-4736

Wheelchair Athletics of the USA
2351 Parkwood Road
Snellville, GA 30278
Phone: 770-972-0763

Wheelchair Sports USA
3595 East Fountain Boulevard, Suite L-1
Colorado Springs, CO 80910
Phone: 719-574-1150
Fax: 719-574-9840

World Wheelchair Sports 3552
George Court
Eugene, OR 97401
Phone: 541-485-1860

Appendix D

DISABILITIES QUIZ

The purpose of this quiz is to see how knowledgeable you are about selected disabilities. *This is not an intelligence test.* You may be quite intelligent regarding disabilities but score low on this quiz, and vice versa. The purpose of this quiz is to challenge and enlighten you regarding specific information. Nothing short of an extensive battery of tests and observations by experts will adequately measure your sensitivity to people who have disabilities. This quiz does not meet these criteria. When supplemented with other information, this quiz can help you to get in touch with your overall knowledge of disabilities.

The *Disabilities Quiz* is designed to be self-administered and self-scored. The degree of your "disability" is presented to remind you that labeling can be self-debasing. What you learn from the quiz is more important than your initial score. There is nothing wrong with not knowing answers to the questions. However, depending on your needs, there may be something wrong if you continually miss the answers. For optimum effectiveness, complete this quiz before reading the text and again after you finish it.

Allow fifteen minutes to answer the questions. Write your answers on a separate sheet of paper. Write the letter of the response that is the most correct answer for each question.

1. Which word does not belong?
   a. Crips
   b. Retards
   c. Gimps
   d. None of the above

2. This disease is characterized by abnormally thick mucus that forms plugs in body organs.
   a. Muscular dystrophy
   b. Cystic fibrosis
   c. Multiple sclerosis
   d. Cerebral palsy

3. All but which of the following are major conditions of cerebral palsy?
   a. Spastic
   b. Deafness
   c. Ataxia
   d. Rigidity

4. Which is the largest open minority group in the United States?
   a. African Americans
   b. Females
   c. Hispanic Americans
   d. People with disabilities

5. The stages of grief in the order they generally occur are
   a. Denial, anger, bargaining, depression, acceptance

b. Anger, denial, depression, bargaining, acceptance
c. Denial, bargaining, anger, depression, acceptance
d. Bargaining, anger, denial, depression, acceptance

6. Being blind in one eye did not prevent him from becoming a famous actor:
   a. Art Carney
   b. Peter Falk
   c. George Kennedy
   d. Raymond Burr

7. Which statement is false?
   a. Physical disabilities are more readily accepted than are mental ones.
   b. A mentally ill middle-class person is less stigmatized than a mentally ill lower-class person.
   c. The basic needs of most people with disabilities are different than those of most people without disabilities.
   d. Except for the limitations imposed by their impairments, people with disabilities are no different than people without disabilities.

8. The positive reference group for most people with disabilities is
   a. Middle-class people with disabilities
   b. Lower-class people with disabilities
   c. Middle-class people without disabilities
   d. Lower-class people without disabilities

9. The largest group of students with disabilities are
   a. Partially sighted
   b. Speech impaired
   c. Orthopedically disabled
   d. Hard of hearing

10. A college graduate with a disability who shifts the responsibility for his alcoholism to nondisabled people is likely to be engaging in which defense mechanism?
    a. Projection
    b. Displacement
    c. Repression
    d. Compensation

11. The primary source of security and support for people with disabilities is
    a. Professional helpers
    b. Peer groups
    c. Employers
    d. The family

12. Which statement is false?
    a. Men with disabilities are more likely to be employed than are women with disabilities.
    b. Males with disabilities are more likely to be referred to vocational training than are females with disabilities.
    c. There is a larger percentage of female heads of households with disabilities than of male heads of households with disabilities.
    d. Women with disabilities are less likely than are women without disabilities to get a divorce.

13. This renowned Roman had epilepsy:
    a. Cicero
    b. Appius Claudius
    c. Pontius Lupus
    d. Julius Caesar

14. Which is not a major kind of barrier for most people with physical disabilities?
    a. Intellectual
    b. Housing
    c. Architectural
    d. Recreation

15. Which person does not belong in this list?
    a. Captain Hook
    b. Richard III
    c. Peter Pan
    d. Quasimoto

16. In ancient Rome infants with disabilities were
    a. Worshipped as gods
    b. Killed by their fathers

c. Drowned in the Ganges River
d. Considered intellectual geniuses

17. Prior to the Civil War, hospitals for the care of persons with physical disabilities were established in
a. New York and Philadelphia
b. Boston and Cleveland
c. St. Louis and Chicago
d. Indianapolis and Detroit

18. The Goodwill Industries was organized in the United States in 1902 by this person:
a. Edgar Helms
b. Helen Keller
c. William Booth
d. Jane Addams

19. The first Board of Vocational Education was founded under this act in 1918:
a. The Smith-Fess Act
b. The Barden-LaFollette Act
c. The Social Security Act
d. The Smith-Sears Act

20. Partial or complete paralysis of two limbs on the same side of the body is called
a. Monoplegia
b. Diplegia
c. Hemiplegia
d. Paraplegia

21. Not even speaking with a stutter detracted from the contribution of this person:
a. Booker T. Washington
b. W. B. DuBois
c. Malcolm X
d. George Washington Carver

22. Physiological causes of deafness include
a. Bad teeth
b. Malnutrition
c. Inflammation of the middle ear
d. All of the above
e. None of the above

23. This disease attacks the brain and spinal cord:
a. Multiple sclerosis
b. Cystic fibrosis
c. Osteoarthritis
d. Cerebral palsy

24. Which of the following are the victims of the most discrimination?
a. Nonwhite females with disabilities
b. White males with disabilities
c. White females with disabilities
d. Nonwhite males with disabilities

25. The inability of an individual to function adequately in a work setting because of barriers created by internal fears is called
a. A physical handicap
b. An emotional disability
c. A social disability
d. A physical disability

26. She was the first deaf person to have a lead role on Broadway, and she won a Tony award in 1980 for her performance in Children of a Lesser God.
a. Helen Hayes
b. Priscilla Rounds
c. Phyllis Frelich
d. Patti LuPone

27. Which physical disability does not belong in this list?
a. Cerebral palsy
b. Paraplegia
c. Diabetes mellitus
d. Spina bifida

28. Most lower-class children with disabilities come from homes characterized as
a. Lacking substantial material objects but receiving enough warmth and parental support
b. Lacking substantial material objects and parental support

c. Having adequate material objects but lacking parental warmth and support
d. Having adequate material objects and parental warmth

29. Antidisability attitudes tend to be well developed in children first around this age:
a. Three
b. Ten
c. Seventeen
d. Twenty

30. Public Law 94-142 is also known as the
a. Vocational Rehabilitation Act
b. Architectural Barriers Act
c. Education for All Handicapped Children Act
d. Veterans' Rehabilitation Act

31. This gifted athlete continued playing baseball after losing a leg in an automobile accident:
a. Bill Toomey
b. Jack Pardee
c. Lou Gehrig
d. Monty Stratton

32. Which is likely to be the most dominant factor in the life of a middle-class, African American woman with a disability?
a. Her ethnic identity
b. Her disability
c. Her social class
d. Her sex

33. Which of the following is the single most difficult aspect of nonverbal communication when helpers are dealing with clients who have disabilities?
a. Eye contact
b. Manner of speaking
c. Touching
d. Smiling

34. Title V, Section 504, of the Rehabilitation Act of 1973 provides for
a. Barrier-free federal buildings
b. Nondiscrimination of the physically disabled in all federally funded programs
c. Establishment of an Interagency Committee on Handicapped Employees
d. None of these

35. Attitudes about people with disabilities are
a. Seldom formed by logic
b. Formed as a function of intelligence
c. Usually formed by personal experience
d. None of the above

36. Which of the following is true?
a. People with disabilities are not seen by high-status people as social and economic threats.
b. People with disabilities are a distinct cultural group.
c. People with disabilities are a unique ethnic group.
d. People with disabilities become handicapped in a way that parallels racial and ethnic characteristics.

37. Most Native Americans with disabilities can be found
a. On reservations
b. In the inner cities
c. In the suburbs
d. In small towns

38. Federal law requires that job applicants with disabilities
a. Fill out separate employment forms
b. Take the same tests as applicants without disabilities
c. Be given a different interview than applicants without disabilities
d. Be hired if the company has not filled its quota of workers with disabilities

39. This famous actress has diabetes:
    a. Mary Tyler Moore
    b. Meryl Streep
    c. Liza Minnelli
    d. Sally Field

40. This U.S. Senator from Hawaii lost his right arm in Italy as a soldier during World War II:
    a. Cooper Brown
    b. Spark Matsunaga
    c. Daniel Inouye
    d. Daniel Akaka

41. This famous composer was blind. Two of his compositions were "Ave Maria" and "Faust":
    a. Franz Schubert
    b. Charles Gounod
    c. George Handel
    d. Peter Tchaikovsky

42. This is a major cause of orthopedic disabilities:
    a. Rheumatic fever
    b. Brain injury
    c. Infantile paralysis
    d. All of the above
    e. None of the above

43. Which is the most crucial factor in determining whether persons with disabilities will make satisfactory adjustment to their disability?
    a. Skilled rehabilitation counselors
    b. Their families
    c. Attitudes of society
    d. Extent of the disabilities

44. Which of the following is normal behavior for parents of children with disabilities?
    a. To want to protect them from emotional hurt
    b. To feel guilty and ashamed
    c. To grieve
    d. All of the above
    e. None of the above

45. This outstanding historian suffered from gout:
    a. Edward Gibbon
    b. Allan Nevin
    c. Edward Channing
    d. William Prescott

46. His deafness was overshadowed by his painting ability:
    a. El Greco
    b. Van Gogh
    c. Goya
    d. Rembrandt

47. Which of the following statements is true?
    a. Men are more likely to have diabetes than are women.
    b. Middle-class people are more likely to have diabetes than are lower-class people.
    c. Whites are more likely to have diabetes than nonwhites.
    d. All of the above are true.
    e. None of the above is true.

48. Within American ethnic minority families, persons with physical disabilities generally are
    a. Treated like cripples
    b. Loved as persons
    c. Considered bad omens
    d. Not wanted

49. Which of the following statements is true?
    a. Workers with disabilities are likely to injure themselves.
    b. Insurance companies will not let employers hire workers with disabilities.
    c. As a group, workers with disabilities are absent from their jobs more than workers without disabilities.
    d. All of the above are true.
    e. None of the above is true.

50. Ray Charles is to music what Henry Luce is to
    a. Journalism
    b. Law
    c. Mathematics
    d. Theatre

ANSWERS

1. d	18. a	35. a
2. b	19. d	36. a
3. b	20. c	37. a
4. d	21. d	38. b
5. a	22. d	39. a
6. b	23. a	40. c
7. c	24. a	41. b
8. c	25. b	42. d
9. b	26. c	43. b
10. a	27. c	44. d
11. d	28. a	45. a
12. d	29. b	46. c
13. d	30. c	47. e
14. a	31. d	48. b
15. c	32. b	49. e
16. b	33. c	50. a
17. a	34. b	

SCORE

45–50	No disability in terms of this quiz
40–44	Slight disability
35–39	Moderate disability
30–34	Severe disability
Less than 30	Profound disability

A word of caution: Your disability, if any, will become a handicap if the information you do not know adversely affects your interactions with persons with disabilities.

Appendix E

MEDICAL TERMINOLOGY AND DEFINITIONS

INTRODUCTION

The following glossary of terms represent terminologies used in this text as well as some that have not been used. All terminologies discussed are ones that health-related rehabilitation helping professionals will encounter at various times in the helping process. The discussion of each term is relatively brief; space does not permit a detailed discussion of each. If more detailed information is needed, we recommend that the reader consult the following sources: (1) professional disability-related resources (*see* Appendices B and C for listings), and (2) the *Encyclopedia of Disability and Rehabilitation* (Dell Orto & Marinelli, 1995). Finally, space also does not permit a discussion of every term or condition a health-related professional helper would encounter; thus, the omission of terms should not be interpreted as our evaluation of them as being unimportant.

-A-

Advocacy

Advocacy is an active process designed to make any system–public, community-based, or private–more responsive to the needs of each individual served by that system (Dell Orto & Marinelli, 1995). Advocacy can take many forms, such as self-advocacy, in which a person with a disability or groups of individuals with disabilities advocate for their rights. Advocacy often occurs in what is called *system advocacy,* in which a professional association (e.g. muscular dystrophy) advocates for the rights of its members and all persons who have that disability.

Additionally, there are organizations or committees, such as the Office of Disability Policy (formerly the President's Committee for Employment of Persons with Disabilities), which advocate for increased employment opportunities for all persons with disabilities, and the Disability Rights Education and Defense Fund (DREDF), which advocates for the civil rights of all persons with disabilities.

Affective Disorder

Affective refers to one's feelings and emotions, thus affective disorder relates to mood disorders. Therefore, affective disorder is an umbrella term for a variety of mood disorders such as depression and bipolar disorder; both of these and other affective disorders will be discussed in their appropriate sections.

Affirmative Action

Currently, the words affirmative action cause considerable debate with regard to their meaning and the intent of their user. Some have strong beliefs that affirmative action programs create discrimination by giving an advantage to a specific group over another group; others view affirmative action programs as creating opportunities for persons who have been in a disadvantaged situation for considerable periods of time.

The various debates notwithstanding, the term affirmative action refers to taking affirmative or positive steps to help ensure equal or fair treatment. With regard to persons with disabilities, the term was first mentioned in the 1973 Rehabilitation Act section 503. Dell Orto and Marinelli (1995) contend that "affirmative action in employment of individuals with disabilities means elimination of disability factors from decision making and the provision of reasonable accommodation as needed to assure that each protected individual receives the opportunities he or she would have received had there been no disability. It differs in one significant way from other affirmative action laws and programs; unlike the others, disability affirmative action is not based on numbers. It set no goals, quotas, or timetables" (p. 22). For the most part, this statement is accurate, particularly the fact there are no quotas established; however, the specific goal of eliminating barriers to employment of persons with disabilities is evident. Additionally, a timetable for compliance with Title I of the Americans with disabilities act (employment) was established. Effective July 26, 1992, all private employers who had twenty-five or more employees became subject to this title, and effective July 26, 1994, all private employers who had fifteen or more employees became subject to Title I. Taking this information into consideration, it is accurate to state that Title I does not require employers to hire a given number of persons with disabilities; rather, it promotes the hiring of the best-qualified persons.

Allied Health Professionals

The term allied health professions generally refers to health professionals who are not physicians or dentists. Physical therapists, physician assistants, occupational therapists, medical technologists, speech pathologists, audiologists, nurses, psychologists, and rehabilitation counselors are some of the major allied health professionals who work with persons with disabilities.

Alzheimer's Disease

Alzheimer's disease is a form of dementia. Dementia is a condition in which one's intellectual abilities decrease to the point that daily functions are impaired. Alzheimer's accounts for approximately 60 percent of diagnosed cases of dementia. Dementia generally affects the elderly; therefore, the projection for the next 50 years is an increase in diagnosed Alzheimer cases, given the fact that the number of persons age seventy and above is expected to increase during this same period.

Americans with Disabilities Act

The Americans with Disabilities Act is a civil rights law that prohibits discrimination of persons on the basis of them having a disability. The law was enacted July 26, 1990, and has five titles: Title I, Employment; Title II, Public Service; Title III, Public Accommodations; Title IV, Telecommunications Relay Services; and Title V, Miscellaneous Provisions. (See Chapter 7 for more information with regard to the ADA.)

Anorexia Nervosa

Anorexia nervosa and bulimia nervosa are eating disorders and will be discussed under "Eating Disorders."

Anxiety Disorder

Each of us experiences anxiety at some time in our life. In most cases, anxiety creates psychological discomfort for a short period of time, then we utilize various coping mechanisms to eliminate whatever is creating the anxiety. Problems occur when fear of a situation or reaction to a situation is out of proportion to the threat. In these cases, the reaction is called anxiety disorder. According to the National Institute of Mental Health, the following list summarizes the various kinds of anxiety disorders:

Panic disorder is represented by intense fear that recurs without warning. Some of the symptoms are chest pain, heart palpitation, shortness of breath, and fear of dying.

Obsessive-compulsive disorder is characterized by repeated involuntary thoughts and/or repeated behaviors seemingly uncontrollable.

Posttraumatic stress disorder displays persistent symptoms, such as nightmares, depression, and flashbacks, to mention only three that occur while experiencing a traumatic event.

Phobias involve two major categories: (1) social phobia, which is a fear of social situations such as parties and other social gatherings, and (2) specific phobia, which is an irrational fear of things that pose no threat.

Generalized anxiety disorder is characterized by constant worry over most situations, expecting the worst to happen. The worry is exaggerated out of proportion to the event or perceived threat.

Treatment of anxiety disorders is often handled by medication or psychotherapy. With regard to psychotherapy, behavioral psychotherapy has proven to be effective.

Aphasia

Aphasia is an impairment of the ability to use or comprehend words, usually as a result of a stroke or other brain injury. Often people with aphasia will have difficulty in expressing themselves and may also have problems with reading and writing. Dell Orto and Marinelli (1995) classify aphasia into two groups: (1) nonfluent aphasia, which is characterized by speech that has a considerable amount of pauses. The rate of speech is slow and sometimes sentences are incomplete. The severity of the aphasia influences how well sentences are formed and the extent of the person's vocabulary. (2) Fluent aphasia is characterized by a normal rate of speech, but the aphasia may be evident as a result of the person's inability to retrieve specific nouns. As an example, instead of being able to immediately say cup, the person may say the thing you drink coffee from. As one can tell, it is difficult for a layperson to determine whether a person is affected by aphasia; therefore, professionals, such as speech pathologists, who are trained to detect and diagnosis aphasia, should be consulted.

Art Therapy

Art therapy is a very versatile therapy being used by trained art therapists, occupational therapists, and psychotherapists. Some professionals use art as a means for the client to express emotions; others may use art as both an expression of emotions and a way to observe the clients' perception of their environment.

Art therapy has been reported to be useful in a variety of ways, including working with emotionally disturbed children, the elderly, persons with learning disabilities, persons with physical disabilities, and persons who are chemically dependent, to mention only a few.

Arthritis

Arthritis means inflammation of one or more joints. Arthritis is one of the most common human ailments, and there are several forms of the disorder. Some of the disorders are:

Gout, which occurs as a result of uric acid deposits in the joints. The joints that are most often affected are in the feet, hands, and wrists. Pain and inflammation may occur in any joint,

Rheumatoid arthritis is characterized by inflammation of joints and surrounding tissue stiffness; muscular aches may also be present.

Osteoarthritis causes deterioration of joint cartilage and the creation of bone spurs. Osteoarthritis is the most common of the various types of arthritis, primarily affecting the elderly.

Lupus is a chronic inflammatory autoimmune disorder that may affect internal organs (kidney, heart, lung), the skin (rashes), as well as joints of the body (in the fingers, knees, wrists, etc.). Women are affected more than are men.

Because there are a number of forms of arthritis, a physician is required to diagnose type and prescribe treatment. Helping professionals such as physical and occupational therapists frequently are involved in the treatment of patients with arthritis. Vocational rehabilitation counselors may be called upon to assist clients with training to secure employment compatible with abilities.

Assistive Technology

Assistive technology can mean any device used to assist persons with limitations in regard to accomplishing their activities of daily living. Activities of daily living can mean more than eating, and clothing oneself; it may mean performing one's work, if work is part of the persons daily activities. The Technology Related Assistance for Individuals with Disabilities Act of 1988 offers the following definition of Assistive Technology device: "Any item, piece of equipment or product system, whether acquired commercially, off the shelf, modified or customized, that is used to increase, maintain, or improve functional capabilities of individuals with disabilities."

Attention Deficit Disorder (ADD) and Attention Deficit Hyperactivity Disorder (ADHD)

There is considerable discussion with regard to ADD and ADHD. To be more specific, questions arise with regard to what ADD is. Are ADD and ADHD the same? Additionally, there are varying opinions with respect to treatment of the disorder. Perhaps a small minority of people question whether ADD and ADHD are in fact disorders, especially in children or are these children simply "disobedient."

At the present time, the consensus is that attention deficit is a legitimate disorder. It is a behavioral disorder manifesting itself as difficulty in concentrating. Additionally, the consensus appears to be that when discussing ADD and ADHD, we are referring to the same disorder. Some clinicians prefer to use ADHD because it includes hyperactivity, which is often part of the observed behavior, especially in children. Adults also have the disorder. ADHD is classified as a learning disability. Behavioral therapy has been used to successfully treat clients with attention disorders.

Audiology/Audiologist

Audiology is the prevention, diagnosis, and remediation of hearing impairments. Persons who need to be tested for possible hearing limitation are referred to an audiologist. In the United States, audiologists generally have a masters degree and are certified by the American Speech Language and Hearing Association. Some academic institutions have begun offering doctorates in audiology.

Autism

Autism is a developmental disability that is usually manifested in the form of poor verbal and nonverbal communication as well as poor imaginative play in children, generally under the age of three. Children diagnosed with autism frequently have difficulty in having appropriate social interaction with other children, frequently displaying overly aggressive behavior toward their peers. Ranging from mild to severe these children do not develop their verbal and nonverbal communication at a level equivalent to other children at that same age. Boys are three times more likely to be diagnosed with autism than are girls. Some of the more common and observable behaviors associated with autism are repeated actions, such as rocking back and forth and clapping of hands.

Currently, there are no firm statistics with regard to the extent of the disorder among children; the estimate range from one half million to one and a half million. This wide range is an indication of the difficulty and uncertainty of the diagnosis. According to some US government statistics, Autism is growing in the United States at a rate of 10 to 17 percent per year.

-B-

Bipolar Disorder

Bipolar disorder, frequently referred to as manic depression, is characterized by mood swings from states of elation in which the person presents signs of euphoria to depression in which the person experiences feelings of hopelessness. The mood swings are not always from one extreme to the other; there may be times when the person's mood returns to what may be considered normal before moving to one of the extremes. Of course, each person is an individual; therefore, the pattern of mood swings differs by individual. Likewise, there are varying degrees of severity of the mood swings that individuals experience. According to the *Diagnostic and Statistical Manual of Mental Disorders* (4th edition) *(DSM IV)*, bipolar disorder is a mental illness characterized by the presence of one or more of the following: manic episode, mixed episode and hypomanic episode. The manic phase is characterized by periods of an elevated mood. To be more specific, the person may become hyperactive; his or her mind is flooded with ideas; the belief that one can accomplish almost anything is quite often one of the predominant feelings; additionally, he or she generally experiences a heightened self-esteem as well as a decreased need for sleep.

The depressive phase tends to be the opposite side of life's coin in that the person's mood is depressed, with loss of energy and ambition. The person may experience insomnia, and, in this case, it is a result of feelings of hopelessness. Low self-esteem and a decreased interest in what once were daily activities are also major characteristics of this phase of the illness.

The mixed episode phase refers to the person's experiencing mixed symptoms of both mania and depression; the hypomanic phase refers to a milder form of the manic phase.

Currently it is estimated that from one to three percent of the U.S. population has a bipolar disorder, and the onset of the disorder is generally between the ages of fifteen and twenty-five. Generally, bipolar disorders can be effectively treated with medication; however, sometimes patients refuse to take their medication, especially when they are in the manic phase, because they have a feeling that they are in control of themselves. Conversely, some patients discontinue medication because they feel the medication controls their lives.

Treatment of persons with bipolar disorder is often with medication and in severe cases with electroconvulsive therapy.

Dell Orto and Marinelli (1995), in their edited work, identify three steps of psychiatric rehabilitation for persons with bipolar disorder. The first step is a comprehensive assessment of assets and impairments. The second step is planning based on the finding in the first step. In the planning stage, the helping professional formulates goals and organizes treatment and the rehabilitation plan, taking into consideration the results of the assessment and the environment in which the patient will interact. The third step involves putting the treatment plan into motion. The involvement of vocational rehabilitation counselors and occupational therapists may include getting the patient ready for vocation and/or skill development.

Behavior Therapy

Behavior therapy is based on the principles and procedures of the scientific method, experimentally derived principles of learning and systematically applied to help people change their maladaptive behaviors. Research methods are used to evaluate the effectiveness of both assessment and treatment procedures. Thus behavioral concepts and procedures are stated explicitly and tested empirically and continually (Corey, 2001).

Body Image

Body image refers to how one perceives his or her body and how one thinks others perceive his or her body. Certainly all humans have some perception of their bodies, and to some extent this perception affects how the person interacts with the environment. The perception of one's body *may* (we emphasize may) have a major impact on some persons with disabilities, especially if the condition of the person's body has a negative impact on her or his interaction with the environment. In these cases, a helping professional's skills can be valuable, particularly counseling skills.

Bulimia Nervosa

See Eating Disorders.

-C-

Caregiver

Caregiver refers to anyone who provides assistance on a continual or consistent basis to someone in need of such assistance. Caregivers can be professional helpers, paraprofessionals, and/or family members. The care can range from minimal assistance such as grocery shopping for a person to assisting the person with all major daily activities of living.

Carpal Tunnel Syndrome

Carpal tunnel syndrome refers to a pain in the hand and/or wrist caused by compression of the median nerve in the wrist. Currently, we hear the diagnosis of carpal tunnel syndrome with regard to people who do considerable keyboard work, such as typing or manipulating a computer keyboard, or persons who experience repetitive movement that causes considerable impact to the wrist, such as persons who consistently play racquetball. Additionally, some diseases, such as rheumatoid arthritis, diabetes, and high blood pressure, to mention a few, may contribute to the onset of the syndrome.

Cerebral Palsy

Cerebral palsy is a group of disorders that are caused by damage to the brain. The disorder affects movement and/or nerve functions. Cerebral palsy is not just one disorder but consists of several forms. Spastic cerebral palsy affects approximately 70 percent of those persons with cerebral palsy. This form of cerebral palsy is characterized by stiff and contracted muscles. If a single limb on one side of the body is affected, it is referred to as spastic hemiplegia; if both legs are involved, it is referred to as spastic diplegia; if both arms and legs are affected, it is termed spastic quadriplegia. Another form of cerebral palsy is called athetoid or dyskinetic, which is characterized by uncontrolled movement and may affect the hands, feet, arms, facial muscles, and tongue (resulting in drooling).

Athetoid cerebral palsy affects approximately 10 percent of persons with cerebral palsy. Yet another form of cerebral palsy is referred to as ataxic and it affects 5 to 10 percent of persons with cerebral palsy. This form is characterized by poor coordination, unsteady walking gait, and sometimes uncontrollable tremors. The final type of cerebral palsy is called mixed form and may be a combination of the previously mentioned forms of cerebral palsy.

Cerebral palsy is generally diagnosed in a child before the age of three. Additionally, cerebral palsy is not a progressive disorder. Muscles may weaken not because of the disease progress but as a result of lack of use and exercise of the muscles. Muscles will weaken in persons without cerebral palsy if they are not used regularly.

It has been reported that approximately one third of children who have cerebral palsy have mild intellectual impairment, another one third are considered moderately to severely impaired, and the remaining one third are considered intellectually normal.

Some helping professionals frequently used in the treatment of persons with cerebral palsy are physicians, physical therapists, occupational therapists, speech pathologists, audiologists, nurses, social workers, psychologists, vocational rehabilitation counselors, and vocational evaluators.

Civil Rights

In the United States, civil rights refer to the legal rights of persons that are afforded by the Constitution and laws of the United States of America. Quite often, civil rights are associated with rights of ethnic minorities; however, every American has civil rights. The 1990 ADA and the 2008 Amendments is a civil rights law that prohibits discrimination against persons on the basis of having a disability.

Communication Disorder

From the context of the rehabilitation helping professional, communication disorder refers to impairments and/or limitations of communicating with other humans. Human communication may take various forms, such as verbal (spoken words) and nonverbal (gestures, body posture, etc). For communication disorders there are rehabilitation helping professionals such as speech therapists, speech pathologists, and audiologists who specialize in working with persons who have communication limitations.

-D-

Deinstitutionalization

The institutionalization of persons with disabilities, particularly those who were considered mentally ill or mentally retarded, has been somewhat of a mixed bag. In some cases, institutionalization is for the purpose of removing the "unwanted" from the view of the general public. In other cases, institutionalization was considered "moral" treatment. Regardless of the intent, over the decades, institutionalization for those who were no harm to themselves or society became synonymous with restricting the rights and opportunities of persons with disabilities. In the 1960s and 1970s, through legislation and advocacy, efforts were put forth to establish mental health facilities as well as transition homes for persons who were institutionalized. Thus, deinstitutionalization for those deemed to be able to live outside of an institution gained momentum. Therefore, the term deinstitutionalization refers to moving persons who have been institutionalized out of institutions and into communities.

Dementia

Dementia refers to impairment of brain function. Dementia may be either progressive or treatable. However, most dementia is progressive. There are many symptoms of dementia, and some of the most common are memory loss, severe confusion, and decrease in problem-solving ability. As dementia progresses, frequently personality changes are noted, such as depression and irritability.

Depression

Depression has been referred to by some researchers as the common cold of mental health. This description is used because depression is so common. Everyone at some time feels depressed. The depth of these feelings, as well as the length of time that one experiences the feelings, has an influence on whether the person is considered to be ill with depression. Depression is characterized by feelings of sadness and a general feeling of being unhappy. Again, all humans experience these feelings; however, if the feelings deepen to the point that one's appetite is affected and the person's normal sleep habit is altered and there is a loss of interest in activities that normally bring pleasure, it may be a sign that the person is in a state of depression that goes beyond the normal low-grade depression most people experience. Generally, if the person experiences these symptoms as well as other feelings of helplessness for a two-week period, it is a sign that the depression has exceeded the normal range of depressed moods.

Developmental Disabilities

The Developmental Disabilities Services and Facilities Construction Amendment of

1970 offers the following definition of developmental disabilities: a severe, chronic disability of a person that (a) is attributable to a mental or physical impairment or combination of mental or physical impairments; (b) is manifested before the person attains age twenty-two years; (c) is likely to continue indefinitely, (d) results in substantial functional limitations in three or more of the following areas of major life activities: self-care, receptive and expressive language, learning, mobility, self-direction, capacity for independent living, and economic sufficiency; and (e) reflects the person's need for a combination and sequence of special interdisciplinary or generic care, treatment, or other services that are lifelong or of extended duration and are individually planned and coordinated. Developmental disability is frequently thought to be only mental retardation or the currently acceptable label intellectual disability. Certainly intellectual disability is a developmental disability; however, as one can see from the previously mentioned definition, other conditions are considered to be developmental disabilities.

Diabetes Mellitus

Diabetes refers to the body's inability to produce insulin or properly use the insulin that is produced. Insulin is a hormone that helps convert food into energy. There are two main types of diabetes. Type 1 often begins in childhood and has been referred to as juvenile diabetes. Type 2 is referred to as adult onset; there are an estimated 23.6 million persons with this type of diabetes. A third type is called gestational, which develops during pregnancy and generally disappears following birth. It is believed there are several factors that contribute to a person's developing diabetes, such as obesity and a sedentary lifestyle. The rate of diabetes is high among the ethnic minority groups of African Americans and American Indians.

Diabetes is a major cause of death in American Indians. There are several complications that may occur as a result of uncontrollable diabetes including renal disease. Amputation is another risk. Persons with diabetes are at significant risk for lower extremity amputations. Persons with diabetes account for 50 percent of all nontraumatic amputations performed in the United States. Persons with diabetes are more at risk for blindness than is the general population. The leading cause of morbidity and mortality among persons with diabetes is cardiovascular disease. The annual risk for death or disability from cardiovascular disease is two to three times greater for persons with diabetes than for persons without diabetes.

-E-

Eating Disorders

Eating disorders may include compulsive overeating, in which the person continually overeats during the day and evening. A result of this generally is obesity, especially if the person does not engage in appropriate exercise.

Anorexia nervosa is another eating disorder that is characterized by a fixation on weight loss. In many cases, the person is of normal weight; however, she (the majority of anorexia nervosa cases are females) has a distorted body image and believes that she is fat and/or gaining weight. To remove the perceived excessive weight, the person may engage in a great deal of exercise, excessive dieting, and abuse of laxatives. In some instances, the person may also induce vomiting.

Another eating disorder is bulimia nervosa, which is characterized by binge eating, frequently followed by self-induced vomiting. During the period of binge eating, the person often takes in enormous amounts of food and calories, followed by guilt feelings and a fear of becoming obese, thus leading to the self-induced vomiting.

In most cases of eating disorders, the exact cause is not known. It is believed that psychological and emotional problems are part of the cause. It is further believed that the psychological and emotional problems are precipitated by social pressure to have the perfect body.

Epidemiology/Epidemiologist

The term epidemiology refers to the study of the distribution of diseases within a population. Most state health departments employ epidemiologists who frequently issue reports of the distribution of diseases by age, sex, and ethnicity, to mention only three variables.

Two words that are frequently used in reports distributed by epidemiologists are prevalence, which is generally referring to the percentage of a population that is affected by the disease or disorder being discussed and incidence, which refers to the rate of occurrence of a disease or disorder. An epidemiologist can be either a physician or a nonphysician. Most will have a doctoral degree from a school of public health or a medical doctor's degree, or both.

Empowerment

A simplified definition of empowerment is being able to help oneself accomplish desired tasks and/or goals. Frequently, the goal of advocates for persons with disabilities is to cause the person to become as self-reliant as possible.

End-Stage Renal Disease

End-stage renal disease refers to the loss of all or most of kidney functions. Stated in other terms, the kidneys are no longer able to adequately filter the waste in the body so that the individual can carry on with normal activities of daily living. Generally, an individual is considered to be in end-stage renal failure when the kidney function is below 10 percent of normal.

Persons with severe kidney disorders such as end-stage renal disease often have three choices for treatment: (1) filtering of the blood to remove toxins through a process called hemodialysis, (2) removal of body waste through the process called peritoneal dialysis, and (3) kidney transplant. A variety of rehabilitation helping professionals, such as nurses, physical therapists, occupational therapists, vocational rehabilitation counselors, and psychologists, may be involved in the rehabilitation process of persons with a kidney disorder. Rehabilitation counselors and psychologists can be valuable members of the rehabilitation team as the patient works through emotional reactions to adjustment to the disability. Among the major causes of kidney disease are hypertension, diabetes, and abusive use of certain drugs, both over the counter and prescription.

Epilepsy

Epilepsy refers to seizures that occur as a result of irregular electrical impulses discharged in the brain. There are primarily two types of seizures: (1) grand mal, which involves the loss of consciousness, and (2) petit mal, which occurs without loss of consciousness.

Ergonomics

There are numerous definitions of ergonomics, depending on the discipline attempting to define the term. For our purposes, ergonomics means engineering the work environment so the worker can be safe and productive to his or her potential. Given this definition, reasonable accommodations can be considered a type of ergonomic effort.

-H-

Hemophilia

Hemophilia, often referred to as the bleeding disease, occurs as a result of the blood taking a long time to clot. Blood has clotting factors and they have been named factor I through XIII based on the order of their discovery. There are two major types of hemophilia, A and B. Hemophilia A is the most common and is a result of a lack of clotting factor VIII. Hemophilia B results from a lack of factor IX. Another important fact to know is that hemophilia is sex linked. To be more specific, mostly men are affected. Women are primarily carriers.

Human Immunodeficiency Virus (HIV)

Dickson (2001) provides the following explanation of HIV: The disease follows a predictable and, as of today, an unalterable course. Once a person is infected with HIV, the virus invades different cells in the blood and body tissues. Certain white blood cells, known as helper T-lymphocytes or CD4+ cells, are particularly vulnerable to HIV. The virus attaches to the CD4 receptor site of the target cell and fuses its membrane to the cell's membrane. HIV is a retrovirus, which means it uses an enzyme to convert its own genetic material into a form indistinguishable from the genetic material of the target cell. The virus' genetic material migrates to the cell's nucleus and becomes integrated with the cell's chromosomes. Once integrated, the virus can use the cell's own genetic machinery to replicate itself. Additional copies of the virus are released into the body and infect other cells in turn. Although the body does produce antibodies to combat HIV infection, the antibodies are not effective in eliminating the virus.

The initial stage of the HIV infection is known as acute or primary HIV infection. In a typical case, this stage lasts three months. The virus concentrates in the blood. The assault on the immune system is immediate. After the symptoms associated with the initial stage subside, the disease enters what is referred to sometimes as the asymptomatic phase. The term is a misnomer in some respects for clinical features persist throughout, including lymphodenopathy, dermatological disorder, oral lesions, and bacterial infections. Although it varies with each individual, in most instances, this stage lasts from seven to eleven years (Dickson, 2001, p. 7).

The ways that HIV can be transmitted are also misunderstood. The belief that the infection can be transmitted by casual contact such as touching is held by some individuals. Today there are three known methods of transmission: exchange of body fluid in sexual intercourse, exposure to infected blood products, and transmission interutero, from an infected mother to a fetus (Dickson, 2001, p. 9).

Hospice

Hospice is an organized system of care provided to persons who have been diagnosed as terminally ill.

Huntington's Disease

Huntington's disease is an inherited disease that involves the degeneration of nerve cells in the brain. As the nerve cells die, there is a progressive loss of mental function, a decrease in cognitive function that may affect speech. The disease is also characterized by abnormal facial and body movements, frequently of a jerking nature.

-I-

Independent Living

From the standpoint of rehabilitation, independent living can mean several things. The meaning will depend on the persons' circumstances. To be more specific, in some cases, independent living may mean living with the support of personal assistance, individuals (either professional and/or family member), and assistive technology. The independence that this individual has may be his or her ability to make choices. In other cases, independent living may mean the person takes care of his or her activities of daily living with a minimum of assistance.

Inclusion

As much as is possible, including persons with disabilities in society's daily activities is a global definition of inclusion. In many instances, the term inclusion, when used with regard to persons with disabilities, refers to including students who are considered to be intellectually disabled in classroom activities with nondisabled students. This has been a major thrust of educators in recent times; however, from the vantage point of the universe of persons with disabilities, inclusion goes beyond public and private school classrooms. Inclusion in social, religious, employment, and family activities are equally important.

-J-

Job Accommodation

The term job accommodation refers to making the employment environment accessible to persons with disabilities.

-L-

Learning Disability

Learning disability is the overall name for a variety of limitations to one's ability to effectively learn, such as ADA, and dyslexia, to mention only one.

-M-

Mainstreaming

Mainstreaming is a term that has been used to refer to involving persons with disabilities in the daily activities of society. Mainstreaming encompasses several activities such as deinstitutionalization of persons with mental disabilities. The term also includes intergrating persons who are considered to be intellectually disabled in classroom settings and activities with the nondisabled students. Today, the word inclusion is most often used to refer to these activities.

Mental Illness

Mental illness is a general term used for a variety of psychiatric, psychological, and mood disorders, many of which are described in the *DSM-IV.*

Mental Retardation or Intellectual Disability

The American Association of Mental Retardation (AAMR) defines mental retardation as significantly subaverage intellectually functioning existing concurrently with related limitations in two or more of the following applicable adaptive skill areas: communication, self-care, home living, social skills, community use, self-direction, health and safety, functional academics, leisure, and work. The Association believes mental retardation becomes apparent before age eighteen. In its *DSM-IV*, the American Psychiatric Association provides the following definition of mental retardation: (1) significantly subaverage general intellectual functioning for children and adults with an IQ of 70 or below on an individually administered IQ test; for infants, a clinical judgment of significantly subaverage intellectual functioning; (2) concurrent deficits or impairments in adaptive functioning, in other words, the person's effectiveness in meeting the age and cultured standards in areas such as communication, daily living skills, personal independence, and self-sufficiency; and (3) onset before age eighteen (Dell Orto & Marinelli, 1995, p. 457).

According to Dell Orto and Marinelli (1995), mental retardation is categorized by level of severity: IQ between 55 and 69, mildly retarded; IQ between 40 and 54, moderately retarded; IQ between 25 and 39, severely retarded; and IQ between 0 and 24, profoundly retarded. The authors, however, point out that in the educational area a three-category system is often used that differs somewhat from the previously mentioned psychological categorization. The education category system is as follows: educable mentally retarded, IQ 50 to 70; trainable mentally retarded, IQ 30 to 50; and severely retarded, IQ below 30, (p. 457).

Multiple Sclerosis

The exact origin of multiple sclerosis is not known, and currently there is no known cure. Multiple sclerosis involves inflammation of the central nervous system. It is believed the inflammation destroys the covering of nerve cells and the resulting scar tissue interrupts and/or blocks transmission of nerve impulses in the affected area. Some of the symptoms and results of multiple sclerosis can be weakness of one or more extremities, paralysis of one or more extremities, spasticity of muscles, and pain in an extremity, to mention only a few.

Muscular Dystrophy

Muscular dystrophy is not one disorder but a group of inherited disorders that generally leads to muscular weakness and atrophy. Some of the inherited disorders are Duchenne's dystrophy, which affects primarily males (primarily boys); Becker's muscular dystrophy, which also affects boys and is a milder form of Duchenne that progresses at a slower rate. both cause muscle weakness of the legs. Another form of muscular dystrophy is Emery-Dreifuss; it primarily involves weakness and wasting of muscles in the shoulder, upper arms, and calves. Additionally, stiffness of joints may occur as well as some heart problems.

Musculoskeletal Disorders

The term musculoskeletal disorders applies to a number of disorders, including the various forms of arthritis, bursitis, and tendon and ligament damage, to mention a few. Musculoskeletal disorders have negatively affected the soft tissue and bones of the body to the point that they alter the normal functions of the affected areas.

-N-

Neurological Disorders

Neurological disorders are caused by impairment of the nervous system, such as strokes, epilepsy, Alzheimer's disease, Parkinson's disease, multiple sclerosis, and muscular dystrophy.

Neurology/Neurologist

Neurology is a medical specialty dealing with illness and injuries affecting the brain, spinal cord, peripheral nerves, and muscles. Examples of conditions treated by neurologists include epilepsy, headache, stroke, multiple sclerosis, cerebral palsy, dementia, disorders of the peripheral nerves, and muscular disorders (Dell Orto & Marinelli, 1995). A neurologist is a medical doctor.

Neuromuscular Disorders

Neuromuscular disorders involve the nerves (motor neurons) that connect the brain and spinal cord to muscles, the junction of the nerves and muscles (neuromuscular junction), or the muscles themselves. Since motor neurons provide central and growth regulation for muscles, any disorder that damages these nerves will impair the muscles as well. Disorders that strike nerves are primarily known as neuropathies. Disorders that affect the connection between nerve and muscles are known as neuromuscular junction disorders (Dell Orto & Marinelli, 1995). Poliomyelitis is an example of a neuromuscular disorder.

-O-

Obsessive-Compulsive Disorder

Obsessive-compulsive disorder is a psychological anxiety disorder characterized by obsessive or compulsive behavior. Obsession may be described as the mind being stuck on a particular thought(s) and, in a manner of speaking, replaying those thoughts over and over. Compulsion may be described as being similar to the replay button on a video cassette. The individual repeats behavior(s) over and over. In both obsessive and compulsive behaviors there generally is some type of ritual associated with the action. To be more specific, the person repeats the behavior or thoughts in a certain pattern or order. In most cases, the person having the thoughts or performing the behavior has a difficult time in controlling them, given the fact the thoughts and/or behavior is designed to avoid or eliminate anxiety.

Occupational Therapy/Occupational Therapist

Occupational therapy is a very versatile and valued part of the rehabilitation program for persons with disabilities. In general, the occupational therapy program is designed to assist the person with a disability in learning to handle activities of daily living, taking into consideration the limitations that have occurred from the disability. Occupational therapy services are beneficial to children and the elderly as well as all age groups in between. As previously mentioned, the occupational therapy services may include teaching a person with a disability how to handle daily life activities, such as eating, preparing food, dressing, and general household duties. The service may also involve helping the person with a disability adjust to and learn new ways of handling a work environment such as manipulating a computer terminal with limited or no use of hands. Similarly, the service may include teaching a patient how to effectively use a mobility aid. Use of adaptive technology is also a major role of occupational therapy. One can see that occupational therapy is an important component of the rehabilitation team.

Occupational therapists are the human side of occupational therapy. To be more specific the therapist is the professional who puts the therapy program into action. An occupational therapist will have a minimum of a bachelor's degree and be certified by the American Occupational Therapy Association. There are occupational therapy assistants who will generally have a two-year college degree.

-P-

Personality Disorder

Personality disorders are reflected in a person's distorted beliefs and/or actions with regard to self-worth, distorted views of the worth of others, as well as the person's distorted concepts and interaction with his or her environment. Arthur Dell Orto and Marinelli (1995) inform us that personality disorders are grouped clinically into three major clusters: "Cluster A includes paranoid schizoid and schizoid-typed personality disorders. Cluster B includes antisocial, borderline, histrionic and narcissistic personality disorders. Cluster C includes avoidant, dependent and obsessive-compulsive personality disorders" (p. 546).

Physical Therapy/Physical Therapist

Physical therapy is the examination, treatment, and instruction of human beings to detect, assess, prevent, correct, alleviate, and limit physical disability, movement dysfunction, bodily malfunction and pain from injury, disease, and any other physical or mental condition. It includes the administration interpretation, evaluation, and modification of treatment (Dell Orto & Marinelli, 1995).

The physical therapist is the allied health professional responsible for administering the physical therapy program and treatment. Physical therapists have a minimum of a bachelor's degree and are certified by the American Physical Therapy Association. The requirement for becoming a physical therapist is being increased to a master's degree.

Physician

In most cases, the physician is the leader of the health care team. Most physicians will have completed a bachelor's degree, and all will have completed a medical doctor's degree, generally four years of medical school beyond the undergraduate program. There are a number of specialties in medicine. The physician, once he or she has completed the medical degree, will specialize in one or more specialty areas; therefore, the length required to complete varies based upon the specialty area requirement. All physicians are required to become licensed by the state in which they practice. Additionally, many become certified by a board of examiners relating to the areas of specialty.

Poliomyelitis

Polio is the weakening and/or paralysis of muscles of the body. Generally, all muscles and nerves of the body are affected. The weaker muscles and/or paralysis may be in one or more limbs. Poliomyelitis is caused by a viral infection. There is medication and a vaccine that is very effective in preventing one from becoming infected. In the United States, since the 1950s, very few persons have contracted the virus that causes polio.

Prosthesis

Prosthesis means an artificial limb.

Psychiatry/Psychiatrist

Psychiatry is one of the medical specialties and has as its emphasis working with people who have mental and or emotional problems. Psychiatrists are medical doctors trained in a psychological/psychiatry specialty.

Psychology/Psychologist

Psychology is the study of human behavior. To be more specific, it is the study of how humans think and the way humans behave with regard to their thoughts.

Psychologists are mental health professionals who study human behavior and apply intervention strategies with the goal of helping a person overcome mental and/or emotional problems. There are a number of specialties in psychology, such as clinical, experimental, educational, and counseling to mention a few. A psychologist may be trained at the masters or doctoral level. Additionally, most psychologists take additional training in an area of specialty (e.g. family counseling) and become licensed and/or certified. Psychologists and psychiatrists do very similar things from a psychological prospective, with one notable exception: psychiatrist are medical doctors and as such are able to prescribe medication to assist in the psychological adjustment, whereas psychologists cannot prescribe medication.

Psychotherapy

Psychotherapy is the treatment of mental and emotional problems through the use of various psychological theories and techniques with the goal of helping the client/patient gain insight into his or her behavior, thus promoting positive change in behavior.

Psychosocial Aspects of Disabilities

A compact definition of psychosocial aspects of disabilities is a study of the psychological and social factors that have an impact on the life of a person with a disability.

-Q-

Quadriplegia

Quadriplegia means paralysis that has some involvement in all four limbs. The spinal cord has thirty segments: eight cervical, twelve thoracic, five lumbar, and five sacral. Injury to any of the eight cervical segments will cause quadriplegia.

-R-

Reasonable/Accommodations

A key requirement of the ADA of 1990 is that employers must make reasonable accommodations for the person with a disability to help enable her or him to be successful in completing the required job functions. The employer does not have to provide the requested accommodation(s) if he or she can prove that the accommodations would create an undue hardship. Therefore, according to the ADA, a reasonable accommodation means:

• Modification or adjustments to a job application process that enables a qual-

ified applicant with a disability to be considered for the position said qualified applicant desires
- Modifications or adjustments to the work environment, or to the manner or circumstances under which the position held or desired is customarily performed to enable a qualified individual with a disability to perform the essential functions of the position
- Modifications or adjustments that enable an employee with a disability to enjoy equal benefits and privileges or employment as are enjoyed by other similarly situated employees without disabilities

Rehabilitation

Rehabilitation is a term that is difficult to adequately define in that it is a concept defined by each individual and his or her needs. To be more specific, what rehabilitation means to one individual may not be accurate for another person. What ultimately determines rehabilitation is the level of the individual's limitations and/or problems. Therefore, if one has minor injuries and limitations, rehabilitation may mean full or 90 percent return to former levels of functioning. Another person may have significant limitations and recovery may be 50 percent or less of former level of functioning; however, through adaptation and motivation the person is able to assist with his or her activities of daily living. Is this person not also rehabilitated, albeit not at 100 percent?

Taking these facts into consideration, we believe a reasonable definition of rehabilitation is returning the individual back to as much of former function as possible.

Respite Care

Respite care refers to any program that provides service to persons with disabilities so that family members, who often are the primary caregivers, can receive temporary relief from the daily care. The respite care can range from a few hours to several weeks. Respite care service may be provided in the home, or the patient may be temporarily relocated to a health-care facility.

-S-

Schizophrenia

The definition of schizophrenia is provided by the symptoms of the disorder, and they are delusions, hallucinations, disorganized speech, and grossly disorganized or catatonic behavior; these must last at least one month.

Sheltered Employment

Sheltered workshops generally provide employment for persons who have significant disabilities and are unable to work in a competitive work environment. Through innovation and creativity, rehabilitation personnel have begun to develop different work environments such as supported employment to help meet the employment needs of persons with significant disabilities. Additionally many sheltered workshops have begun to offer training and employment that goes beyond what has traditionally been called their role of providing menial employment.

Sickle Cell Anemia

Sickle cell anemia is an inherited blood disease caused by abnormally shaped (sickle-shaped) red blood cells. Because of the shape of the red blood cells, oxygen-carrying capacity is reduced. The disorder can be fatal, especially if there is an insufficient oxygen supply to tissue and vital organs. The disorder is prevalent among African Americans, with approximately 10 percent of the African American population being carriers of the disorder. If two persons with the sickle cell trait have offspring, there is a one in four risk of the children having the disorder.

Special Education

Special education represents services designed to assist students who have special instructional needs. Those receiving these services may be persons who are considered to be to have an intellectual disability and those who have other learning disabilities. In 1975, the Education for All Handicapped Children Act (name later changed to Individuals with Disabilities Education Act) required that all children with disabilities be provided a free and appropriate education in the least restrictive environment. Although this did not eliminate segregating students with disabilities from the nondisabled students, the legislation and subsequent acts and amendments have increased the inclusion of students with disabilities into a somewhat integrated educational setting.

Stroke

A stroke occurs when the blood supply to part of the brain is interrupted, resulting in the death of brain tissue. There are numerous factors that may contribute to the interrupted supply of blood to the brain. Some of these factors are hypertension, diabetes, heart disease, smoking, and blood clots.

Results of a stroke, in part, are determined by the part of the brain that is affected. In some cases, speech is impaired and there is paralysis of one or more limbs. Rehabilitation efforts such as speech therapy and physical and occupational therapy often are very beneficial in assisting the person to regain as much former function as possible.

Supported Employment

According to the Developmental Disabilities Act of 1984, supported employment is for persons with developmental disabilities for whom competitive employment at or above the minimum wage is unlikely and who, because of their disabilities, need intensive ongoing support to perform in a work setting; conducted in a variety of settings, particularly worksites in which persons without disabilities are employed; and supported by an activity needed to sustain paid work by persons with disabilities, including supervision, training, and transportation.

By definition, supported employment has three essential feature: (1) opportunities for paid productive work, along with (2) ongoing support and training to enssure continued employment, and (3) employment in socially integrated environments (Sinnott-Oswald, Gliner, & Spencer, 1991, p. 103).

-U-

Undue Hardship

As was stated in the explanation of reasonable accommodation, the 1990 ADA requires an employer to provide accommodations for an employee with a disability unless the employer can prove the accommodation creates an undue hardship. An undue hardship means an action requiring significant difficulty or expense, one that is unduly costly, extensive, disruptive, or that will fundamentally alter the nature of the employment. The definition is very broad so that undue hardship can be determined on a case by case basis. What is an undue hardship for a small local grocery store probably will not be a hardship for a multi-million dollar company.

SUMMARY

The explanation of the terminology and definitions presented are not intended to provide a comprehensive review of medical terms. This is in most cases written to provide a beginner's overview of terms and definitions. We hope that these explanations will stimulate your desire to learn more about the subjects discussed; thus you will do additional research.

Because statistics change over periods of time, and given the current state of technology the statistics are changing rather quickly, in most cases, we deliberately avoid providing statistics. The reader is encouraged to research the appropriate statistics for your state and location as well as national statistics.

POINTS OF DISCUSSION AND/OR SUGGESTED ACTIVITIES

In explaining most of the terms, no statistics were given as to prevalence of a disease in the United States population because statistics frequently change. Take any five terms that relate to a disease or disability and obtain the latest statistics of prevalence and any other relevant facts that relate to the nation, your state, and/or local community.

As previously stated, space did not permit an all-inclusive listing of relevant terms. Identify at least five diseases, disabilities, and/or terms in which you have an interest (not listed in this chapter) and develop an informational sheet on each.

REFERENCES

Dickson, D.T. (2001). *HIV, AIDS and the Law.* New York: Aldine de Gruytei.

Dell Orto, A.E., and Marinelli, R.P. (Eds.). (1995). *Encyclopedia of Disability and Rehabilitation.* New York: Simon and Schuster Macmillan.

Corey, G. (2001). *Theory and Practice of Counseling and Psychotherapy* (6th ed.). Pacific Grove, CA: Brooks/Cole.

INDEX

A

Attitudes and behaviors, 35-44
   Social attitudes, 36, 37
   Attitudes learned, 38-41
   How attitudes are formed, 41-44

B

Beliefs and Treatments, 17-29
   Ancient beliefs and practices, 18, 19
      Religious beliefs, 18
      Abandonment and death, 18, 19
      Literature, 20-22
   Early American views, 22-25
      Pioneering spirit, 23
      Humanitarian and rehabilitation activities, 23-25
   Elizabethan English poor laws, 22, 23
   Social Cleansing, 25-28
      Social Darwinism, 25, 26
      Eugenics, 26-28
Burnout, 129, 130

C

Caring, 127, 128
Childhood development, 54-57
   Middle childhood, 54
   Preadolescence or puberty, 54, 55
   Adolescence, 55, 56
   Adulthood, 56, 57
Communication, 59, 60
   Understanding, 60
   Listening, 60
   Organizing one's thoughts, 60
   Wait for reaction, 60
   Open mind, 60

Conference etiquette, 161
Coping styles, 153-165
   Methods of coping, 157-164
      Depression, 157, 158
      Denial, 158, 159
      Repression, 159
      Projection, 159, 160
      Displacement, 160
      Sublimation, 161
      Aggression, 161
      Dependency, 161, 162
      Self-abasement, 162
      Regression, 162
      Compensation, 162, 163
      Fantasy, 163
      Passing, 163
      Transference, 164
      Countertransference, 164
Cultural Sensitivity, 183-193
   Defining culture, 184, 185
   Disability culture, 187, 188
   Disability culture sensitivity, 188-191
   Deaf culture, 191, 192

D

Disability issues for the twenty-first century, 209-217
   When is disability a disability? 210, 211
   Fate of persons with severe disabilities, 212, 213
   Inclusion, 213
   End of life decisions, 213, 214
   Personal assistive services, 214
   Are accommodations preferential treatment? 214, 215
   How much should be spent on rehabilitation? 215, 216
   Prenatal testing and genetics, 216, 217

Disability models, 6-14
  Moral/religion model, 7, 14
  Charity model, 7, 8, 14
  Social paternalistic model, 8, 9, 14
  Medical/functional limitation/rehabilitation model, 9, 10, 14
  Minority/cultural group model, 11, 12, 14
  Empowerment model, 12, 13, 14
  Sociopolitical concept model, 13, 14
Disability politics, 99-118
  Advocacy, 100-102
  League of physically handicapped protest, 101, 102
  Independent living center movement, 102-105
  Legislative action, 105-116
    Smith-Fess Act, 105
    Barden-LaFollotte Act, 105, 106
    Vocational Rehabilitation Act Amendment (1965), 106
    Rehabilitation Act of 1973, 106, 107
    Education of All Handicapped Children Act of 1975, 107
    Individuals with Disability Education Act, 107, 108
    Americans with Disability Act of 1990, 108-113
    Americans with Disability Act Amendments of 2008, 113-115
    Rehabilitation Act Amendments of 1992, 115, 116
    Rehabilitation Act Amendments of 1993, 116
    Rehabilitation Act Amendments of 1998, 118

E

Empowerment, 67-77
  Actions, 68-71
    Wheel of justice protest, 68
    Deaf president now protest, 68, 69
    Section 504 protest, 69, 70
    League of Physically Handicapped Protest, 70, 71
  Benefits of, 71, 72
  Becoming empowered, 72-74
    Self-acceptance, 72, 73
    Education/training, 72, 73
    Employment, 73, 74
  Persons with disabilities empowering themselves, 75-77
    Breaking act of overdependence, 76
    Becoming engaged in community activities, 76,77
Employment, 79-95
  Protestant work ethic, 80, 81
  Self-esteem, 81-83
  Disability and, 83
  Obstacles to, 83-85
  Myths, 85-87
    Safety, 85
    Insurance, 85
    Liability, 85
    Productivity, 86
    Attendance, 86
    Accommodation, 86
    Acceptance, 87
  Preparing for, 87, 88
  Laws that aid, 89
    Americans with Disability Act, 89
    Workforce Investment Act, 89, 90
    Rehabilitation Act Amendment (Section 508), 90
    Ticket to Work Act, 90, 91
  Agencies that aid, 91, 92
    Vocational Rehabilitation, 91
    Veterans Administration, 91
    Social Security Administration, 91, 92
    Sheltered Workshops, 92
  Supported Employment, 92, 93
    What is, 93
    Purpose of, 93
    Philosophy of, 93
    Models of, 93, 94
    Job coach, 94
Eugenics, 26-28
  Maintaining Employment, 94, 95

F

Family, 119-131
  Members of, 120
  Members roles, 120-122
    Mother, 120, 121
    Father, 121
    Others, 121, 122
Feelings, 50
Feelings and behaviors, 122-125
  Self-pity, 122, 123
  Magic cures, 123

Guilty and shame, 123, 124
Overprotection, 124
Resentment, 124, 125
Children, 125
Marital problems, 126, 127

H

Helping Professionals, 167-181
  The helping relationship, 168-173
    Establishing trust and rapport, 168, 169
    Confidentiality, 169
    Identifying and clarifying issues, 169
    Establishing goals, 170, 171
    Identifying and implementing solutions, 171, 172
    Termination, 172, 173
  Becoming an effective helper, 175-180
    Trustworthy, 174
    Effective communicator, 174-176
    Caring and compassionate, 176, 177
    Empathic, 177
    Understanding self, 177, 178
    Understanding human behavior, 178
    Understanding resources, 178
    Understanding family dynamics, 178
    Understanding cultural differences, 178, 179
    Understanding disabilities, 179, 180
Human Rights for All, 197-206
Human Service Personnel, 135-151

I

Interview, 136-141
  Gestures, 139, 140
  Manner of speaking, 140
  Zones of territory, 140
  Touching, 140
  Listening, 140, 141

P

Positive thought, 58
Pride, 61, 62
Professional helpers, 147-149

R

Rapport, establishing, 141-143
Realism, 58, 59
Responsibility, 59
Review of related literature, 34, 35

S

Self-acceptance, 57, 58
Self-actualization, 149, 150
Self-improvement, 61
Social Darwinism, 25, 26
Social development, 50-57
  Havinghurst's Development Tasks, 52
    Early childhood, 52
    Middle childhood, 52
    Later maturity, 52
  Erikson's Life Cycle Stages, 52, 53
    Trust v mistrust, 52
    Autonomy v doubt, 52, 53
    Initiative v guilt, 53
    Industry v inferiority, 53
    Identity v role confusion, 53
    Intimacy v self-absorption, 53
    Generalivity v self-absorption, 53
    Integrity v despair, 53
  Piaget's Intellectual Development Stages, 53
    Sensorimotor, 53
    Preoperational, 53
    Concrete operational, 53
    Formal operational, 53
  Bruner's Stages of Concept Development, 53
    Preoperational, 53
    Concrete operational, 53
    Formal operational, 53
Societal Responsibility, 74, 75
Stress, 155-157

W

What is considered a disability? 33
Who are persons with a disability? 32, 33
Why are we prejudice? 32
Why is the population of persons with disabilities increasing? 33, 34